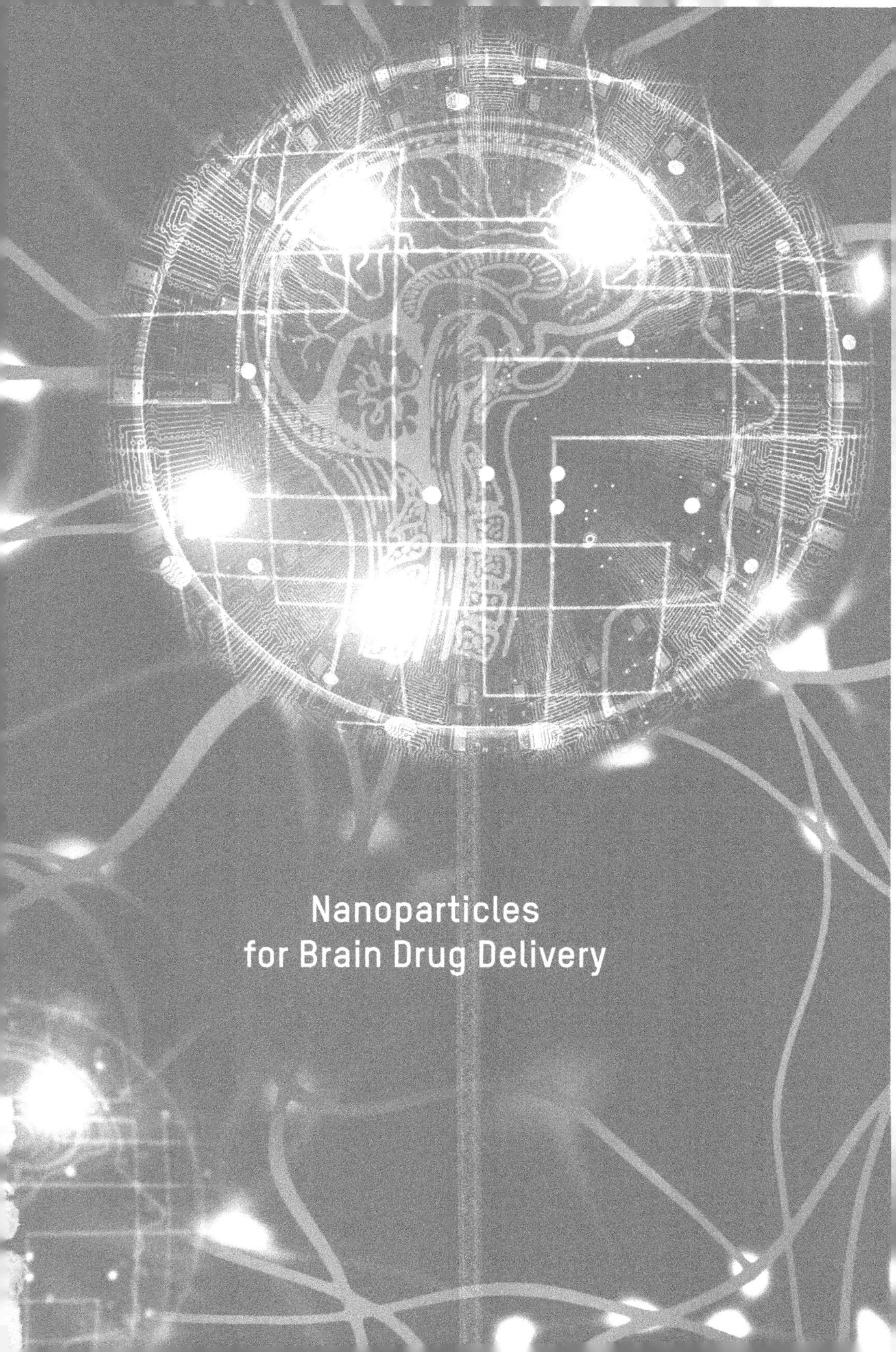

Nanoparticles for Brain Drug Delivery

Nanoparticles for Brain Drug Delivery

Edited by

Carla Vitorino | Andreia Jorge | Alberto Pais

JENNY STANFORD
PUBLISHING

Published by

Jenny Stanford Publishing Pte. Ltd.
Level 34, Centennial Tower
3 Temasek Avenue
Singapore 039190

Email: editorial@jennystanford.com
Web: www.jennystanford.com

British Library Cataloguing-in-Publication Data
A catalogue record for this book is available from the British Library.

Nanoparticles for Brain Drug Delivery

ISBN 978-981-4877-31-2 (Hardcover)
ISBN 978-1-003-11932-6 (eBook)

Contents

Part II: Nanomedicines

Preface

This book gathers contributions from experts in different, complementary fields, having in common their interest in developing new strategies for brain drug delivery based on nanotechnologies. It encompasses general aspects pertaining to fundamental development, including in silico, in vitro, and in vivo approaches. It also covers a diversity of nanomedicines applied in treatment and/or diagnosis and monitoring of central nervous system disorders. Aspects concerning their translation from the bench to clinical practice are also seamlessly discussed. It is expected that this book will inspire readers to discover possible approaches to holistically delivering drugs into the brain.

Carla Vitorino
Andreia Jorge
Alberto Pais
2021

Part I
Fundamentals

Chapter 1

Recent Trends in Nanotechnology for Brain Delivery: A Brief Outlook

Carla Vitorino,[a,b,c] Andreia Jorge[c] and Alberto Pais[c]
[a]*Faculty of Pharmacy, University of Coimbra, Pólo das Ciências da Saúde, Azinhaga de Santa Comba, 3000-548 Coimbra, Portugal*
[b]*Centre for Neurosciences and Cell Biology (CNC), University of Coimbra, Faculty of Medicine, Rua Larga, Pólo I, 1st Floor, 3004-504 Coimbra, Portugal*
[c]*Coimbra Chemistry Centre, Department of Chemistry, University of Coimbra, Rua Larga, 3004-535 Coimbra, Portugal*
csvitorino@ff.uc.pt

Brain targeting still represents a major therapeutic challenge: drug delivery to the brain is strictly regulated by the blood–brain barrier (BBB), which imposes an overwhelming obstacle for many central nervous system (CNS) active drugs. The BBB is responsible for the homeostatic mechanism of defence of the brain against foreign substances, including toxic molecules and pathogens. However, drug penetration is only one among several difficult challenges. These stem from the complexity and heterogeneity of cell brain composition, affecting both the prevalence and the response to simple drug targets, and also the respective pharmacokinetics and stability [1, 2].

Nanoparticles for Brain Drug Delivery
Edited by Carla Vitorino, Andreia Jorge and Alberto Pais

ISBN 978-981-4877-31-2 (Hardcover), 978-1-003-11932-6 (eBook)
www.jennystanford.com

The increasing incidence of brain-related pathologies and the hurdles which undermine the development of efficient and effective strategies have pushed both researchers and the pharmaceutical industry to search for novel therapeutic alternatives. Nanotechnology undoubtedly offers a broad bunch of options to circumvent the multiple challenges imposed for brain drug delivery [3].

Recent solutions from nanotechnology encompass a wide diversity of nanocarriers, ranging from organic to inorganic, and systems combining materials from both natures, known as hybrid nanosystems. Synthetic particulate delivery systems (e.g. liposomes, solid lipid matrix nanoparticles, polymeric nanoparticles, micelles, gold, iron oxide particles) can be presented in multiple designs, with different compositions, stabilities and solubilities, supported by flexible and often up-scalable production methods, while offering versatile loading capacities for a variety of therapeutics [4]. However, and despite the evident progress in the development of effective drug delivery nanocarriers, their clinical application still remains conditioned by delivery, targeting and safety concerns [5]. These include unknown tissue interactions and adsorption of serum proteins, resulting in unpredicted outcomes which include rapid clearance, inefficient loading, nonbiodegradability, and essentially a lack of specific and active targeting to the tissue/organ of interest.

To overcome these shortcomings, a variety of advanced surface chemistry engineering strategies have been proposed, directed at either improving stability and circulation or enhancing tissue targeting and cellular uptake. Such approaches take into consideration the overexpressed receptors in cells to mediate the internalisation of specific ligands and their associated therapeutic cargoes. Taking advantage of the cell-type-specific fingerprint, many smart nanosystems have been hierarchically decorated to incorporate specific moieties able to bind to receptor-docking sites. Candidates acting as recognition anchors may include aptamers, antibodies, peptides, proteins, carbohydrates, and small molecules, such as folate and vitamins [6].

Alternatively, carrier cells have been equated as drug delivery vehicles on the basis of their intrinsic tropism toward a site of interest and their capability to release a desired therapeutic agent. Different cargo types can be transported, such as antibodies, therapeutic genes and proteins, microRNA, oncolytic viruses, or even nanoparticles. Some examples include mesenchymal stem cells, macrophages, endothelial cells, or cancer cells [4].

Exosomes, as extracellular vesicles which bud from various cells through spontaneous or inducible biological processes, have also sparked particular interest as a natural, yet nonviral, alternative to synthetic vectors [7, 8]. Notwithstanding their somewhat natural active targeting capabilities and ability to traverse physiological barriers, such as the BBB, issues associated with the use of whole cells for drug delivery can be ascribed to the fact that the cells may differentiate and/or actually trigger pathologies, including cancer and possible metastasis [4].

Driven by these principles, more recently the use of biomimeting materials has become a reality in the form of cell membrane–camouflaged nanoparticles. These biohybrid systems essentially combine the technological advantages of nanomaterials with the stealth and biocompatibility characteristics of, for example, erythrocytes, leukocytes, or stem cell ghosts [9]. Cell ghosts, as nanosize biosystems devoid of their intracellular components, retain, however, the majority of their membrane proteins and lipids, which can be channeled to active or passive targeting [10].

Note, however, that the versatility of nanocarrier systems is not confined to the challenges imposed by intravenous administration. Physiological surrogates, such as the intranasal route, are pointed out as a reliable and direct pathway to surpass the BBB. Indeed, owing to the unique direct connection between the brain and the nasal cavity mediated by the olfactory epithelium, intranasal administration is the only route through which the brain is in connection with the outside environment, thus considerably enlarging the application of nanotechnology for brain delivery [11, 12].

The use of nanoscale systems does not hamper the respective combination with physical methods such as ultrasound, commonly employed to reversibly perturb the BBB and facilitate transport into the brain, allowing a complementary non-invasive boosting strategy for CNS drug delivery [13].

Apart from the therapeutic purposes, nanotechnology can also be fine-tuned to serve diagnosis, giving rise to its application in the theranostic area. Nanotheranostics, by integrating diagnostic and therapeutic functions in a single system, holds the benefits of nanotechnology and opens avenues in oncology and the personalised medicine research field [14].

All these aspects will be detailed and expanded throughout the subsequent chapters.

Acknowledgments

The Coimbra Chemistry Centre (CQC) is supported by the Fundação para a Ciência e Tecnologia (FCT) through Project UID/QUI/00313/2020. A.F.J. acknowledges FCT, Portugal, for financial support regarding the postdoctoral grant SFRH/BPD/104544/2014.

References

1. Dong, X. (2018). Current strategies for brain drug delivery. *Theranostics*, **8**(6), 1481–1493.
2. Miranda, A., Blanco-Prieto, M., Sousa, J., Pais, A., Vitorino, C. (2017). Breaching barriers in glioblastoma. Part I: Molecular pathways and novel treatment approaches. *Int. J. Pharm.*, **531**(1), 372–388.
3. Alyautdin, R., Khalin, I., Nafeeza, M. I., Haron, M. H., Kuznetsov, D. (2014). Nanoscale drug delivery systems and the blood–brain barrier. *Int. J. Nanomed.*, **9**, 795–811.
4. Schoen, B., Machluf, M. (2016). Cell ghosts: cellular membranes for drug delivery, in *Perspectives in Micro- and Nanotechnology for Biomedical Applications*, World Scientific Publishing, pp. 225–273.
5. Soares, S., Sousa, J., Pais, A., Vitorino, C. (2018). Nanomedicine: principles, properties, and regulatory issues. *Front. Chem.*, **6**, 360.
6. Jorge, A., Pais, A., Vitorino, C. (2020). Targeted siRNA delivery using lipid nanoparticles. *Methods Mol. Biol.*, **2059**, 259–283.
7. Zheng, M., Huang, M., Ma, X., Chen, H., Gao, X. (2019). Harnessing exosomes for the development of brain drug delivery systems. *Bioconjugate Chem.*, **30**(4), 994–1005.
8. Bunggulawa, E. J., Wang, W., Yin, T., Wang, N., Durkan, C., Wang, Y., et al. (2018). Recent advancements in the use of exosomes as drug delivery systems. *J. Nanobiotechnol.*, **16**(1), 81.
9. Chen, M., Chen, M., He, J. (2019). Cancer cell membrane cloaking nanoparticles for targeted co-delivery of doxorubicin and PD-L1 siRNA. *Artif. Cells Nanomed. Biotechnol.*, **47**(1), 1635–1641.
10. Toledano Furman, N. E., Lupu-Haber, Y., Bronshtein, T., Kaneti, L., Letko, N., Weinstein, E., et al. (2013). Reconstructed stem cell nanoghosts: a natural tumor targeting platform. *Nano Lett.*, **13**(7), 3248–3255.

11. Vitorino, C., Silva, S., Bicker, J., Falcao, A., Fortuna, A. (2019). Antidepressants and nose-to-brain delivery: drivers, restraints, opportunities and challenges. *Drug Discov. Today*, **24**(9), 1911–1923.

12. Mistry, A., Stolnik, S., Illum, L. (2009). Nanoparticles for direct nose-to-brain delivery of drugs. *Int. J. Pharm.*, **379**(1), 146–157.

13. Teleanu, D. M., Chircov, C., Grumezescu, A. M., Volceanov, A., Teleanu, R. I. (2018). Blood-brain delivery methods using nanotechnology. *Pharmaceutics*, **10**(4), 269.

14. Mendes, M., Sousa, J., Pais, A., Vitorino, C. (2018). Targeted theranostic nanoparticles for brain tumor treatment. *Pharmaceutics*, **10**(4), 181.

Chapter 2

Understanding Brain Delivery

Joana Bicker,[a,b] Ana Fortuna,[a,b] Gilberto Alves[c] and Amílcar Falcão[a,b]

[a]*Laboratory of Pharmacology, Faculty of Pharmacy, University of Coimbra, Azinhaga de Santa Comba, 3000-548 Coimbra, Portugal*

[b]*Coimbra Institute for Biomedical Imaging and Translational Research (CIBIT), University of Coimbra, Azinhaga de Santa Comba, 3000-548 Coimbra, Portugal*

[c]*CICS-UBI – Health Sciences Research Centre, University of Beira Interior, Av. Infante D. Henrique, 6200-506 Covilhã, Portugal*

joana.bicker@gmail.com

The development of new treatments for central nervous system (CNS) pathologies is being hampered by an insufficient comprehension of the mechanisms behind brain disorders, a lack of predictiveness of preclinical models and misinterpretation of pharmacokinetic parameters regarding brain exposure. This chapter begins by describing the barriers which separate the blood from the CNS and its fluids, namely the blood–brain barrier (BBB), between the blood and brain parenchyma, and the blood–cerebrospinal fluid barrier, formed by epithelial cells of the choroid plexus and the

Nanoparticles for Brain Drug Delivery
Edited by Carla Vitorino, Andreia Jorge and Alberto Pais

ISBN 978-981-4877-31-2 (Hardcover), 978-1-003-11932-6 (eBook)
www.jennystanford.com

arachnoid epithelium. The restrictiveness of these barriers can be attributed not only to the presence of tight junctions between brain endothelial cells and choroid plexus cells but also to the existence of a cooperative efflux system at the BBB, that is, P-glycoprotein and breast cancer resistance protein. For this reason, the identification of efflux liabilities is advised by regulatory guidelines. Furthermore, the fact that the BBB is dynamic and undergoes physiological or pathological changes adds another layer of complexity to the optimisation of models required for drug development. Overall, a thorough understanding of CNS pathophysiology is essential to surpass these obstacles and achieve efficient drug delivery.

2.1 The Central Nervous System in Drug Discovery and Development

Investigating the access of a molecule to the central nervous system (CNS) is always a fundamental step, regardless of whether the therapeutic target is central or peripheral. CNS restriction can be interpreted as a hurdle or an opportunity, depending on the specific purpose of the drug discovery and development program.

CNS exposure of drugs aimed at peripheral targets may be problematic and cause adverse effects in two situations: first, if the drug reaches sufficient concentrations in the CNS to result in off-target action and second, if the modulated target is also located in the CNS, in which case adverse effects will be an outcome of on-target engagement (right target/wrong tissue) [1]. Pharmacological selectivity could be a solution to off-target liabilities; nevertheless, when the target exists both peripherally and centrally, the key would be to design compounds with a limited access to the CNS [1, 2].

Peripheral selectivity can be achieved by developing compounds with a low rate of passive permeability, acidic functional groups or affinity to efflux transporters at the blood–brain barrier (BBB) [3]. These molecules display unbound brain-to-plasma concentration ratios ($K_{p,uu}$) below 1, such as second-generation histamine-H1 receptor antagonists (e.g. (*S*)-cetirizine: $K_{p,uu}$ = 0.22) which have better tolerability profiles than first-generation antagonists, due to a more restricted access to the CNS [4]. Designing dual efflux substrates is an efficient strategy to minimise CNS penetration [3] since the lower $K_{p,uu}$ is, the higher will be the dose necessary to obtain active concentrations in the CNS, maintaining an unaltered potency [5]. Estimates of brain exposure should always consider potency, since efflux substrates can still be centrally active, provided there is sufficient potency [6].

In the last few years, the development of innovative treatments directed at CNS pathologies has been generally unsuccessful despite the increasing global burden of disease attributed to these disorders [7] and existent commercial opportunities. The high attrition rates and expensive late-stage failures led larger pharmaceutical companies to down-scale their CNS development programs and smaller companies to abandon this therapeutic area [8].

This occurs because making go/no-go decisions during CNS drug development is particularly difficult (Fig. 2.1). For instance, the high complexity of the human CNS contributes to an insufficient understanding of the aetiology and pathophysiology of many CNS disorders, making it difficult to develop targeted and validated therapies [9]. However, even the optimisation of a molecule with affinity for an identified target does not necessarily ensure success, because the target may not be as relevant in the disease process as it was initially anticipated [10]. The solution may reside in the simultaneous modulation of more than one relevant target [10, 11]. In this context, phenotypic screening was pointed out as an alternative strategy to target-based screening, because it does not require previous knowledge about the molecular targets involved in CNS diseases. Nevertheless, it is still necessary to continue the investigation of disease-relevant cellular phenotypes with improved assay throughput, and the target(s) must be identified later in the process (target deconvolution) [12, 13]. A recent phenotype-based screen was developed for the discovery of drugs directed at multiple sclerosis [14].

Additional obstacles and recommended measures are described in Fig. 2.1. Animal models used in drug discovery often lack adequate predictive power to estimate efficacy in humans [15]. Although a particular aspect of a disease can be mimicked in an animal model, an entire disorder can rarely be recapitulated, in part due to an incomplete knowledge of the molecular mechanisms of the disease, but also due to genetic differences between species [9, 10].

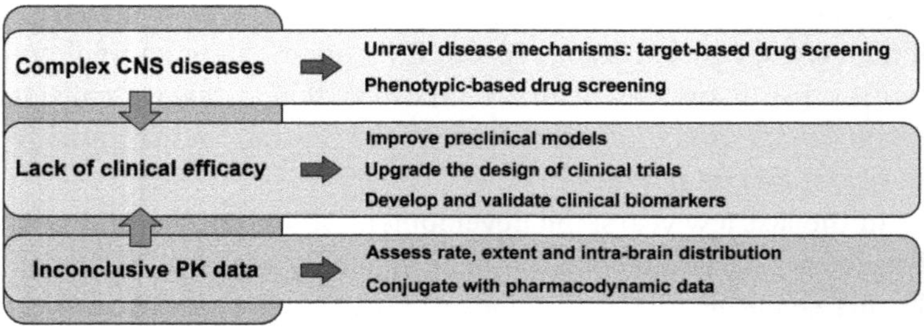

Figure 2.1 Main problems encountered during central nervous system (CNS) drug development and suggested measures [9–11, 16, 17]. PK, pharmacokinetics.

In addition to improving or creating new animal models, it has been suggested to associate nonrodent (e.g. zebrafish) or non-animal (e.g. induced pluripotent stem cells, computational neuroscience) models of disease mechanisms to facilitate translation [9, 18].

The existence of inconclusive pharmacokinetic data is another hindering factor in CNS drug discovery. Until recently, the rate and extent of drug transfer across the BBB were used interchangeably and total drug concentrations in plasma and brain were estimated, instead of free and pharmacologically relevant concentrations [11]. The determination of total brain-to-plasma ratios (K_p) or their logarithm (log BB) is misleading and generates excessively lipophilic molecules. While lipophilicity may increase the permeability (rate) with which molecules cross the BBB, it can also cause nonspecific binding to the brain parenchyma, decrease unbound drug concentrations in the brain interstitial fluid, increase affinity to efflux transporters and reduce aqueous solubility, thereby complicating drug formulation [4, 10]. Therefore, it is advisable to evaluate the extent of exposure based on $K_{p,uu}$, as previously mentioned, and combine physicochemical properties which improve not only the rate but also the extent and intrabrain distribution [4, 6].

2.2 CNS Barriers and Fluids

Molecular traffic between the blood and the CNS is regulated by protective barriers: the BBB, formed by brain endothelial cells (BECs) and other elements of the neurovascular unit, that is, astrocytes, pericytes, microglia, neurons and extracellular matrix;

the blood–cerebrospinal fluid barrier (BCSFB), formed by epithelial cells of the choroid plexus, which secrete cerebrospinal fluid (CSF) into the cerebral ventricles; and the avascular arachnoid epithelium, which does not significantly contribute to exchanges between the blood and the CNS due to a smaller surface area [19].

These barriers preserve the microenvironment of the CNS by limiting the paracellular diffusion of hydrophilic solutes and ions between the blood, the CSF and the brain parenchyma. The restrictiveness is conferred by tight junctions between BECs of the BBB and choroid epithelial cells of the BCSFB [20]. It creates distinct apical and basolateral domains and leads to high cell polarisation, which, in turn, causes a differential distribution of influx and efflux transporters across membranes [21, 22].

The choroid plexus in each ventricle is separated from the brain parenchyma by ependymal cells which outline the ventricles. In the adult, most of the ependymal surface, with the exception of the choroid plexus, is not connected by tight junctions but by leakier gap junctions [23]. Moreover, the capillaries in the choroid plexus are fenestrated (Table 2.1) and separated from the epithelial cells by a layer of connective tissue named stroma [23]. Supposedly, the higher endothelial permeability of the basement membrane surrounding the choroidal capillary walls is caused by the absence of astrocytic foot processes, which in contrast are present at the BBB and contribute to its higher restrictiveness [24].

Furthermore, choroid epithelial cells display well-developed microvilli projected into the CSF in the ventricular lumen, which increase the surface area for an effective delivery of the CSF and other transport functions [23]. Early literature data indicated that the surface area of the choroid plexus was only 0.021 m^2 or 0.1% compared with 20 m^2 of the reported surface area of the BBB [25]. Nevertheless, this information has been rectified, and more recently assessed data demonstrated a significant underestimation of the surface area of the human choroid plexus, pointing towards 2–5 m^2 [26].

Compared to peripheral endothelial cells, BECs display a much lower rate of transcellular vesicular traffic (i.e. transcytosis) (Table 2.1). This is possibly related to a pericyte-induced down-regulation [27] or to the different lipid composition of BECs, which suppresses the formation of caveole vesicles [28]. On the other hand, choroid epithelial cells have shown a high density of vesicles, suggesting an intense endocytotic activity at the BCSFB [29].

Table 2.1 Physiological differences between the two main CNS barriers [19, 23, 29]

BBB	BCSFB
Nonfenestrated capillaries	Fenestrated capillaries
Few cytoplasmic vesicles	High number of cytoplasmic vesicles
More mitochondria than peripheral endothelial cells	Abundant mitochondria (higher than BBB)
Enzymatic activity under investigation	High enzymatic activity
Main efflux transporters (blood-facing side): P-glycoprotein (P-gp) and breast cancer resistance protein (BCRP)	Main efflux transporters (blood-facing side): multidrug resistance–associated protein (MRP)1 and MRP4

In BECs, receptor-mediated transcytosis (RMT) and adsorptive-mediated transcytosis (AMT) enable the access of larger molecules such as proteins and peptides into the CNS [30]. While RMT implies ligand binding to a receptor, internalisation, subcellular routing, exocytosis and dissociation from the receptor, AMT is receptor-independent and encompasses binding of cationic protein residues with the anionic glycocalyx [31]. RMT also occurs at the BCSFB, together with additional specific transcytosis pathways [29].

Another aspect in which the BBB and BCSFB diverge is the expression and location of efflux transporters (Table 2.1). At the human BBB, P-glycoprotein (P-gp; MDR1; ABCB1) and breast cancer resistance protein (BCRP; ABCG2) form a team of gatekeepers on the blood-facing surface of BECs [32], as will be discussed in greater detail in Section 2.3. Conversely, at the BCSFB, P-gp was found in the apical or CSF-facing surface of choroid epithelial cells, indicating that it engages in epithelial cell-to-CSF efflux and prevents the traffic of substrates out of the CSF. In the blood-facing surface of choroidal epithelial cells, the traffic is barred by multidrug resistance–associated proteins (MRP; ABCC), MRP1 and MRP4 [33]. Western blot studies revealed that in the adult rat brain, the expression levels of

P-gp in the choroid plexus are 0.5% of those found in BECs, whereas MRP1 levels in BECs are only 4% of those in the choroid plexus of the fourth ventricle. These differences were also confirmed in human samples. Thus, it has been speculated that P-gp at the BCSFB could prevent the accumulation of neurotoxic lipophilic substances in the brain, while MRP1 is responsible for the basolateral efflux of drug conjugates formed in the choroid plexus [34].

Indeed, choroid plexus epithelial cells possess drug-metabolising enzymes with especially high activity, namely epoxide hydrolases, UDP-glucurono-, sulfo- or glutathione *S*-transferases (GSTs). The association of metabolic reactions with the efflux of drug conjugates establishes another neuroprotective barrier which limits drug distribution into the CSF [22]. In BECs there are phase I and phase II enzymes, such as cytochrome P450 (CYP) CYP1B1 and CYP2U1, monoamine oxidase A and B, catechol-*O*-methyltransferase and GSTs [35]. Although these enzymes inhibit the transport of neurotransmitters from the brain to blood and vice versa [31], additional evidence concerning their impact on drug access to the CNS is necessary.

As previously mentioned, about two-thirds of the CSF are secreted at high capacity by four choroid plexuses in the lateral right, lateral left, third and fourth brain ventricles [36, 37]. The CSF circulates from the lateral to the third ventricle via the interventricular foramina and then to the fourth ventricle through the cerebral aqueduct. Afterwards, it flows down the central canal of the spinal cord and circulates in the subarachnoid space, where it is reabsorbed by arachnoid villi or granulations, which are valve-like structures which enable the CSF to flow out into cerebral veins when its pressure is higher than venous pressure [36]. Lastly, the CSF is directed into the systemic venous circulation or to regional and cervical lymph nodes through cranial and spinal nerves [38, 39]. Regular CSF flow is critical for balanced cerebral metabolism and propelled by several mechanisms, including arterial pulsations in the choroid plexus, a hydrostatic pressure gradient from the CSF to venous blood and the movement of ciliary processes which extend from the apical surfaces of ependymal cells [24]. The rate of production and the composition of the CSF are altered by circadian oscillations [40, 41].

Consequently, the CSF ensures efficient neuronal function through the removal of unnecessary metabolites from the brain interstitial fluid (ISF), which fills the extracellular space between neurons and glia within the brain parenchyma [19, 42]. The CSF acts as a sink by lowering concentration gradients and taking substances to drainage sites for extrusion, namely at the arachnoidal–lymphatic–venous interfaces [37]. Nevertheless, the exact drainage process remains controversial. The glymphatic system hypothesis supports the existence of subarachnoid CSF influx into the brain along arterial perivascular spaces, followed by the convective flow of the ISF in the extracellular space into venous perivascular spaces, for clearance into the systemic circulation. The convective flow was attributed to aquaporin-4 (AQP4) channels on astrocytic-end feet [43]. Despite agreeing with the existence of a perivascular fluid system, the glymphatic system hypothesis was recently reassessed by questioning the role of AQP4 and suggesting that CSF–ISF exchanges occur mostly by diffusion, rather than flow, at the brain extracellular space [39]. In addition to CSF–ISF exchanges at perivascular spaces, other exchanges occur at ependymal and pia-glial surfaces of the brain through gap junctions [37, 44]. CSF–ISF exchanges are important for substances required by the CNS which do not significantly cross the BBB, including compounds which use the CSF for a wider CNS distribution (e.g. melatonin), compounds which enter the CNS via choroid plexus (e.g. vitamin C and folate) or compounds secreted by the choroid plexus, for CNS use [39].

Drug delivery to the CNS through the BCSFB has been discouraged due to the larger surface area of the BBB, little mixing within the CSF, high CSF turnover and larger diffusion distance from the CSF to brain tissue than between brain capillaries [3, 45, 46]. It has also been referred that drugs injected into the CSF by the intrathecal route distribute to the blood and superficial brain areas but do not reach deep brain parenchyma [45]. However, Pizzo et al. [47] achieved the delivery of a macromolecule (immunoglobulin G [IgG]) into deep brain regions following intrathecal infusion in rats. The distribution occurred along perivascular spaces, probably through stomata on leptomeningeal cells in the subarachnoid space. This discovery created another possible route for drug delivery into the CNS.

Due to previously mentioned reasons, CSF samples may not be a good surrogate of unbound drug concentrations in the ISF, particularly for efflux substrates. The concentrations of P-gp and/or BCRP substrates in the ISF may be overpredicted by unbound CSF concentrations [6]. This has been justified by the different location and expression of these transporters at the BBB and BCSFB. Since at the BCSFB, P-gp is located in the CSF-facing surface of choroid epithelial cells, drugs which are P-gp substrates would be pumped into the CSF, leading to higher CSF concentrations and to an overestimation of unbound ISF concentrations [3]. Another possible explanation is that P-gp at the BCSFB is less expressed and may be less efficient than P-gp at the BBB, indicating that the estimated unbound CSF concentrations would be higher than actual ISF concentrations, which would be decreased by P-gp efflux at the BBB [48]. Associated with this are disadvantages of the CSF sampling procedure which may affect the results, namely alterations of CSF volume and ventricular pressure, regional differences, inflammation and others [39, 49].

2.3 Efflux Transporters at the BBB

P-gp and BCRP form a potent efflux team at the BBB by limiting the entry of several drugs into the CNS. Both transporters are part of the adenosine triphosphate (ATP)-binding cassette (ABC) superfamily and participate in the regulation of the absorption, distribution and elimination of several xenobiotics, including drugs and their metabolites [50]. The overexpression of these transporters in cancer cells contributes to the development of drug resistance, responsible for chemotherapeutic failure or malignant tumour progression, but it was also reported at the BBB in refractory epilepsy (transporter hypothesis), leading to increased extrusion of antiepileptic drugs from the CNS or decreasing their uptake in epileptic tissue [50, 51].

While P-gp is a full transporter composed of two homologous halves connected by a linker sequence, each containing six transmembrane sequences and one cytoplasmic nucleotide-binding domain, BCRP is a half-transporter and requires dimerisation to attain functionality [52]. They are ubiquitously expressed in several tissues and possess broad and often overlapping substrate specificity, including structurally unrelated compounds [50]. The precise location of P-gp at the BBB is under discussion, but most published data reveal that in mammals, P-gp is mainly expressed at the apical membrane of BECs [53] although it can also be found in astrocytes [54, 55], microglia [56], neurons [57] and intracellularly [58]. BCRP levels in human brain microvessels (8.14 fmol μg^{-1} protein) and cynomolgus monkey microvessels (14.2 fmol μg^{-1} protein) are 1.85- and 3.22-fold higher, respectively, than BCRP levels in mice (4.41 fmol μg^{-1} protein). In contrast, mice express 2.56 and 3.29 times more P-gp than humans and monkeys [59–61]. Therefore, P-gp appears to be the main transporter in rodents, while BCRP is more predominant in humans and primates. It should be noted, however, that a higher transporter expression may not necessarily imply higher functionality. There are conflicting results regarding P-gp expression and functionality at the BBB in epilepsy models. Using different approaches, Uchida et al. [62] found a relation between these concepts, whereas Lange et al. [63] did not. Thus, alterations of transporter expression should be interpreted carefully and complemented with an analysis of functionality.

Table 2.2 Examples of P-gp and BCRP inhibitors [69–78]

<table>
<tr><th>P-gp</th><th>BCRP</th></tr>
<tr><td>First generation: verapamil, nifedipine, diltiazem, amiodarone, quinidine, prazosin, cyclosporine A, tacrolimus, erythromycin, tamoxifen, ibuprofen</td><td rowspan="3">Fumitremorgin C and analogues (Ko143, Ko132, Ko134), novobiocin, triclabendazole and metabolites, HIV protease inhibitors (nelfinavir, saquinavir, ritonavir), tyrosine kinase inhibitors (imatinib, nilotinib, apatinib), elacridar (GF120918), tariquidar (XR9576), tariquidar-derived BCRP inhibitors</td></tr>
<tr><td>Second generation: dexverapamil, MM36, valspodar, biricodar, toremifene</td></tr>
<tr><td>Third generation: zosuquidar (LY-335979), elacridar (GF120918), tariquidar (XR9576), laniquidar (R101933), ontogen (OC-144-093), HM30181</td></tr>
</table>

As previously stated, P-gp and BCRP operate in synergy, limiting drug penetration across the BBB [32, 64–67], and when one is inhibited, the other compensates its loss of function [68]. To improve target exposure and/or overcome drug resistance, several P-gp and

BCRP inhibitors have been developed throughout the years (Table 2.2).

First-generation P-gp inhibitors are pharmacologically active compounds, which were already in clinical use or under investigation for other therapeutic indications when the ability to inhibit P-gp was revealed [70]. Nevertheless, several of these compounds are substrates for other transporters and enzymes, leading to pharmacokinetic interactions [79]. Furthermore, these compounds have low affinity for P-gp, demanding the use of high doses, which, together with their nonselective activity, result in toxicity. Second-generation P-gp inhibitors are analogues of first-generation inhibitors with improved efficacy, tolerability and potency due to structural modifications [79, 80] but still retain some properties which limit their use as P-gp modulators, namely the interaction with CYP3A4 enzymes [51, 70]. Lastly, third-generation P-gp inhibitors were developed aiming at higher potency [79], less drug interactions and toxicity [81], some of which also inhibit BCRP, such as tariquidar and elacridar. Notwithstanding, despite their promising characteristics, many third-generation inhibitors revealed unexpected toxicity or lack of efficacy in clinical trials [70]. A possible explanation is that indiscriminate blockage in several tissues may prevent substrates from being eliminated from the organism and cause toxicity [82]. Therefore, it has been recommended to shift the focus from identifying increasingly potent or specific inhibitors to developing strategies for targeting the inhibitors to specific sites of action [83]. For instance, Gomes et al. [84] developed an innovative method to transiently silence P-gp at the BBB. It involved BBB-targeted nanoparticles using transferrin-mimetic peptides and loaded with silencing RNA, which enabled a temporary reduction of P-gp messenger RNA (mRNA) up to 52% [84].

The identification of P-gp and BCRP substrates and/or inhibitors is recommended by international guidelines during drug development in order to prevent potential transporter-mediated drug–drug interactions (DDIs) [71, 85]. Although DDIs in the intestine, liver and kidneys are more common, BBB drug transporter interactions are rarer. For instance, Sadeque et al. [86] reported an interaction involving P-gp inhibition at the BBB of healthy volunteers, between loperamide (victim) and quinidine (perpetrator), which resulted in respiratory depression. Sasongko et al. [87] and Muzi et al. [88] also described P-gp inhibition at the BBB by cyclosporine A (perpetrator) with consequent increase of the CNS penetration of verapamil (victim). Notwithstanding, the concentrations of the perpetrators used in these studies were high, and consequently, DDIs are unlikely to occur in therapeutic doses. Furthermore, the higher brain concentrations of the victim drug could be a result of higher plasma concentrations originated from a DDI in another place of the body [2]. The International Transporter Consortium (ITC) considers that currently available drugs which are P-gp or BCRP inhibitors do not attain sufficient unbound concentrations in plasma to increase CNS exposure, meaning that the risk of DDIs at the human BBB is low [89].

Drug-induced activation or induction of ABC transporters at the BBB has been less studied compared to efflux inhibition. Nonetheless, there is interest in this field concerning possible induction-mediated DDIs at the BBB and also induction for therapeutic purposes, namely the removal of amyloid-beta peptides from the CNS by P-gp at the BBB [90]. Chan et al. [91] assessed P-gp induction by dexamethasone (ligand of the pregnane X receptor) at the BBB of mice, using quinidine as P-gp substrate. Unbound quinidine concentrations in the brain ISF were 2.5-fold lower, while P-gp expression was 1.5-fold higher in dexamethasone-treated animals compared with vehicle-treated animals [91]. P-gp and BCRP induction has also been studied in human brain microvessel endothelial cells (hCMEC/d3). P-gp expression and function were induced following a 72 h exposure to antiretroviral drugs [92, 93], while selective ligands of the peroxisome proliferator-activated receptor alpha (PPAR-α) induced BCRP expression. The intracellular accumulation of mitoxantrone, a BCRP substrate, was significantly reduced after 72 h of exposure to PPAR-α ligands [94]. The upregulation of P-gp/BCRP expression at the BBB has also been reported following chronic exposure to opioids, which may lead to tolerance and pharmacoresistance [95]. Nevertheless, after 11–29 days of treatment of healthy human volunteers with rifampicin, a known P-gp inducer, there was no induction of P-gp at the BBB, using clinical doses which normally induce P-gp in the intestine. It was explained that rifampicin may not achieve sufficient concentrations in BECs to induce P-gp, in contrast to the high concentrations attained in the intestine. Additionally, P-gp at the human BBB may already be maximally induced by environmental or endogenous factors, meaning that further induction may not be feasible [96]. For these reasons, the ITC considers that the induction of efflux transporters at the human BBB appears improbable [89].

2.4 BBB Evolution in Physiological and Pathological States

The BBB is a dynamic interface which undergoes physiological changes through life. These include modifications which take place during development and maturation, as well as alterations resulting from circadian oscillations, pregnancy, physical exercise and ageing.

Circadian rhythms are the outcome of a series of neuronal and hormonal inputs generated by endogenous clocks in order to regulate several physiological processes during the 24 h day [97]. Although much is yet unknown concerning the role of circadian oscillations on BBB properties, it was found that the BBB permeability of *Drosophila* is circadian-dependent and higher at night, while P-gp effluxes at higher rates during the day (active phase). Consequences on drug delivery were shown by a more efficient phenytoin administration during this period [98].

Pregnancy has been associated with an increase of BBB permeability as a result of hemodynamic changes in the brain. It does not appear to be related with differences of tight junction expression but with a higher hydrostatic pressure on the BBB [99]. The main adaptations of cerebral circulation and BBB to pregnancy were described by Cipolla et al. [100] and include the protective role which the BBB exerts against peripherally activated leucocytes, microglia and tumour necrosis factor alpha (TNF-α), which could provoke neuronal hyperexcitability and seizures in pregnant women. In addition, there are a few studies concerning potential alterations in foetal BBB related to efflux transporters. Viral infections during pregnancy [101] and short-term exposure to sertraline (4 h) [102] resulted in P-gp inhibition in foetal and maternal BBB. In opposition, placental P-gp was activated after sertraline exposure, suggesting a tissue-specific effect [102]. This tissue-specific effect has also been observed for norbuprenorphine, a P-gp substrate. P-gp had a minor role in its foetal exposure but highly restricted its brain distribution [103]. On the other hand, chronic exposure to zidovudine induced BCRP expression in both foetal brain and placenta [104].

Moderate and high-intensity physical exercise on the treadmill led to an increase of BBB permeability in healthy men as a consequence of higher oxidative stress, contrary to low-intensity physical exercise [105]. Similarly, it was found that obesity (body mass index $\geq$5 kg/m^2) can induce BBB dysfunction by reducing serum neurotrophic factor levels and increasing oxidative stress. This can be counteracted through the practice of regular aerobic exercise, in opposition to acute and excessively intense physical exercise, in order to correct the oxidant–antioxidant imbalance [106, 107]. In disease situations such as autoimmune encephalomyelitis, chronic cerebral hypoperfusion and ischaemic stroke, physical exercise appears to decrease BBB dysfunction by promoting angiogenesis and cerebral vascular remodelling [108], improving cognitive impairment and white matter injury [109] and inhibiting disease progression through immunomodulatory effects [110]. Nevertheless, additional studies are necessary to clarify the effect of quantity and different kinds of physical exercise in the modulation of BBB permeability in disease states [111].

Before examining BBB alterations underlying ageing, it is important to define physiological or normal ageing as a deterioration of functions without cognitive decline or dementia [112]. Briefly, some of the age-related differences observed in humans encompass a decrease of capillary density and surface area; an increase in capillary wall thickness, accompanied by a decrease in the number of BECs and respective mitochondria; a reduced expression of tight junctions and P-gp; accumulation of extracellular matrix components and an increase of the thickness of the basal lamina; production of neurotoxic pro-inflammatory mediators by microglia; pericyte degeneration; and deterioration of neuronal plasticity with increased apoptosis [112, 113]. Reports on astrocytic modifications during ageing are varied. Some authors affirm that astrogliosis takes place with ageing, that is, an augmented proliferation and reactivity of astrocytes characterised by a higher expression of glial fibrillary acidic protein as a response to an inflammatory and oxidative state [114]. In parallel, other authors describe a loss of astrocytic endfeet contact with BECs in aged mice caused by a depletion of AQP4 [115] as well as an accumulation of iron in astrocytes which can generate free radicals and harm cells [116]. Although there are controversial data, ageing has been associated with a higher permeability of the human BBB, according to a meta-analysis of 31 studies with 1953 individuals [117]. Indeed, albumin extravasation has been observed, together with increased brain leakage. It is believed that this leakiness may play a role in the development of age-related dementias [118].

There are numerous studies in the literature concerning the effect of pathological conditions on the BBB, particularly Alzheimer's disease (AD) but also Parkinson's disease (PD), epilepsy, multiple sclerosis, schizophrenia, depression and hypertension, among others [119–124].

To this day, very little is known about role of the BBB in PD. Initially, it was speculated that the BBB remained intact during PD due to the successful use of aromatic amino acid decarboxylase (AADC) inhibitors. AADC inhibitors like carbidopa and benserazide were developed to increase the availability of levodopa (L-DOPA) to the brain by preventing its peripheral conversion to dopamine. This means that if the BBB was compromised, AADC inhibitors would cause central inhibition and prevent the formation of dopamine in the brain, thereby reducing the potency of L-DOPA [125]. Notwithstanding, studies found that benserazide does inhibit central AADC in the rat at 10 mg/kg, which, according to the authors, indicates BBB breakdown in PD [125, 126]. Furthermore, modifications of [^{11}C]-verapamil brain uptake were also reported in patients with early-stage or advanced-stage PD in 37 different brain regions. In early-stage PD, a lower uptake of [^{11}C]-verapamil was observed in midbrain and frontal regions, whereas in late-stage PD, a higher uptake was verified in frontal white matter regions. Therefore, it was suggested that there may be a regional upregulation of P-gp in early-stage PD and a downregulation of P-gp in late-stage PD [127]. This P-gp dysfunction could be a part of PD pathogenesis by facilitating the entrance of neurotoxins to the brain [128]. Likewise, BCRP expression in brain capillaries appears to be decreased in an animal model of PD [129], in contrast to AD, for which increased BCRP expression and activity has been reported in vivo [130]. Another possible cause which has been explored for PD pathogenesis is the passage of metals through the BBB, namely iron

[116], explaining the interest in iron-chelating therapies for PD [131]. It was proposed to exploit BBB disruption for PD or AD treatment in order to facilitate the delivery of nanocarriers according to the degree of disease severity [132]. Once again, it is important to resort to targeted nanocarriers for the BBB and also specific brain regions, thereby preventing drug delivery to several parts of the body, which could result in systemic toxicity [133]. For example, brain-targeted liposomes were recently developed for PD treatment, revealing the capacity to cross the BBB and reach the striatum and substantia nigra, while maintaining a restricted off-target distribution [134].

As previously mentioned, the overexpression of ABC transporters at the BBB has been associated with pharmacoresistant epilepsy [51]. Other epilepsy-related BBB modifications which have been investigated encompass a decrease in tight junction expression, tight junction opening and albumin extravasion [124, 135], important indicators of BBB leakage. Indeed, cerebrovascular dysfunction is one of the mechanisms behind seizure activity and epilepsy perpetuation, but it is thought to extend beyond BBB breakdown and may also imply impaired CSF–ISF circulation. Changes in CSF–ISF circulation can affect the pharmacology of antiepileptic drugs through the impediment of drug distribution as a result of a reduced ISF flow, or through the potentiation of side effects caused by decreased brain clearance. Therefore, BBB damage, increased vascular permeability and pathological changes in ISF–CSF circulation can be synergistically involved in the pathogenesis of neurological diseases [136].

In fact, cerebrovascular dysfunction has not only been associated with epilepsy but is acknowledged to play a role in several diseases, including depression, schizophrenia and hypertension [137, 138]. Hypertension is a common cause of BBB lesions, given that it impacts the structure of blood vessels and particularly the arterioles which deliver blood to central regions of the brain. Vascular remodelling caused by hypertension modifies not only the vessel wall but the surrounding extracellular matrix as well, leading to blood vessel fibrosis, vascular stiffening, cerebral blood flow impairment and, ultimately, hypoperfusion and hypoxia. In turn, hypoxia triggers neuroinflammation, which activates the release of proteases by microglia which open the BBB by loosening tight junctions and breaking down the basal lamina [139]. Similar consequences have been found in rats with acute hypertension, namely BBB breakdown and an increase of brain microvascular permeability [140]. Another proposed mechanism for BBB disruption in hypertension was the elevated circulating level of angiotensin-II, which contributes to an exacerbated sympathoexcitation [141]. Nevertheless, in spite of the described neuroprotective effects of angiotensin-II blockers, inclusively of the BBB [142] a conducted study with candesartan (and ursodeoxycholic acid) failed to prevent the deterioration of BBB integrity and cognitive function in dietary-induced obese mice, even though blood pressure was successfully reduced [143].

2.5 Conclusions

CNS barriers and the BBB, in particular, constitute a major obstacle to the delivery of small-molecule drugs and therapeutic macromolecules to the brain. Its low paracellular permeability together with the expression of efflux transporters on the blood-facing surface of BECs restrict molecular traffic and hinder progress in the treatment of CNS diseases. This led to great interest in drug delivery strategies which bypass the BBB (e.g. intranasal drug delivery) or take advantage of its inward transport routes (e.g. targeted nanocarriers).

Furthermore, the structural complexity and dynamic alterations of the BBB in health and disease states complicate the creation of predictive BBB models, most necessary during drug development stages.

In the future, a greater understanding of the pathological mechanisms behind CNS diseases and the improvement of drug delivery systems will be essential for the development of innovative treatments directed at several CNS disorders.

References

1. Bagal, S., Bungay, P. (2014). Restricting CNS penetration of drugs to minimise adverse events: role of drug transporters. *Drug Discov. Today Technol.*, **12**, 79–85.

2. Cole, S., Bagal, S., El-Kattan, A., Fenner, K., Hay, T., Kempshall, S., Lunn, G., Varma, M., Stupple, P., Speed, W. (2012). Full efficacy with no CNS

side-effects: unachievable panacea or reality? DMPK considerations in design of drugs with limited brain penetration. *Xenobiotica*, **42**, 11–27.

3. Di, L., Rong, H., Feng, B. (2013). Demystifying brain penetration in central nervous system drug discovery. *J. Med. Chem.*, **56**, 2–12.
4. Rankovic, Z. (2015). CNS drug design: balancing physicochemical properties for optimal brain exposure. *J. Med. Chem.*, **58**, 2584–2608.
5. Hammarlund-Udenaes, M. (2009). Active-site concentrations of chemicals - are they a better predictor of effect than plasma/organ/tissue concentrations? *Basic Clin. Pharmacol. Toxicol.*, **106**, 215–220.
6. Loryan, I., Sinha, V., Mackie, C., Van Peer, A., Drinkenburg, W., Vermeulen, A., Morrison, D., Monshouwer, M., Heald, D., Hammarlund-Udenaes, M. (2014). Mechanistic understanding of brain drug disposition to optimize the selection of potential neurotherapeutics in drug discovery. *Pharm. Res.*, **31**, 2203–2219.
7. Feigin, V. L., Vos, T. (2019). Global burden of neurological disorders: from global burden of disease estimates to actions. *Neuroepidemiology*, **52**, 1–2.
8. Yokley, B. H., Hartman, M., Slusher, B. S. (2017). Role of academic drug discovery in the quest for new CNS therapeutics. *ACS Chem. Neurosci.*, **8**, 429–431.
9. Pankevich, D. E., Altevogt, B. M., Dunlop, J., Gage, F. H., Hyman, S. E. (2014). Improving and accelerating drug development for nervous system disorders. *Neuron*, **84**, 546–553.
10. Gribkoff, V. K., Kaczmarek, L. K. (2017). The need for new approaches in CNS drug discovery: why drugs have failed, and what can be done to improve outcomes. *Neuropharmacology*, **120**, 11–19.
11. de Lange, E. C. M., van den Brink, W., Yamamoto, Y., de Witte, W. E. A., Wong, Y. C. (2017). Novel CNS drug discovery and development approach: model-based integration to predict neuro-pharmacokinetics and pharmacodynamics. *Expert Opin. Drug Discov.*, **12**, 1207–1218.
12. Khurana, V., Tardiff, D. F., Chung, C. Y., Lindquist, S. (2015). Toward stem cell-based phenotypic screens for neurodegenerative diseases. *Nat. Rev. Neurol.*, **11**, 339–350.
13. Wagner, B. K. (2016). The resurgence of phenotypic screening in drug discovery and development. *Expert Opin. Drug Discov.*, **11**, 121–125.
14. Lariosa-Willingham, K., Leonoudakis, D. (2018). A central nervous system axonal myelination assay for high-throughput screening. *Methods Mol. Biol.*, **1791**, 179–192.

15. Goetghebeur, P. J., Swartz, J. E. (2016). True alignment of preclinical and clinical research to enhance success in CNS drug development: a review of the current evidence. *J. Psychopharmacol.*, **30**, 586–594.

16. Kesselheim, A. S., Hwang, T. J., Franklin, J. M. (2015). Two decades of new drug development for central nervous system disorders. *Nat. Rev.*, **14**, 1–2.

17. Butlen-Ducuing, F., Pétavy, F., Guizzaro, L., Zienowicz, M., Haas, M., Alteri, E., Salmonson, T., Corruble, E. (2016). Challenges in drug development for central nervous system disorders: a European medicines agency perspective. *Nat. Rev. Drug Discov.*, **15**, 813–814.

18. Meshalkina, D. A., Song, C., Kalueff, A. V (2017). Better lab animal models for translational neuroscience research and CNS drug development. *Lab Anim. (NY)*, **46**, 91–92.

19. Abbott, N. J., Patabendige, A. A. K., Dolman, D. E. M., Yusof, S. R., Begley, D. J. (2010). Structure and function of the blood-brain barrier. *Neurobiol. Dis.*, **37**, 13–25.

20. Whish, S., Dziegielewska, K. M., Møllgård, K., Noor, N. M., Liddelow, S. A., Habgood, M. D., Richardson, S. J., Saunders, N. R. (2015). The inner CSF-brain barrier: developmentally controlled access to the brain via intercellular junctions. *Front. Neurosci.*, **9**, 1–15.

21. Chow, B. W., Gu, C. (2015). The molecular constituents of the blood-brain barrier Brian. *Trends Neurosci.*, **38**, 598–608.

22. Ghersi-Egea, J.-F., Strazielle, N., Calata, M., Silva-Vargas, V., Doetsch, F., Engelhardt, B. (2018). Molecular anatomy and functions of the choroidal blood-cerebrospinal fluid barrier in health and disease. *Acta Neuropathol.*, **135**, 337–361.

23. Kaur, C., Rathnasamy, G., Ling, E. A. (2016). The choroid plexus in healthy and diseased brain. *J. Neuropathol. Exp. Neurol.*, **75**, 198–213.

24. Johanson, C. E., Stopa, E. G., McMillan, P. N. (2011). The blood-cerebrospinal fluid barrier: structure and functional significance. *Methods Mol. Biol.*, **686**, 101–131.

25. Dohrmann, G. J., Bucy, P. C. (1970). Human choroid plexus: a light and electron microscopic study. *J. Neurosurg.*, **33**, 506–516.

26. Spector, R., Keep, R. F., Robert Snodgrass, S., Smith, Q. R., Johanson, C. E. (2015). A balanced view of choroid plexus structure and function: focus on adult humans. *Exp. Neurol.*, **267**, 78–86.

27. Armulik, A., Genové, G., Mäe, M., Nisancioglu, M. H., Wallgard, E., Niaudet, C., He, L., Norlin, J., Lindblom, P., Strittmatter, K., Johansson,

B. R., Betsholtz, C. (2010). Pericytes regulate the blood-brain barrier. *Nature*, **468**, 557–561.

28. Andreone, B. J., Chow, B. W., Tata, A., Lacoste, B., Ben-Zvi, A., Bullock, K., Deik, A. A., Ginty, D. D., Clish, C. B., Gu, C. (2017). Blood-brain barrier permeability is regulated by lipid transport- dependent suppression of caveolae-mediated transcytosis. *Neuron*, **94**, 581–594.
29. Strazielle, N., Ghersi-Egea, J.-F. (2016). Potential pathways for CNS drug delivery across the blood-cerebrospinal fluid barrier. *Curr. Pharm. Des.*, **22**, 5463–5476.
30. Abbott, N. J. (2013). Blood-brain barrier structure and function and the challenges for CNS drug delivery. *J. Inherit. Metab. Dis.*, **36**, 437–449.
31. Erickson, M. A., Banks, W. A. (2018). Neuroimmune axes of the blood–brain barriers and blood–brain interfaces: bases for physiological regulation, disease states, and pharmacological interventions. *Pharmacol. Rev.*, **70**, 278–314.
32. Agarwal, S., Hartz, A. M. S., Elmquist, W. F., Bauer, B. (2011). Breast cancer resistance protein and P-glycoprotein in brain cancer: two gatekeepers team up. *Curr. Pharm. Des.*, **17**, 2793–2802.
33. Rao, V. V, Dahlheimer, J. L., Bardgett, M. E., Snyder, A. Z., Finch, R. A., Sartorelli, A. C., Piwnica-Worms, D. (1999). Choroid plexus epithelial expression of MDR1 P-glycoprotein and multidrug resistance-associated protein contribute to the blood-cerebrospinal-fluid drug-permeability barrier. *Proc. Natl. Acad. Sci. U. S. A.*, **96**, 3900–3905.
34. Gazzin, S., Strazielle, N., Schmitt, C., Fevre-Montange, M., Ostrow, J. D., Tiribelli, C., Ghersi-Egea, J. F. (2008). Differential expression of the multidrug resistance-related proteins ABCb1 and ABCc1 between blood-brain interfaces. *J. Comp. Neurol.*, **510**, 497–507.
35. Shawahna, R., Uchida, Y., Decleves, X., Ohtsuki, S., Yousif, S., Dauchy, S., Jacob, A., Chassoux, F., Daumas-Duport, C., Couraud, P. O., Terasaki, T., Scherrmann, J. M. (2011). Transcriptomic and quantitative proteomic analysis of transporters and drug metabolizing enzymes in freshly isolated human brain microvessels. *Mol. Pharm.*, **8**, 1332–1341.
36. Abbott, N. J. (2004). Evidence for bulk flow of brain interstitial fluid: significance for physiology and pathology. *Neurochem. Int.*, **45**, 545–552.
37. Johanson, C. E., Duncan, J. A., Klinge, P. M., Brinker, T., Stopa, E. G., Silverberg, G. D. (2008). Multiplicity of cerebrospinal fluid functions: new challenges in health and disease. *Cerebrospinal Fluid Res.*, **5**, 1–32.

38. Lun, M. P., Monuki, E. S., Lehtinen, M. K. (2015). Development and functions of the choroid plexus–cerebrospinal fluid system. *Nat. Rev. Neurosci.*, **16**, 445–457.

39. Abbott, N. J., Pizzo, M. E., Preston, J. E., Janigro, D., Thorne, R. G. (2018). The role of brain barriers in fluid movement in the CNS: is there a "glymphatic" system? *Acta Neuropathol.*, **135**, 387–407.

40. Nilsson, C., Stahlberg, F., Thomsen, C., Henrikssen, O., Herning, M., Owman, C. (1992). Circadian variation in human cerebrospinal fluid production measured by magnetic resonance imaging. *Am. J. Physiol.*, **262**, 20–24.

41. Harrington, M. G., Salomon, R. M., Pogoda, J. M., Oborina, E., Okey, N., Johnson, B., Schmidt, D., Fonteh, A., Dalleska, N. F. (2010). Cerebrospinal fluid sodium rhythms. *Cerebrospinal Fluid Res.*, **7**, 1–9.

42. Lei, Y., Han, H., Yuan, F., Javeed, A., Zhao, Y. (2016). The brain interstitial system: anatomy, modeling, in vivo measurement, and applications. *Prog. Neurobiol.*, **157**, 230–246.

43. Illiff, J. J., Wang, M., Liao, Y., Plogg, B. A., Peng, W., Gundersen, G. A., Benveniste, H., Vates, G. E., Deane, R., Goldman, S. A., Nagelhus, E. A., Nedergaard, M. (2012). A paravascular pathway facilitates CSF flow through the brain parenchyma and the clearance of interstitial solutes, including amyloid β. *Sci. Transl. Med.*, **4**, 1–13.

44. Spector, R., Robert Snodgrass, S., Johanson, C. E. (2015). A balanced view of the cerebrospinal fluid composition and functions: focus on adult humans. *Exp. Neurol.*, **273**, 57–68.

45. Pardridge, W. M. (2016). CSF, blood-brain barrier, and brain drug delivery. *Expert Opin. Drug Deliv.*, **13**, 963–975.

46. Hammarlund-Udenaes, M., Fridén, M., Syvänen, S., Gupta, A. (2008). On the rate and extent of drug delivery to the brain. *Pharm. Res.*, **25**, 1737–1750.

47. Pizzo, M. E., Wolak, D. J., Kumar, N. N., Brunette, E., Brunnquell, C. L., Hannocks, M. J., Abbott, N. J., Meyerand, M. E., Sorokin, L., Stanimirovic, D. B., Thorne, R. G. (2018). Intrathecal antibody distribution in the rat brain: surface diffusion, perivascular transport and osmotic enhancement of delivery. *J. Physiol.*, **596**, 445–475.

48. Fridén, M., Winiwarter, S., Jerndal, G., Bengtsson, O., Hong, W., Bredberg, U., Hammarlund-Udenaes, M., Antonsson, M. (2009). Structure-brain exposure relationships in rat and human using a novel data set of unbound drug concentrations in brain interstitial and cerebrospinal fluids. *J. Med. Chem.*, **52**, 6233–6243.

49. de Lange, E. C., Danhof, M., de Boer, a G., Breimer, D. D. (1997). Methodological considerations of intracerebral microdialysis in pharmacokinetic studies on drug transport across the blood-brain barrier. *Brain Res. Brain Res. Rev.*, **25**, 27–49.

50. Chen, Z., Shi, T., Zhang, L., Zhu, P., Deng, M., Huang, C., Hu, T., Jiang, L., Li, J. (2016). Mammalian drug efflux transporters of the ATP binding cassette (ABC) family in multidrug resistance: a review of the past decade. *Cancer Lett.*, **370**, 153–164.

51. Tang, F., Hartz, A. M. S., Bauer, B. (2017). Drug-resistant epilepsy: multiple hypotheses, few answers. *Front. Neurol.*, **8**, 1–19.

52. Sanchez-Covarrubias, L., Slosky, L. M., Thompson, B. J., Davis, T. P., Ronaldson, P. T. (2014). Transporters at CNS barrier sites: obstacles or opportunities for drug delivery? *Curr. Pharm. Des.*, **20**, 1422–1449.

53. Löscher, W., Potschka, H. (2005). Role of drug efflux transporters in the brain for drug disposition and treatment of brain diseases. *Prog. Neurobiol.*, **76**, 22–76.

54. Schlachetzki, F., Pardridge, W. M. (2003). P-glycoprotein and caveolin-1alpha in endothelium and astrocytes of primate brain. *Neuroreport*, **14**, 2041–2046.

55. Golden, P. L., Pardridge, W. M. (1999). P-glycoprotein on astrocyte foot processes of unfixed isolated human brain capillaries. *Brain Res.*, **819**, 143–146.

56. Lee, G., Schlichter, L., Bendayan, M., Bendayan, R. (2001). Functional expression of P-glycoprotein in rat brain microglia. *J. Pharmacol. Exp. Ther.*, **299**, 204–212.

57. Volk, H. A., Burkhardt, K., Potschka, H., Chen, J., Becker, A., Löscher, W. (2004). Neuronal expression of the drug efflux transporter P-glycoprotein in the rat hippocampus after limbic seizures. *Neuroscience*, **123**, 751–759.

58. Rajagopal, A., Simon, S. M. (2003). Subcellular localization and activity of multidrug resistance proteins. *Mol. Biol. Cell.*, **14**, 3389–3399.

59. Uchida, Y., Ohtsuki, S., Katsukura, Y., Ikeda, C., Suzuki, T., Kamiie, J., Terasaki, T. (2011). Quantitative targeted absolute proteomics of human blood-brain barrier transporters and receptors. *J. Neurochem.*, **117**, 333–345.

60. Ito, K., Uchida, Y., Ohtsuki, S., Aizawa, S., Kawakami, H., Katsukura, Y., Kamiee, J., Terasaki, T. (2011). Quantitative membrane protein expression at the blood-brain barrier of adult and younger cynomolgus monkeys. *J. Pharm. Sci.*, **200**, 3939–3950.

61. Agarwal, S., Uchida, Y., Mittapalli, R. K., Sane, R., Terasaki, T., Elmquist, W. F. (2012). Quantitative proteomics of transporter expression in brain capillary endothelial cells isolated from P-glycoprotein (P-gp), breast cancer resistance protein (Bcrp), and P-gp/Bcrp knockout mice. *Drug Metab. Dispos.*, **40**, 1164–1169.

62. Uchida, Y., Ohtsuki, S., Terasaki, T. (2014). Pharmacoproteomics-based reconstruction of in vivo P-glycoprotein function at blood-brain barrier and brain distribution of substrate verapamil in pentylenetetrazole-kindled epilepsy, spontaneous epilepsy, and phenytoin treatment models. *Drug Metab. Dispos.*, **42**, 1719–1726.

63. De Lange, E. C. M., vd Berg, D. J., Bellanti, F., Voskuyl, R. A., Syvänen, S. (2018). P-glycoprotein protein expression versus functionality at the blood-brain barrier using immunohistochemistry, microdialysis and mathematical modeling. *Eur. J. Pharm. Sci.*, **124**, 61–70.

64. Polli, J. W., Olson, K. L., Chism, J. P., John-williams, L. S., Yeager, R. L., Woodard, S. M., Otto, V., Castellino, S., Demby, V. E. (2009). An unexpected synergist role of P-glycoprotein and breast cancer resistance protein on the central nervous system penetration of the tyrosine kinase inhibitor lapatinib. *Drug Metab. Dispos.*, **37**, 439–442.

65. Kodaira, H., Kusuhara, H., Ushiki, J., Fuse, E., Sugiyama, Y. (2010). Kinetic analysis of the cooperation of P-glycoprotein (P-gp/Abcb1) and breast cancer resistance protein (Bcrp/Abcg2) in limiting the brain and testis penetration of erlotinib, flavopiridol, and mitoxantrone. *J. Pharmacol. Exp. Ther.*, **333**, 788–796.

66. Oberoi, R. K., Mittapalli, R. K., Elmquist, W. F. (2013). Pharmacokinetic assessment of efflux transport in sunitinib distribution to the brain. *J. Pharmacol. Exp. Ther.*, **347**, 755–764.

67. Laramy, J. K., Kim, M., Parrish, K. E., Sarkaria, J. N., Elmquist, W. F. (2018). Pharmacokinetic assessment of cooperative efflux of the multitargeted kinase inhibitor ponatinib across the blood-brain barrier. *J. Pharmacol. Exp. Ther.*, **365**, 249–261.

68. Bauer, M., Römermann, K., Karch, R., Wulkersdorfer, B., Stanek, J., Philippe, C., Maier-Salamon, A., Haslacher, H., Jungbauer, C., Wadsak, W., Jäger, W., Löscher, W., Hacker, M., Zeitlinger, M., Langer, O. (2016). Pilot PET study to assess the functional interplay between ABCB1 and ABCG2 at the human blood–brain barrier. *Clin. Pharmacol. Ther.*, **100**, 131–141.

69. Staud, F., Ceckova, M., Micuda, S., Pavek, P. (2010). Expression and function of P-glycoprotein in normal tissues: effect on pharmacokinetics. *Methods Mol. Biol.*, **596**, 199–222.

70. Palmeira, A., Sousa, E., Vasconcelos, M. H., Pinto, M. (2012). Three decades of P-gp inhibitors: skimming through several generations and scaffolds. *Curr Med Chem.*, **19**, 1946–2025.

71. Food and Drug Administration (2012). Guidance for industry: drug interaction studies—study design, data analysis, implications for dosing, and labeling recommendations, pp. 1–79.

72. Gameiro, M., Silva, R., Rocha-Pereira, C., Carmo, H., Carvalho, F., de Lourdes Bastos, M., Remião, F. (2017). Cellular models and in vitro assays for the screening of modulators of P-gp, MRP1 and BCRP. *Molecules*, **22**, 1–48.

73. Kwak, J. O., Lee, S. H., Lee, G. S., Kim, M. S., Ahn, Y. G., Lee, J. H., Kim, S. W., Kim, K. H., Lee, M. G. (2010). Selective inhibition of MDR1 (ABCB1) by HM30181 increases oral bioavailability and therapeutic efficacy of paclitaxel. *Eur. J. Pharmacol.*, **627**, 92–98.

74. Fox, E., Bates, S. E. (2007). Tariquidar (XR9576): a P-glycoprotein drug efflux pump inhibitor. *Expert Rev. Anticancer Ther.*, **7**, 447–459.

75. Xia, C. Q., Yang, J. J., Gan, L.-S. (2005). Breast cancer resistance protein in pharmacokinetics and drug-drug interactions. *Expert Opin. Drug Metab. Toxicol.*, **1**, 595–611.

76. Mao, Q., Unadkat, J. D. (2015). Role of the breast cancer resistance protein (ABCG2) in drug transport. *AAPS J.*, **7**, 118–133.

77. Köhler, S. C., Wiese, M. (2015). HM30181 derivatives as novel potent and selective inhibitors of the breast cancer resistance protein (BCRP/ABCG2). *J. Med. Chem.*, **58**, 3910–3921.

78. Barrera, B., Otero, J. A., Egido, E., Prieto, J. G., Seelig, A., Álvarez, A. I., Merino, G. (2012). The anthelmintic triclabendazole and its metabolites inhibit the membrane transporter ABCG2/BCRP. *Antimicrob. Agents Chemother.*, **56**, 3535–3543.

79. Loscher, W., Potschka, H., Löscher, W., Potschka, H. (2005). Blood-brain barrier active efflux transporters: ATP-binding cassette gene family. *NeuroRx*, **2**, 86–98.

80. Silva, R., Vilas-Boas, V., Carmo, H., Dinis-Oliveira, R. J., Carvalho, F., De Lourdes Bastos, M., Remião, F. (2015). Modulation of P-glycoprotein efflux pump: induction and activation as a therapeutic strategy. *Pharmacol. Ther.*, **149**, 1–123.

81. Varma, M. V. S., Ashokraj, Y., Dey, C. S., Panchagnula, R. (2003). P-glycoprotein inhibitors and their screening: a perspective from bioavailability enhancement. *Pharmacol. Res.*, **48**, 347–359.

82. Peña-Sol6rzano, D., Stark, S. A., Konig, B., Sierra, C. A., Ochoa-Puentes, C. (2016). ABCG2/BCRP: specific and nonspecific modulators. *Med. Res. Rev.*, 1–64.

83. Padowski, J. M., Pollack, G. M. (2010). Pharmacokinetic and pharmacodynamic implications of P-glycoprotein modulation. *Methods Mol. Biol.*, **596**, 359–384.

84. Gomes, M. J., Kennedy, P. J., Martins, S., Sarmento, B. (2017). Delivery of siRNA silencing P-gp in peptide-functionalized nanoparticles causes efflux modulation at the blood-brain barrier. *Nanomedicine*, **12**, 1385–1399.

85. European Medicines Agency (2012). Guideline on the investigation of drug interactions: CPMP/EWP/560/95/Rev. 1 Corr. 2**, pp. 1–59.

86. Sadeque, A. J. M., Wandel, C., He, H., Shah, S., Wood, A. J. J. (2000). Increased drug delivery to the brain by P-glycoprotein inhibition. *Clin. Pharmacol. Ther.*, **68**, 231–237.

87. Sasongko, L., Link, J. M., Muzi, M., Mankoff, D. A., Yang, X., Collier, A. C., Shoner, S. C., Unadkat, J. D. (2005). Imaging P-glycoprotein transport activity at the human blood-brain barrier with positron emission tomography. *Clin. Pharmacol. Ther.*, **77**, 503–514.

88. Muzi, M., Mankoff, D. A., Link, J. M., Shoner, S. C., Collier, A. C., Sasongko, L., Unadkat, J. D. (2009). Imaging of cyclosporine inhibition of P-glycoprotein activity using 11C-verapamil in the brain: studies of healthy humans. *J. Nucl. Med.*, **50**, 1267–1275.

89. Kalvass, J. C., Polli, J. W., Bourdet, D. L., Feng, B., Huang, S.-M., Liu, X., Smith, Q. R., Zhang, L. K., Zamek-Gliszczynski, M. J. (2013). Why clinical modulation of efflux transport at the human blood-brain barrier is unlikely: the ITC evidence-based position. *Clin. Pharmacol. Ther.*, **94**, 80–94.

90. Hartz, A. M. S., Miller, D. S., Bauer, B. (2010). Restoring blood-brain barrier P-glycoprotein reduces brain amyloid-beta in a mouse model of Alzheimer's disease. *Mol. Pharmacol.*, **77**, 715–723.

91. Chan, G. N. Y., Saldivia, V., Yang, Y., Pang, H., de Lannoy, I., Bendayan, R. (2013). In vivo induction of P-glycoprotein expression at the mouse blood-brain barrier: an intracerebral microdialysis study. *J. Neurochem.*, **127**, 342–352.

92. Zastre, J. A., Chan, G. N. Y., Ronaldson, P. T., Ramaswamy, M., Couraud, P. O., Romero, I. A., Weksler, B., Bendayan, M., Bendayan, R. (2009). Up-regulation of p-glycoprotein by HIV protease inhibitors in a human brain microvessel endothelial cell line. *J. Neurosci. Res.*, **87**, 1023–1036.

93. Chan, G. N. Y., Patel, R., Cummins, C. L., Bendayan, R. (2013). Induction of P-glycoprotein by antiretroviral drugs in human brain microvessel endothelial cells. *Antimicrob. Agents Chemother.*, **57**, 4481–4488.

94. Hoque, M. T., Robillard, K. R., Bendayan, R. (2012). Regulation of breast cancer resistant protein by peroxisome proliferator-activated receptor in human brain microvessel endothelial cells. *Mol. Pharmacol.*, **81**, 598–609.

95. Chaves, C., Remiao, F., Cisternino, S., Decleves, X. (2017). Opioids and the blood-brain barrier: a dynamic interaction with consequences on drug disposition in brain. *Curr. Neuropharmacol.*, **15**, 1156–1173.

96. Liu, L., Collier, A. C., Link, J. M., Domino, K. B., Mankoff, D. A., Eary, J. F., Spiekerman, C. F., Hsiao, P., Deo, A. K., Unadkat, J. D. (2015). Modulation of P-glycoprotein at the human blood-brain barrier by quinidine or rifampin treatment: a positron emission tomography imaging study. *Drug Metab. Dispos.*, **43**, 1795–1804.

97. Pilorz, V., Helfrich-Förster, C., Oster, H. (2018). The role of the circadian clock system in physiology. *Pflugers Arch. Eur. J. Physiol.*, **470**, 227–239.

98. Zhang, S. L., Yue, Z., Arnold, D. M., Artiushin, G., Sehgal, A. (2018). A circadian clock in the blood-brain barrier regulates xenobiotic efflux. *Cell*, **173**, 1–10.

99. Cipolla, M. J., Sweet, J. G., Chan, S.-L. (2011). Cerebral vascular adaptation to pregnancy and its role in the neurological complications of eclampsia. *J. Appl. Physiol.*, **110**, 329–39.

100. Cipolla, M. J. (2013). The adaptation of the cerebral circulation to pregnancy: mechanisms and consequences. *J. Cereb. Blood Flow Metab.*, **33**, 465–478.

101. Bloise, E., Petropoulos, S., Iqbal, M., Kostaki, A., Ortiga-Carvalho, T. M., Gibb, W., Matthews, S. G. (2017). Acute effects of viral exposure on P-glycoprotein function in the mouse fetal blood-brain barrier. *Cell. Physiol. Biochem.*, **41**, 1044–1050.

102. Bhuiyan, M., Petropoulos, S., Gibb, W., Matthews, S. G. (2012). Sertraline alters multidrug resistance phosphoglycoprotein activity in the mouse placenta and fetal blood-brain barrier. *Reprod. Sci.*, **19**, 407–415.

103. Liao, M. Z., Gao, C., Shireman, L. M., Phillips, B., Risler, L. J., Neradugomma, N. K., Choudhari, P., Prasad, B., Shen, D. D., Mao, Q. (2017). P-gp/ABCB1 exerts differential impacts on brain and fetal exposure to norbuprenorphine. *Pharmacol. Res.*, **119**, 61–71.

104. Filia, M. F., Marchini, T., Minoia, J. M., Roma, M. I., De Fino, F. T., Rubio, M. C., Copello, G. J., Evelson, P. A., Peroni, R. N. (2017). Induction of

ABCG2/BCRP restricts the distribution of zidovudine to the fetal brain in rats. *Toxicol. Appl. Pharmacol.*, **330**, 74–83.

105. Roh, H.-T., Cho, S.-Y., Yoon, H.-G., So, W.-Y. (2017). Effect of exercise intensity on neurotrophic factors and blood–brain barrier permeability induced by oxidative–nitrosative stress in male college students. *Int. J. Sport Nutr. Exerc. Metab.*, **27**(3), 239–246.
106. Roh, H. T., So, W. Y. (2017). The effects of aerobic exercise training on oxidant–antioxidant balance, neurotrophic factor levels, and blood–brain barrier function in obese and non-obese men. *J. Sport Heal. Sci.*, **6**, 447–453.
107. Roh, H. T., Cho, S. Y., So, W. Y. (2017). Obesity promotes oxidative stress and exacerbates blood-brain barrier disruption after high-intensity exercise. *J. Sport Heal. Sci.*, **6**, 225–230.
108. Wang, X., Zhang, M., Feng, R., Li, W. B., Ren, S. Q., Zhang, J., Zhang, F. (2014). Physical exercise training and neurovascular unit in ischemic stroke. *Neuroscience*, **271**, 99–107.
109. Lee, J.-M., Park, J.-M., Song, M. K., Oh, Y. J., Kim, C.-J., Kim, Y.-J. (2017). The ameliorative effects of exercise on cognitive impairment and white matter injury from blood-brain barrier disruption induced by chronic cerebral hypoperfusion in adolescent rats. *Neurosci. Lett.*, **638**, 83–89.
110. Souza, P. S., Gonçalves, E. D., Pedroso, G. S., Farias, H. R., Junqueira, S. C., Marcon, R., Tuon, T., Cola, M., Silveira, P. C. L., Santos, A. R., Calixto, J. B., Souza, C. T., de Pinho, R. A., Dutra, R. C. (2016). Physical exercise attenuates experimental autoimmune encephalomyelitis by inhibiting peripheral immune response and blood-brain barrier disruption. *Mol. Neurobiol.*, **54**, 4723–4737.
111. Małkiewicz, M. A., Szarmach, A., Sabisz, A., Cubała, W. J., Szurowska, E., Winklewski, P. J. (2019). Blood-brain barrier permeability and physical exercise. *J. Neuroinflammation*, **16**, 1–16.
112. Erdő, F., Denes, L., de Lange, E. (2017). Age-associated physiological and pathological changes at the blood–brain barrier: a review. *J. Cereb. Blood Flow Metab.*, **37**, 4–24.
113. Pan, Y., Nicolazzo, J. A. (2018). Impact of aging, Alzheimer's disease and Parkinson's disease on the blood-brain barrier transport of therapeutics. *Adv. Drug Deliv. Rev.*, **135**, 62–74.
114. Cotrina, M. L., Nedergaard, M. (2002). Astrocytes in the aging brain. *J. Neurosci. Res.*, **67**, 1–10.
115. Duncombe, J., Lennen, R. J., Jansen, M. A., Marshall, I., Wardlaw, J. M., Horsburgh, K. (2016). Ageing causes prominent neurovascular

dysfunction associated with loss of astrocytic contacts and gliosis. *Neuropathol. Appl. Neurobiol.*, **43**, 477–491.

116. Popescu, B. O., Toescu, E. C., Popescu, L. M., Bajenaru, O., Muresanu, D. F., Schultzberg, M., Bogdanovic, N. (2009). Blood-brain barrier alterations in ageing and dementia. *J. Neurol. Sci.*, **283**, 99–106.

117. Farrall, A. J., Wardlaw, J. M. (2009). Blood-brain barrier: ageing and microvascular disease - systematic review and meta-analysis. *Neurobiol. Aging*, **30**, 337–352.

118. Gorlé, N., Van Cauwenberghe, C., Libert, C., Vandenbroucke, R. E. (2016). The effect of aging on brain barriers and the consequences for Alzheimer's disease development. *Mamm. Genome*, **27**, 407–420.

119. Kealy, J., Greene, C., Campbell, M. (2020). Blood-brain barrier regulation in psychiatric disorders. *Neurosci. Lett.*, **726**, 133664.

120. Pires, P. W., Dams Ramos, C. M., Matin, N., Dorrance, A. M. (2013). The effects of hypertension on the cerebral circulation. *Am. J. Physiol. Circ. Physiol.*, **304**, H1598–H1614.

121. Ortiz, G. G., Pacheco-Moisés, F. P., Macías-Islas, M.Á., Flores-Alvarado, L. J., Mireles-Ramírez, M. A., González-Renovato, E. D., Hernández-Navarro, V. E., Sánchez-López, A. L., Alatorre-Jiménez, M. A. (2014). Role of the blood-brain barrier in multiple sclerosis. *Arch. Med. Res.*, **45**, 687–697.

122. Montagne, A., Zhao, Z., Zlokovic, B. V. (2017). Alzheimer's disease: a matter of blood-brain barrier dysfunction? *J. Exp. Med.*, **214**, 3151–3169.

123. Najjar, S., De Sanctis, V., Chong, D., Pahlajani, S., Najjar, A., Stern, J. N. H. (2017). Neurovascular unit dysfunction and blood–brain barrier hyperpermeability contribute to schizophrenia neurobiology: a theoretical integration of clinical and experimental evidence. *Front. Psychiatry*, **8**, 1–11.

124. Han, H., Mann, A., Ekstein, D., Eyal, S. (2017). Breaking bad: the structure and function of the blood-brain barrier in epilepsy. *AAPS J.*, **19**, 973–988.

125. Desai, B. S., Monahan, A. J., Carvey, P. M., Hendey, B. (2007). Blood-brain barrier pathology in Alzheimer's and Parkinson's disease: implications for drug therapy. *Cell Transplant.*, **16**, 285–299.

126. Jonkers, N., Sarre, S., Ebinger, G., Michotte, Y. (2001). Benserazide decreases central AADC activity, extracellular dopamine levels and levodopa decarboxylation in striatum of the rat. *J. Neural Transm.*, **108**, 559–570.

127. Bartels, A. L., Willemsen, A. T. M., Kortekaas, R., De Jong, B. M., De Vries, R., De Klerk, O., Van Oostrom, J. C. H., Portman, A., Leenders, K. L. (2008). Decreased blood-brain barrier P-glycoprotein function in the progression of Parkinson's disease, PSP and MSA. *J. Neural Transm.*, **115**, 1001–1009.

128. Kortekaas, R., Leenders, K. L., Van Oostrom, J. C. H., Vaalburg, W., Bart, J., Willemsen, A. T. M., Hendrikse, N. H. (2005). Blood-brain barrier dysfunction in Parkinsonian midbrain in vivo. *Ann. Neurol.*, **57**, 176–179.

129. Vautier, S., Milane, A., Fernandez, C., Bourasset, F., Chacun, H., Lacomblez, L., Farinottti, R. (2009). Role of two efflux proteins, ABCB1 and ABCG2, in blood-brain barrier transport of bromocriptine in a murine model of MPTP-induced dopaminergic degeneration. *J. Pharm. Pharm. Sci.*, **12**, 199–208.

130. Xiong, H., Callaghan, D., Jones, A., Bai, J., Rasquinha, I., Smith, C., Pei, K., Walker, D., Lue, L.-F., Stanimirovic, D., Zhang, W. (2009). ABCG2 is up-regulated in Alzheimer's brain with cerebral amyloid angiopathy and may act as a gatekeeper at the blood-brain barrier for Aβ1-40 peptides. *J. Neurosci.*, **167**, 1171–1181.

131. Wang, N., Jin, X., Guo, D., Tong, G., Zhu, X. (2017). Iron chelation nanoparticles with delayed saturation as an effective therapy for Parkinson disease. *Biomacromolecules*, **18**, 461–474.

132. Umlauf, B. J., Shusta, E. V. (2019). Exploiting BBB disruption for the delivery of nanocarriers to the diseased CNS. *Curr. Opin. Biotechnol.*, **60**, 146–152.

133. Caruso, F., Furtado, D., Björnmalm, M., Kempe, K., Ayton, S., Bush, A. I. (2018). Overcoming the blood-brain barrier: the role of nanomaterials in treating neurological diseases. *Adv. Mater.*, **30**, 1–66.

134. Qu, M., Lin, Q., He, S., Wang, L., Fu, Y., Zhang, Z., Zhang, L. (2018). A brain targeting functionalized liposomes of the dopamine derivative N-3,4-bis(pivaloyloxy)-dopamine for treatment of Parkinson's disease. *J. Control. Release*, **277**, 173–182.

135. Seiffert, E., Dreier, J. P., Ivens, S., Bechmann, I., Tomkins, O., Heinemann, U., Friedman, A. (2004). Lasting blood-brain barrier disruption induces epileptic focus in the rat somatosensory cortex. *J. Neurosci.*, **24**, 7829–7836.

136. Marchi, N., Banjara, M., Janigro, D. (2016). Blood-brain barrier, bulk flow, and interstitial clearance in epilepsy. *J. Neurosci. Methods*, **260**, 118–124.

137. Vasilevko, V., Passos, G. F., Quiring, D., Head, E., Kim, R. C., Fisher, M., Cribbs, D. H. (2010). Aging and cerebrovascular dysfunction: contribution of hypertension, cerebral amyloid angiopathy, and immunotherapy. *Ann. N. Y. Acad. Sci.*, **1207**, 58–70.

138. Qosa, H., Miller, D. S., Pasinelli, P., Trotti, D. (2015). Regulation of ABC efflux transporters at blood-brain barrier in health and neurological disorders. *Brain Res.*, **1628**, 298–316.

139. Rosenberg, G. A. (2017). Extracellular matrix inflammation in vascular cognitive impairment and dementia. *Clin. Sci.*, **131**, 425–437.

140. Mohammadi, M. T., Dehghani, G. A. (2014). Acute hypertension induces brain injury and blood-brain barrier disruption through reduction of claudins mRNA expression in rat. *Pathol. Res. Pract.*, **210**, 985–990.

141. Biancardi, V., Stern, J. (2016). Compromised blood-brain barrier permeability: novel mechanism by which circulating angiotensin II signals sympathoexcitatory centers during hypertension. *J. Physiol.*, **594**, 1591–1600.

142. Villapol, S., Saavedra, J. M. (2015). Neuroprotective effects of angiotensin receptor blockers. *Am. J. Hypertens.*, **28**, 289–299.

143. Mamo, J. C. L., Lam, V., Giles, C., Coulson, S. H., Fimognari, N., Mooranian, A., Al-Salami, H., Takechi, R. (2017). Antihypertensive agents do not prevent blood–brain barrier dysfunction and cognitive deficits in dietary-induced obese mice. *Int. J. Obes.*, **41**, 926–934.

Chapter 3

Novel Routes to Accessing the Brain: Intranasal Administration

Ana Serralheiro,[a] Joana Bicker,[b,c] Gilberto Alves,[d] Amílcar Falcão[b,c] and Ana Fortuna[b,c]

[a]*Department of Chemistry and Pharmacy, Faculty of Science and Technology, University of Algarve, Campus de Gambelas, 8005-139, Faro, Portugal*
[b]*Laboratory of Pharmacology, Faculty of Pharmacy, University of Coimbra, Pólo das Ciências da Saúde, Azinhaga de Santa Comba, 3000-548 Coimbra, Portugal*
[c]*Coimbra Institute for Biomedical Imaging and Translational Research (CIBIT), University of Coimbra, Coimbra, Portugal*
[d]*CICS-UBI – Health Sciences Research Centre, University of Beira Interior, Av. Infante D. Henrique, 6200-506 Covilhã, Portugal*
anacfortuna@gmail.com

Direct drug brain delivery with minimal systemic exposure attracted great interest and became one of the most challenging research areas with regard to the treatment of central nervous system (CNS)-related diseases. In opposition to invasive methods like intraparenchymal, intracerebroventricular or intrathecal injections/infusions, non-invasive intranasal delivery has stood out with high drug target efficacy of chronically administered drugs.

Nanoparticles for Brain Drug Delivery
Edited by Carla Vitorino, Andreia Jorge and Alberto Pais

ISBN 978-981-4877-31-2 (Hardcover), 978-1-003-11932-6 (eBook)
www.jennystanford.com

In this chapter, nose-to-brain delivery mechanisms are explained, as well as experimental in vivo models which have been used to exploit them, specifying central drugs which have been administered by the intranasal route.

3.1 Introduction

According to a recent World Health Organization report [1], neurological disorders, such as epilepsy, migraine, stroke, multiple sclerosis, Alzheimer's disease and Parkinson's disease, are currently estimated to affect as many as a billion people worldwide, being one of the leading causes of disability. Their intricate pathophysiology and the difficulty of systemically administered therapeutics in accessing the brain represent a great challenge in the development of efficacious agents for central targets [2]. In spite of intense research efforts, many drugs are still not being effectively and efficiently delivered to the central nervous system (CNS), mainly due to the restrictive nature of the blood–brain barrier (BBB) which restricts substances from entering the brain, depending on their lipophilicity, molecular size and charge [3–6].

In the last decades, several different strategies have been attempted in order to circumvent the BBB and improve the delivery of drugs to the brain for therapeutic and diagnostic purposes [7–12]. Intranasal administration, especially to the olfactory region located in the upper portion of the nasal passages, has been shown to non-invasively deliver a wide variety of compounds from the nasal cavity directly to the CNS, bypassing the BBB within a few minutes [13–16]. Increasing evidence of nose-to-brain transport has been reported by numerous research studies wherein the levels of certain drug molecules determined in the cerebrospinal fluid (CSF) and olfactory bulb, after intranasal administration to rodents and rhesus macaques, were considerably higher than those observed following intravenous injection [16–18]. The rapid and preferential distribution of drugs to the brain via the intranasal route may lead to the reduction of systemic exposure and peripheral side effects. Similarly, the dose and frequency of dosing could be decreased, the toxicity minimised and the therapeutic efficacy improved by achieving desired drug concentrations at the biophase [19–21].

Up to date, the investigations have attracted researchers to place the intranasal delivery option for CNS drug targeting under the 'microscope'. Even though the clinical potential of this drug administration avenue still remains controversial, there is substantial curiosity in exploring the nasal route for the treatment of common intracerebral diseases.

To deepen the comprehension of the phenomena inherent to the ability of the intranasal route to directly deliver therapeutic compounds to the CNS, this chapter will provide thorough information with emphasis on this specific topic.

3.2 Nose-to-Brain Drug Delivery

Traditionally, the management of neurological disorders is predominantly performed through peripheral administration of medicines via the oral or intravenous route. However, there are a variety of troublesome issues concerning the use of systemic drug delivery to treat CNS diseases. Many drugs, and in particular macromolecules, are generally degraded in the gastrointestinal tract and/or metabolised in the liver, severely reducing their bioavailability to the point where only a small fraction of the active compound actually reaches the circulatory system and ultimately the brain [2, 22]. Increasing the oral dose to compensate drug loss and the direct delivery of therapeutics into the blood via intravenous injection seem to be obvious alternatives to overcome these limitations. Notwithstanding, the former option may cause unacceptable peripheral adverse events, and the latter remains rather impractical and unattractive, especially for treatments requiring frequent dosing or home administration [2]. Beyond these inconveniences, systemic administration of drugs towards the CNS invariably predicates the passage of the compounds from the bloodstream to the brain by crossing the BBB, which is not always an easy process, mainly for large and/or charged molecules. In addition, plasma protein binding, another consequence of systemic delivery, can also affect both the duration and the intensity of a drug's action, diminishing its ability to efficiently permeate the BBB [22].

Although invasive strategies, such as intracerebroventricular injection, have been stated as a viable solution to defeat the BBB through the introduction of therapeutics directly into the brain, these methods are not realistic for clinical applications. Besides being risky, they involve expensive techniques, demand surgical expertise and are not somehow appropriate for multiple dosing regimens [4, 23]. In view of this fact, intranasal administration has been proposed as a promising non-invasive, practical, safe and convenient delivery method which may allow increased CNS penetration of compounds which otherwise display limited brain uptake, by providing a potential and efficient way to circumvent the BBB while minimising systemic exposure [3, 13, 14, 24]. The exploitation of the nasal cavity as a means of delivering therapeutic agents preferentially to the brain has recently gained significant interest. Detailed pharmacokinetic and pharmacodynamic studies, following intranasal delivery in both animals and humans, have shown that a broad spectrum of compounds not only reach specific areas of the brain but also have effects on CNS-mediated behaviours within a short period of time [23]. Curiously, this route of administration has long been adopted by individuals who consume cocaine illicitly. In fact, it is well known that after sniffing, cocaine is rapidly absorbed from the nasal mucosa, allowing the achievement of a state of euphoria within only 3–5 min [25]. Apart from quick nasal absorption of the narcotic to the systemic circulation, it was hypothesised that such rapid cocaine effects on the CNS were probably due to the presence of a direct pathway from the nasal cavity to the brain. Chow et al. [26] performed a study to determine whether cocaine could be directly transported from the nose to the brain by comparing drug concentration–time profiles in plasma and different brain regions, following both intranasal and intravenous administrations to rats. This work revealed that, unlike what was found by the intravenous route, cocaine concentration in samples collected within 60 min after intranasal administration was considerably different among distinct brain regions, showing the highest level in the olfactory bulb. Moreover, it was also observed that brain-to-plasma ratios of cocaine in the olfactory bulb following intranasal administration were significantly higher than those in other brain areas up to 60 min postdose. Inclusively, at 1 min after intranasal instillation, this parameter exhibited an order of magnitude about 3 times greater compared to intravenous injection. Thus, on the basis of these results, the authors concluded that a direct pathway from the nasal cavity to the brain was probably involved in the delivery of cocaine when it was administered nasally, and the transport of the referred abuse substance from the nose to the brain may have presumably been carried out via the olfactory system.

3.2.1 Pathways and Mechanisms of Nose-to-Brain Transport

While the precise mechanisms governing direct intranasal drug delivery to the CNS are still not completely understood, an accumulating body of evidence has demonstrated that pathways involving nerves connecting the nasal passages to the brain play an important role. In general, there are mainly three possible pathways along which a drug administered into the nasal cavity may travel and attain the CNS. One of these routes includes the systemic pathway by which part of the drug is absorbed to the blood circulation and subsequently reaches the brain by crossing the BBB. The other two enclose direct transfer of the compounds from the nose to the CSF or brain tissue via neuronal transport, which can be accomplished either through olfactory or trigeminal nerves [27–29].

When a drug formulation is nasally applied, it can be deposited in the respiratory region, from where, after escaping enzymatic degradation and the normal rapid clearance by the mucociliary clearance (MCC) system, it may be absorbed to the bloodstream by successfully traversing the mucus and nasal epithelial layers. Once in the systemic circulation, therapeutic compounds can freely diffuse through the BBB and enter the CNS. Nevertheless, as mentioned before, the systemic delivery of drugs to the brain is highly conditioned by the permeability of the molecules across the BBB, which is subsequently dependent on their lipid solubility, molecular size and charge. Hence, the absorption of substrates to the systemic circulation after intranasal administration constitutes an indirect pathway for delivering nasally administered drugs to the brain, and therefore it does not afford any preferential advantage on CNS targeting [3, 30]. Moreover, some limiting factors such as plasma protein binding, plasma protease degradation, systemic dilution and potential peripheral side effects also contribute to make it not ideal for nose-to-brain delivery [23].

Taking into account that the olfactory region is a well-recognised direct portal of entry for drug substances into the brain, several investigations have been made in order to describe the mechanisms involved in the transport of molecules across the olfactory epithelium. In theory, therapeutic agents can be transported from the nasal cavity directly to the CSF or brain parenchyma via two possible routes along the olfactory neurons: the olfactory nerve pathway (intracellular axonal transport) and the olfactory epithelial pathway (extracellular perineural transport) [27, 31].

The *olfactory nerve pathway* has been proposed as a feasible route to transfer drugs directly to the brain via intracellular axonal transport along the olfactory sensory neurons. Consistent evidence has been described by several authors for the uptake of different substances into the olfactory neurons with subsequent distribution to the olfactory bulb and other brain areas by the anterograde axoplasmic flow. Axonal internalisation of numerous metal compounds, such as gold, nickel, mercury, aluminium, manganese and cadmium, was reported to occur by passive diffusion or different mechanisms of endocytosis. A study carried out in rats to assess the possibility of transneuronal transport of wheat germ agglutinin–horseradish peroxidase, after intranasal application, revealed that such substance was intra-axonally delivered to the olfactory bulb, following neuronal uptake through surface receptor binding and subsequent adsorptive endocytosis [32]. Notwithstanding, despite the ability of the intracellular axonal route to deliver agents to the olfactory bulb, distribution to other CNS regions beyond the olfactory system is unclear. Furthermore, it is believed that such transport is slow, taking hours or even days for drugs to reach the brain parenchymal tissue, which, therefore, cannot account for the rapid delivery of some therapeutics to the CNS which exhibit considerably high concentrations in both the CSF and brain almost immediately after or within an hour postintranasal dosing [2, 22, 23]. Hence, this pathway is not likely to explain the observed sudden appearance of certain drugs in the CNS, like, for example, cocaine [26], carbamazepine [33], phenobarbital [34] and testosterone [35], after nasal administration. Accordingly, as an alternative to intracellular axonal uptake, it was suggested that drugs, after traversing the olfactory epithelium, either by transcellular or by paracellular mechanisms, could make their way by entering into the lamina propria and then diffusing into the perineural channels, which appear to be the result of continuous subarachnoid extensions which surround the olfactory nerves from the base of the epithelium to the brain by crossing the cribriform plate.

This extracellular mechanism, also known as *olfactory epithelial pathway*, is considered a faster route of nose-to-brain transfer as compounds are able to paracelullarly cross the perineural epithelium into the fluid-filled perineuronal space, requiring only a few minutes (<30 min) for drugs to travel, most likely by a bulk flow transport phenomenon, along the olfactory axon up to the subarachnoid space filled with the CSF [23]. Nevertheless, some controversial facts have been questioning the viability of this pathway since distinct directions and rates are ascertained between the desired drug diffusion and the CSF flow, which creates a functional barrier against the free movement of molecules from the subarachnoid space to the brain tissue [3, 36]. Furthermore, diffusion decreases exponentially with the distance [36], and in humans, the CSF is continuously renewed approximately every 5 h, being totally replaced more than four times a day [37]. Thus, after reaching the CSF, drugs can be rapidly cleared by drainage into the lymphatic vessels and thereafter into the systemic circulation, hindering their penetration into the brain parenchyma. On the basis of these facts, despite the intimate contact of the CSF and the brain, one cannot be sure that a thorough dynamic balance exists between both compartments, and therefore the drug concentrations will not be equivalent [3].

More recently, a trigeminal nerve pathway has been suggested as another valid route for the transport of molecules directly from the nasal cavity to the brain [27, 38]. The trigeminal nerve is the largest cranial nerve with both sensory and motor functions, and its name derives from the fact that it has three major branches: the mandibular, the maxillary and the ophthalmic nerve divisions. The last two are particularly involved in nose-to-brain drug delivery, since their branches are directly connected to the nasal mucosa, in contrast with the mandibular division, which extends to the lower jaw and teeth, away from the nasal cavity [23, 24]. The maxillary ramification allows the innervation of the lateral walls of the nasal mucosa, whereas the ophthalmic branch innervates both the dorsal segment of the nasal mucosa and the anterior portion of the nose [23, 39]. The three peripheral trigeminal branches meet at the trigeminal ganglion, yielding in a single incoming nerve which ends in the brainstem, at the level of the pons [39].

The transport of nasally administered therapeutic agents via the *trigeminal nerve pathway* was firstly demonstrated by Thorne et al. [40] for insulin-like growth factor I. Since then, a similar mode of transport was also evidenced for other proteins and peptides, including interferon-β1b [38] and hypocretin-1 [23]. Following intranasal instillation of the referred radiolabelled compounds to animal models, higher levels of radioactivity were observed in the trigeminal branches, trigeminal ganglion and pons, strongly indicating the involvement of the trigeminal nerve in the delivery of drugs from the nasal passages to the CNS. Even though no factual data have been reported on the unsheathing cells and channels associated with the trigeminal nerve comparable to those observed with the olfactory ones, there is a substantial conviction that these anatomical features may likewise be present along the trigeminal pathway [24]. Interestingly, unlike the *fila olfactori*a, the trigeminal nerve extends from the respiratory epithelium and enters the brain at two different sites: (1) the anterior lacerated foramen near the pons and (2) the cribriform plate near the olfactory bulb, which allows drug delivery to both caudal and rostral areas of the brain [22, 24].

Although several hypothetic mechanisms were described for the direct delivery of drugs from the nasal cavity to the CNS, the contributions underlying each one have not been yet enlightened. Generally, the rapid appearance of a drug in the brain and CSF indicates preferential involvement of the extracellular transport pathway rather than the olfactory intraneural route. However, the possibility of axonal drug internalisation occurring later cannot be entirely ruled out. In fact, the vast majority of the studies performed in animal models was often conducted for limited periods of time (<240 min) [41], therefore preventing the opportunity to assess whether, beyond the olfactory epithelial pathway, the molecules would also explore the axonal transport to travel within the neurons and reach the brain. On the basis of these considerations, it is likely that drugs may use one or a combination of various pathways in the transport from the nose to the CNS; notwithstanding, so far, the extent of each mechanism still remains experimentally hard to define.

3.3 Nose-to-Brain Delivery Assessment: Experimental Issues

The neuronal connection between the nasal cavity and the brain has been extensively investigated on the hypothesis for CNS targeting of drugs. Albeit the numerous examples that support the success and potential of intranasal administration to rapidly deliver a great diversity of neurotherapeutics into the brain, direct transport following intranasal dosing is not always consistently demonstrated. Beyond that, some contradictory results are occasionally encountered for the same tested molecule and using equal experimental models. For instance, while van den Berg et al. [42] concluded that intranasal estradiol held no advantage in drug targeting to the CSF over intravenous injection, another research group has shown that, after intranasal application, the same compound was transported into the CSF via olfactory neurons, confirming, for this particular case, the existence of a direct transport route from the nasal cavity to the CSF [43]. Opposing results concerning the involvement of a direct nose-to-brain pathway were likewise accounted for melatonin following intranasal administration to rats [44, 45]. These contrasting conclusions for similar drugs may be due to differences in the methodologies employed which raise important issues in what concerns to experimental and formulation factors which can significantly influence the outcome of the studies and the interpretation of the obtained results. Therefore, the distinct methodologies used to study drug transport via the nasal route to the CNS will be discussed later. Some relevant considerations will be given regarding the choice of the experimental models, the definition of the study design and the application of the assessment parameters.

3.3.1 Experimental Models

Many different experimental models are used in nasal drug delivery research, including in vitro, in situ and in vivo techniques [46–49]. Each model has its advantages and limitations which affect how the obtained results can be interpreted and, more importantly, how they can be extrapolated to the human situation.

In effect, it must not be forgotten that the ultimate goal of exploration of the nose-to-brain pathway is to be able to apply this administration route to humans, promoting efficient delivery of drugs to the CNS and, as a consequence, improving their therapeutic efficacy.

With the intent of formulating a successful novel nasal drug delivery system, testing with reliably in vitro, in situ and in vivo models is crucial, their application being dependent on the aim of the study and the phase of the drug discovery and development program [50–53]. In vitro techniques present the ability to control a lot of variables, are cheap, use low amounts of drug and animals and allow high-throughput screening of a large number of compounds. These approaches comprise the use of nasal cell cultures or excised tissues from different animal species and are extremely helpful in evaluating the mechanistic aspects of nasal drug delivery, such as absorption, metabolism and toxicity of drugs at the level of the nasal epithelium [54, 55]. Aware of the major importance that the determination of drugs' permeability across the nasal mucosal membrane has to address their systemic exposure and, thereby, their therapeutic potential, the usefulness of predictive nasal in vitro models at the early stages of the research and development process is unquestionable, contributing to optimising the selection of drug candidates and formulations prior to further preclinical and clinical phases [47]. However, owing to the simplistic environmental conditions under which these models are frequently performed and their limitation with regard to the absence of several physiologic factors, like, for example, the MCC mechanism, led to the need of complementing the obtained experimental in vitro data with other information generated from in situ models. By perfusing a drug solution through the nasal cavity of an anaesthetised animal and monitoring the changes in drug concentration levels remaining in the perfusate at specified time intervals, it is possible to estimate drug absorption through the nasal mucosa [56–58]. Even though in situ techniques provide detailed information about nasal drug absorption kinetics, they also have some drawbacks related to significant differences between experimental and real physiologic conditions. Among other factors, the mucus layer is gradually eroded by the circulating solution, exposing the epithelium and thus increasing the drug absorption rate. Additionally, comparing to the in vivo situation, the nasal drug residence time is much more prolonged, which would give a false impression of improved absorption and/or increased toxicity of the drug [54].

Granted that the complete pharmacokinetics and pharmacodynamics of a drug can only be evaluated in whole animal models, in vivo approaches have been employed in more advanced stages of drug discovery and development programs. Although they are more expensive and labour-intensive, also involving a bigger number of animals, in vivo techniques provide the most comprehensive pharmacological characterisation of the fate and activity of drug molecules within the body, which is not possible to achieve simply resorting to in vitro or in situ methods. As with any biomedical area of research, the majority of the nasal delivery studies has been preferably accomplished in animal models, such as rats, mice, rabbits, sheep, dogs and monkeys [59]. Due to methodological and ethical limitations, much fewer studies have been conducted in humans, and therefore, to date, very few investigations providing evidence for nose-to-brain drug delivery in humans have been reported. Since sampling of human CSF and brain tissue specimens is difficult and risky, the indirect evaluation of pharmacodynamic effects (e.g. event-related brain potentials, attention and working memory function [60]) have been commonly described rather than absolute measurements of CNS drug concentrations [41]. Specialised techniques like positron emission tomography [61, 62], neurosurgical CSF drainage [63] and intraspinal catheterisation [64] have recently allowed CNS quantitative determinations after nasal administration of drugs in human volunteers, but convincing unequivocal proof of the nose-to-brain pathway via demonstration of mass transport is still lacking [2].

Taking into account the large amount of data obtained from nasal delivery studies carried out in laboratory animals, the key question is based on whether these experimental results can be applied to the human clinical situation [65]. As a matter of fact, there are valid reasons to be sceptical about the potential for nose-to-brain transport in humans on the basis of evidence from animal research, whereby the in vivo model used to study the transfer of drugs from the nasal mucosa to the brain must be properly selected in order to allow a feasible extrapolation of the results [2]. Indeed, substantial differences exist between the nasal anatomy and physiology of humans and animals, which should be carefully considered when the results are interpreted and compared, avoiding misleading conclusions (Table 3.1).

In general, rodents are the most widely used animals for intranasal drug delivery experiments [59, 63, 67, 69]. The amount of nasal epithelium which corresponds to the olfactory mucosa is proportionally smaller in humans (3%–8%) compared to mice or rats (45%–50%). In addition, the olfactory region in such animals covers a large part of the nasal mucosa, whereas in humans, the olfactory epithelium is restricted to a small area in the roof of the nasal cavity [70]. Therefore, it is expected that the predisposition of rodents to olfactory deposition and transport of compounds to the brain via the olfactory route may be significantly more pronounced. On the other hand, the volume and renovation rate of the CSF are likewise distinct between the two species once the CSF turnover in rodents is about five to six times higher relative to humans [2]. These differences may have a considerable impact on nose-to-brain drug delivery, especially when the diffusion of compounds from the CSF into the brain tissue is accounted.

Bearing in mind these considerations, conclusions regarding the bioavailability of a compound and the extent of its delivery to the brain in humans should not be straightforwardly drawn from the results solely obtained in animal models. To verify the actual feasibility of the intranasal route for CNS drug delivery, it is imperative to compare data derived from both animal and human research studies. A realistic comparison between humans and rats was performed using resembling experimental setups [45, 63, 71]. By administering identical intranasal and intravenous drug formulations of melatonin and hydroxocobalamin and employing similar sampling times, analogous results were obtained for both evaluated species. Even though no evidence of direct transport of the compounds from the nasal cavity to the CSF has been found, the comparison of these three studies demonstrated that, in this particular case, rat experiments can be predictive for nose-to-CSF transport in humans, strengthening the basis for extrapolating the results from animals to humans.

Table 3.1 Comparison of the anatomical and physiological characteristics of the nasal cavity and cerebrospinal fluid (CSF) among different animal species [37, 41, 66–68]

Species	Nasal cavity characteristics					CSF characteristics	
	Length (cm)	Volume (mL)	Surface area (cm^2)	Olfactory area (cm^2)	Clearance half-time (min)	Volume (mL)	Turnover rate (mL/h)
Human	7.5	20.0	160.0	10.0	15.0	160.0	21.0
Monkey	5.3	8.0	62.0	9.0	10.0	NF	2.5
Sheep	18.0	114.0	327.0	NF	42.0	14.2	7.1
Dog	10.0	20.0	221.0	150.0	20.0	NF	NF
Rabbit	5.2	6.0	61.0	6.0	10.0	2.3	0.6
Rat	2.3	0.4	14.0	7.0	5.0	0.15	0.18
Mouse	0.5	0.03	2.8	1.3	1.0	0.035	0.018

NF, not found.

3.3.2 Study Design

It is important to consider the different methodologies used in intranasal studies since several experimental aspects such as delivery volume, administration technique, drug formulation and anaesthesia can all influence the distribution and deposition of drugs in the nasal cavity and, consequently, the pathways by which a drug may travel to the CNS after intranasal administration. The deposition of the drug within the nasal chamber should be appropriately optimised for the intended therapeutic goal, whether it may be highly concentrated at the olfactory mucosa for a CNS effect or low-deposited in that area when a systemic outcome is desired. Actually, the distance from the nostril to the olfactory epithelium is very short; however, its location in the slit-like olfactory cleft behind the narrow nasal vestibule and at the end of a complex labyrinth of respiratory turbinates severely complicates the access [2]. Expectably, deposition in adequate innervated regions of the nasal cavity can therefore be a critical component of the overall approach towards realising the full potential of nose-to-brain drug delivery [2].

Typically, the administration of drugs into the nose is most often performed by using either a pipettor for delivering drops to alternating nostrils, a piece of tubing attached to a microsyringe/micropipette for inserting within the nasal cavity, or a nasal spray device [23, 69, 72]. Placing the nasal drops at the opening of the nostrils allows the animal to sniff them into the nasal cavity, but the tendency to deposit on the nasal floor and be subjected to rapid MCC is elevated [23]. Nasal sprays usually provide high reproducibility in terms of the emitted dose and a widespread distribution of the drug within the nasal cavity; nevertheless, the probability of deposition in either the oesophagus and/or lungs is much more augmented [23, 72]. Conversely, the use of flexible tubing, by giving the possibility of being inserted inside the nose, enables precise delivery of the drug formulation on a localised mucosal area, inasmuch the deposition in the respiratory and olfactory epithelia essentially depends on the length of the tube [23, 73].

The selection of the drug formulation is also a fundamental issue which should be taken into account. A big part of the intranasally applied compounds is in the form of simple solutions [59]. Nasal drops are the simplest and the most convenient pharmaceutical dosage form, but the precise dosing of drug delivered is somewhat difficult to control, in addition to also being associated to a rapid nasal drainage [74]. When using liquid formulations, a special concern must be considered regarding the administration volume. Differences in delivery volumes are closely related to the amount of the nasal surface area covered by the formulation, affecting the deposition within the nasal cavity and the distribution to the CNS. Depending on the experimental model used, the administration technique applied and the therapeutic effect intended, the delivery nasal volume should be properly adjusted and defined. Hence, delivery volumes which do not overload the total capacity of the nasal cavity must be used and should not exceed 5–10 μL/nostril in mice, 10–25 μL/nostril in rats and 75–100 μL/nostril in humans [69]. Although small volumes may not be sufficient to reach and cover the desired area of the nasal mucosa, an excessive dosage volume may cause loss of the drug formulation by resulting in deposition at the nasopharynx, with subsequent swallowing or drainage to the lower respiratory tract, which, in the latter case, may give rise to respiratory distress and eventually death [23, 75]. Aiming at preventing drainage of a nasally dosed drug solution, some researchers have employed the nasal cavity isolation technique by applying an established surgical procedure in rodents [26, 76–81]. Briefly, after an incision has been made in the neck, the trachea is cannulated to allow the animal free breathing, the upper part of the oesophagus is tied off to restrain swallowing and the nasopalatine duct is sealed to avoid any drug formulation from being cleared into the mouth. Since this method involves a closed and confined system, the data obtained is very reproducible and reliable, providing more concrete information about the transport of the molecules from the nose to the brain [82]. Nonetheless, the use of such treatment would be unrealistic, even unthinkable in humans, and therefore, one should exercise caution in the interpretation and extrapolation of these animal results to humans [69].

Given the limitations described for liquid formulations, alternate semisolid dosage forms, such as gels, have been developed for more precise drug delivery through the nose. They reduce postnasal drip and anterior leakage by maintaining the drug formulation in the nasal mucosa. This enhances the drug residence time inside the nasal cavity and diminishes the MCC, thereby providing a better chance for the drug to be absorbed and transported to the CNS [6, 83]. Recently, in situ nasal gelling systems have emerged as a promising approach which benefit dual advantages from both sol and gel and present themselves for more accurate dosing [84]. Displaying low viscosity properties at the time of administration, in situ gels are easily handled and precisely delivered. Following intranasal instillation, they should readily undergo phase transition to form a gel which is strong enough to reside within the nasal cavity for a prolonged period of time, thus preventing MCC and enhancing drug bioavailability [84].

Albeit most often depreciated, the influence of anaesthesia on the rate and extent of drug transport from the nose to the brain is another matter of debate. In effect, the majority of the preclinical studies have been carried out in anaesthetised mice and rats in order to facilitate nasal drug administration, so it seems possible that both the category of anaesthetic and its delivery route could affect the drug pharmacokinetic profile [85, 86]. Generally, compared to the conscious condition, the anaesthetic state may result in a more effective contact time of the formulation with the nasal mucosa, as well as higher absorption in the olfactory epithelium, which may further increase brain drug uptake [86]. Even though few published records exist regarding the influence of different types of anaesthesia on intranasal brain drug delivery, some authors claim a probable decrease on nasal mucosa cilia clearance rate with the consequent reduction of mucociliary activity [87]. Ideally, to avoid any interference caused by the anaesthesia, the use of conscious animals is clearly preferred; however, rodents commonly do not tolerate intranasal delivery without being sedated, and therefore, this experimental variable should also be appropriately considered.

The design of the experimental setup to investigate nose-to-brain drug delivery also involves the definition of the biological samples collected, the sampling times analysed, the analytical methodologies used to measure the concentration of drugs in different biocompartments and, finally, the type of control or reference employed to make comparisons. Overall, intranasal studies should include frequent sampling of, at least, both plasma and brain tissue or the CSF to enable calculation of the global drug exposure in those specimens. In practice, the brain tissue is sampled by dissection; the organ is usually used as a whole or divided into different anatomical regions after slicing. The analysis of whole-brain concentrations by treating the tissue as an entire piece may disguise the contribution of direct neurological pathways to transport the drug from the nose to the brain; instead, measuring the levels of drug distribution in specific target areas of the brain may afford a more accurate determination of the routes by which the molecules have travelled [85]. When measurement of drug concentrations in brain tissue is intended, one sample per animal per time point has to be taken, which means that several animals are needed to delineate a complete pharmacokinetic profile, probably increasing the variability in the obtained data. On the contrary, similarly to blood, serial sampling of the CSF is also feasible provided by the replacement of the withdrawn volume with the artificial CSF via infusion into the lateral ventricle [88]. Serial CSF sampling is usually performed in rats by microdialysis [89, 90] or cisternal puncture [91–93], and maximal care should be taken to avoid contamination with blood. Mice are unsuitable for CSF sampling due to its extremely low total volume (approximately 35 μL), but the relatively small amount of CSF samples (< 50 μL) which can be collected from rats generally imposes a major problem with respect to drug analysis, requiring highly sensitive analytical methods (such as mass spectrometry) for drug quantification [69]. Nevertheless, the main advantage of this procedure is the possibility of obtaining a drug concentration–time profile in the CSF from one single subject, which saves animals and reduces variability in data.

The importance of frequent and early sampling is highlighted by a study performed by Chow et al. [26] in which cocaine concentrations in rat brain tissue were evaluated after intranasal and intravenous administrations. Interestingly, the area under the concentration–time curve (AUC) of cocaine in the olfactory bulb following 60 min postdose was lower for intranasal comparatively to intravenous delivery; however, when calculated for times up to 4 min, the AUC values determined after intranasal drug administration exceeded those obtained after intravenous injection [26]. Hence, this indication of direct nose-to-brain transfer could easily have been overlooked if samples had not been taken as soon as 1, 2 and 4 min. Particular attention should be given to the sampling times selected.

By tracking the analytical methodologies commonly utilised in the assessment of intranasal delivery, it was found that the investigation of the potential for direct nose-to-brain transport was accomplished either in a qualitative or in a quantitative way. Several imaging tools such as microscopy, radioactivity, fluorescence and gamma scintigraphy have been frequently employed. Although microscopic analysis of brain tissue provides a qualitative answer to whether there is direct drug transfer, it does not give an indication about the proportion of the administered drug which reaches the brain from the nasal cavity.

More sophisticated imaging techniques like autoradiographic and gamma scintigraphy analysis can otherwise enable a direct visualisation and quantification of where the drug formulation has been delivered, what it is doing and whether it is behaving according to its proposed rationale. However, it should be noted that these imaging methods alone do not confirm the presence of intact, free or biologically active drugs in CNS tissues, besides their inability to distinguish between the parent drug and active/inert metabolites [85]. Furthermore, attaching radioligands to the drug might also alter the physicochemical and pharmacologic properties of the therapeutic agent, which may interfere with the pharmacokinetic and pharmacodynamic outcomes of the experiments [85]. In view of these limitations, more accurate and specific assays such as liquid chromatography coupled with different types of detection could be used, providing more complete and definitive descriptions of the pharmacokinetic profiles of the intranasally administered drug and the corresponding active metabolites formed in vivo. Currently, high-performance liquid chromatography (HPLC)-based techniques are the most commonly applied analytical methods for drug separation and subsequent quantification in a wide variety of biological matrices [59].

Taking into account that intranasal delivery is, in the majority of cases, considered as a new route of drug administration, the experimental protocol should be designed to allow the comparison of the obtained results with other alternative routes. In fact, some compounds, even when administered non-nasally, can be preferentially distributed to the olfactory mucosa and the olfactory bulbs [94], highlighting the need for appropriate controls when designing studies in this field. To discriminate the exact transport pathway by which the drug is transferred from the nose to the brain (either via the BBB or the direct olfactory route), an adequate intravenous pharmacokinetic control has commonly been included in the investigations as an experimental comparator. Intravenous delivery is definitively the most widely used alternative route to make comparisons with intranasal administration [23, 69]. Other parenteral delivery routes like, for instance, intramuscular or intraperitoneal and even oral administration may also serve as comparators as long as the pharmacokinetic profiles are properly measured and matched [2].

3.3.3 Assessment Parameters

Investigating nose-to-brain drug targeting presupposes the assessment of the relative distribution of the drug by determining and comparing its concentrations attained on therapeutic sites of action (i.e. brain and/or CSF) with other nontargeted biocompartments such as blood and other peripheral tissues. Bearing in mind that the concentrations observed in the CNS after intranasal administration of drugs could be due not only to the amount of drug directly transported to the brain via neuronal routes but also the fraction which could be absorbed into the systemic circulation and reach the CNS by crossing the BBB and the blood–CSF barrier, intravenous delivery controls are required to determine the contribution of this indirect vascular pathway on blood-mediated brain drug deposition [23, 69]. Therefore, the measurement of drug exposure (given by the AUC) in both the CNS (brain and/or CSF) and blood (plasma or serum) as well as the comparison of the CNS-to-blood concentration ratios after intranasal and intravenous administrations provide an evaluation of the route of drug transport to the brain [26, 46, 65, 69] (Eq. 3.1). Hence, when CNS-to-blood ratios following intranasal delivery are greater than those after intravenous administration, it indicates that direct transport pathways either via epithelial and/or nerve olfactory routes are primarily involved in the transfer of the compounds from the nasal cavity to the brain. Conversely, when the intranasal ratio is equal or lower than the intravenous one, it is assumed that the concentrations observed in the CNS derive mainly from the absorption into the nasal vasculature with further systemic distribution.

$$\text{CNS} - \text{blood ratio} = \frac{\text{AUC}_{\text{CNS}}}{\text{AUC}_{\text{blood}}} \tag{3.1}$$

With the aim of surveying the extent of drug delivery to the brain, specific indexes have been suggested and broadly adopted by several researchers. In accordance, the drug-targeting efficiency (DTE) quantifies the overall tendency of the drug to accumulate in the brain subsequently to intranasal versus systemic administration [59]. It can be described as the AUC_{brain}/AUC_{blood} ratio following intranasal administration compared to that after intravenous injection [46, 95], and it is calculated conforming to Eq. 3.2.

$$\mathrm{DTE} = \frac{(\mathrm{AUC_{brain}}/\mathrm{AUC_{plasma}})_{\mathrm{IN}}}{(\mathrm{AUC_{brain}}/\mathrm{AUC_{plasma}})_{\mathrm{IV}}} \tag{3.2}$$

The value of the DTE can range from 0 to +∞, exhibiting a proportional relationship to the efficiency of drug targeting to the brain. Thus, it can be ensured that there is direct transport of drugs from the nose to the CNS whenever the DTE is higher than 1, as it was demonstrated by Wang et al. [95] in their experiments with intranasal administration of methotrexate to rats. On the basis of their results, the authors suggested that this agent could be directly delivered from the nasal cavity to the CSF, since the value of DTE achieved was 21.7, far greater than 1. By contrast, van den Berg et al. [45] found a DTE value of only 0.76, demonstrating that there was no additional transport of melatonin via the nose–CSF pathway in rats.

Another valuable used index is the nose-to-brain direct transport percentage (DTP), which can be derived from the DTE expression and estimates the relative amount of the drug which reaches the brain via direct neuronal routes [59]. The DTP represents the percentage of drug directly transported via olfactory and/or trigeminal pathways to the brain, subtracting from the total AUC_{brain}, corresponding to the amount of drug administered intranasally which reaches the brain through the BBB by means of the systemic circulation [23, 46] (Eq. 3.3). In fact, since the extent of a drug in blood is proportional to the AUC, it can be assumed that the AUC_{brain} fraction contributed by systemic circulation divided by AUC_{blood} after nasal administration is equal to the same ratio following the intravenous route [96] (Eq. 3.3).

$$\mathrm{DTP}(\%) = \frac{\mathrm{AUC_{brain\ IN}} - \left[\dfrac{\mathrm{AUC_{brain\ IV}}}{\mathrm{AUC_{plasma\ IV}}} \times \mathrm{AUC_{plasma\ IN}}\right]}{\mathrm{AUC_{brain\ IN}}} \times 100 \tag{3.3}$$

Overall, the DTP can range from $-\infty$ to 100%, with values below 0 indicating more efficient drug delivery to the brain following intravenous injection as compared to the intranasal administration [59].

These indexes are interdependent, so more efficient drug uptake to the brain via direct routes will lead to higher values of both the DTE and the DTP. The calculation of the referred parameters is based on several assumptions which should not be entirely ignored. Specifically, the drug pharmacokinetics is assumed to be linear and the analysed AUC values are pretended to reflect the pharmacologically relevant drug concentrations in the brain and blood, despite the fact that the compound can exist in several forms at these biocompartments (e.g. free, protein-bound or encapsulated) and different brain drug disposition patterns can result from distinct transport pathways from the nose to the brain [59]. Notwithstanding, it seems that these measures are helpful in comparing findings across various studies conducted in different labs, also being useful for assessing the effects of diverse formulations on enhancing intranasal delivery of drugs to the CNS [23].

The determination of brain distribution profiles after intranasal and intravenous drug administration also contributes to elucidate whether direct nose-to-brain transport pathways are involved. The assessment of drug distribution is usually performed in animal models and consists of analysing the drug exposure in different regions of the brain. Following drug administration, animals are sacrificed and the whole brain is removed and sectioned in sequential slices from the rostral to the caudal direction. Depending on drug physicochemical properties and the route of administration, distinct brain distribution patterns are observed. In general, nasal delivery is characterised by preferential exposure in the rostral portions of the brain (i.e. olfactory bulb and frontal cortex), whereas systemic administration results in a more homogenous distribution of the substrate throughout the CNS structures [3, 85]. Interestingly, higher drug concentrations can also be encountered in more distant and specific caudal brain areas.

The quantitative analysis of lidocaine levels in multiple brain regions upon intranasal administration to rats demonstrated that brain tissue drug content decreased in a rostral-to-caudal direction from the cortex to the cerebellum; however, a considerable augment was observed at the level of the olfactory bulb and brainstem, suggesting a direct delivery of lidocaine to the CNS along the olfactory and trigeminal nerve pathways [97]. Similar heterogeneous brain distribution patterns were likewise observed by quantitative autoradiographic analysis after intranasal perfusion of the vasoactive intestinal peptide (VIP) to rats [98]. Unlike the uniform brain distribution profile of the VIP when intravenously administered, an irregular deposition of the peptide in specific areas of the brain was observed following intranasal delivery. Higher drug concentrations were attained in sections corresponding to the cerebellum, midbrain, olfactory bulb and frontal cortex. While elevated VIP levels in the olfactory bulb were due to effective delivery of the peptide via the olfactory pathway, accumulation of the drug in distant brain areas remains to be clarified. Apparently, preferential localisations of the peptide corresponded to the brain structures particularly rich in VIP receptors. The authors hypothesised that intranasally administered VIP could perhaps be redistributed from the nasal absorption site into the brain blood microcirculation, thus reaching these specific regions of the brain. On the contrary, Kaur and Kim [87] concluded that there was no evidence of direct nose-to-brain transport of diazepam, since apart from the lower DTE values, homogenous distribution patterns were observed throughout the various regions of the rat and rabbit brain after both intranasal and intravenous administrations. The high lipophilicity value is probably the cause for this rapid and extensive absorption of the substrate into the nasal vasculature.

3.4 Nose-to-Brain Delivery of Central Drugs

Owing, in part, to extensions in the lifespan, the incidence of neurological, mental and neurodegenerative disorders is considerably increasing [99]. Schizophrenia, depression, epilepsy, dementia, alcohol dependence and other mental and neurological disorders constitute 13% of the global burden of disease, surpassing both cardiovascular disease and cancer [100, 101]. They are all a common cause of morbidity and cognitive impairment in older adults, but there is no cure for any of those diseases, although not for lack of trying. Indeed, several efforts have been made in the last decade in an attempt of pursuing the health-related Sustainable Development Goals for 2030 [102].

Recent advances in the fields of pharmacology and molecular neurobiology have led to a better understanding of the CNS disease processes, allowing the development of new therapeutic approaches. Nevertheless, drug discovery and development programs have been centered on selecting molecules with activity at a particular site or receptor in the brain, disregarding the extent of delivery of the compounds to the biophase. For this reason, many promising molecules are failing in the early stages of clinical trials, simply because they are unable to cross the BBB in sufficient quantity to be therapeutically effective. Amongst the several efforts that are being done towards the improvement of drug delivery and targeting to the brain, intranasal administration emerges as a viable and interesting alternative to other conventional routes due to its potential for direct delivery of therapeutics to the CNS, circumventing the BBB. The current research trend reveals that intranasal administration of drugs has been applied in multiple therapeutic areas, including Parkinson´s disease, Alzheimer´s disease, anxiety, depression and psychosis, among others.

Nevertheless, it is noteworthy that although some drugs reach the brain very easily and efficiently as drug solutions, formulation optimisation brings further benefits to many more drugs, namely those which are low-water-soluble, labile, low-permeant and/or less potent. The development of drug delivery systems for intranasal administration should envision increasing mucoadhesion, providing constant or controlled release of drug, improving drug nasal permeability or increasing deposition at olfactory epithelium to maximise the successful nose-to-brain delivery of the drug [37, 103]. In this regard, triggered formulations and nanosystems seem to be promising approaches.

Triggerable systems are mainly thermoresponsive and include in situ gelling formulations which are liquid and easily measurable at temperatures lower than 20°C, gelifying at the physiological temperature of the nasal cavity (c.a. 32°C). This strategy increases drug residence time in the nasal mucosa deeming from the higher viscosity which led to a better performance when compared to the corresponding solutions. An example wherein this strategy was successfully employed is reported by Serralheiro et al. [20, 21], who co-formulated carbamazepine and lamotrigine with the thermoresponsive polymer Pluronic F-127 and the mucoadhesive polymer Carbopol 974P. Pluronic F-127 is a triblock copolymer of poly(ethylene oxide) and poly(propylene oxide) units which is fluid at or below room temperature but turns to a semisolid gel when the temperature increases, as a consequence of the micelle-packing disorder–order transition phenomenon. Accordingly, the intranasal administration of lamotrigine to mice was considered as a suitable and valuable drug delivery strategy for the chronic treatment of epilepsy, also providing a promising alternative approach for a prospective management of pharmacoresistance. In addition, nose-to-brain delivery of carbamazepine was so fast that it was suggested to be a promising alternative route not only for the chronically use of the drug but also in emergency conditions. More recently, the third-generation antiepileptic drug levetiracetam demonstrated, for the first time, direct nose-to-brain delivery when administered as thermorreversible gel [104].

On the other hand, analysis of recent literature data also confirmed that intranasal carrier nanosystems increase nose-to-brain drug delivery when compared to intranasal solutions. Amongst those systems, microemulsions exhibit the lowest pharmacokinetic ratios values, while polymeric micelles showed the highest. Nevertheless, brain-targeting efficacy comparisons between nanosystem groups had little statistical significance, and the superiority of the polymeric micelles group disappeared when nanosystems were compared to the respective intranasal drug solutions. Importantly, intranasal delivery nanosystems for nose-to-brain transportation of drugs should be designed to provide a longer residence time in the nasal cavity to overcome the nasal MCC and facilitate rapid transport of drug across the olfactory nasal mucosa. In this regard, chitosan-based nanoparticles claim both attributes and are most frequently applied, as well as other chitosan chemical modifications, such as the covalent attachment of thiol groups to the primary amino groups of chitosan, which seem to increase mucoadhesiveness and permeation, along with in situ gelling features, without compromising drug biodegradability [105, 106].

3.5 Conclusions

Considering all its inherent and indisputable advantages, the non-invasive intranasal route has been heralded as one of the most promising approaches to improve drug delivery into the CNS; therefore, it is not surprising tht its potential has been exploited for the development of novel and more efficient drug delivery systems. By circumventing the BBB, the intranasal route is also expected to avoid pharmacoresistance mechanisms expressed at this site which are responsible for the development of several refractory central diseases, such as refractory epilepsy and refractory depression.

References

1. WHO (2006). *Neurological Disorders: Public Health Challenges*, pp. 1–218.
2. Djupesland, P. G., Messina, J. C., Mahmoud, R. A. (2014). The nasal approach to delivering treatment for brain diseases: an anatomic, physiologic, and delivery technology overview. *Ther. Deliv.*, **5**(6), 709–733.
3. Graff, C. L., Pollack, G. M. (2005). Nasal drug administration: potential for targeted central nervous system delivery. *J. Pharm. Sci.*, **94**(6), 1187–1195.
4. Hanson, L. R., Frey, W. H., 2nd (2008). Intranasal delivery bypasses the blood-brain barrier to target therapeutic agents to the central nervous system and treat neurodegenerative disease, *BMC Neurosci.*, **9**(Suppl 3), S5.
5. Marianecci, C., Rinaldi, F., Hanieh, P. N., Di Marzio, L., Paolino, D., Carafa, M. (2017). Drug delivery in overcoming the blood-brain barrier: role of nasal mucosal grafting. *Drug Des. Dev. Ther.*, **11**, 325–335.
6. Pires, A., Fortuna, A., Alves, G., Falcao, A. (2009). Intranasal drug delivery: how, why and what for? *J. Pharm. Pharm. Sci.*, **12**(3), 288–311.
7. Joshi, C. R., Labhasetwar, V., Ghorpade, A. (2017). Destination brain: the past, present, and future of therapeutic gene delivery. *J. Neuroimmune Pharmacol.*, **12**(1), 51–83.
8. Peschillo, S., Caporlingua, A., Diana, F., Caporlingua, F., Delfini, R. (2016). New therapeutic strategies regarding endovascular treatment

of glioblastoma, the role of the blood-brain barrier and new ways to bypass it. *J. Neurointerv. Surg.*, **8**(10), 1078–1082.

9. Azad, T. D., Pan, J., Connolly, I. D., Remington, A., Wilson, C. M., Grant, G. A. (2015). Therapeutic strategies to improve drug delivery across the blood-brain barrier. *Neurosurg. Focus*, **38**(3), E9.
10. Rempe, R., Cramer, S., Qiao, R., Galla, H. J. (2014). Strategies to overcome the barrier: use of nanoparticles as carriers and modulators of barrier properties. *Cell Tissue Res*, **355**(3), 717–726.
11. Crawford, L., Rosch, J., Putnam, D. (2016). Concepts, technologies, and practices for drug delivery past the blood-brain barrier to the central nervous system. *J. Control. Release*, **240**, 251–266.
12. Miyake, M. M., Bleier, B. S. (2015). The blood-brain barrier and nasal drug delivery to the central nervous system. *Am. J. Rhinol. Allergy*, **29**(2), 124–127.
13. Costa, C., Moreira, J. N., Amaral, M. H., Sousa Lobo, J. M., Silva, A. C. (2019). Nose-to-brain delivery of lipid-based nanosystems for epileptic seizures and anxiety crisis. *J. Control. Release*, **295**, 187–200.
14. Erdo, F., Bors, L. A., Farkas, D., Bajza, A., Gizurarson, S. (2018). Evaluation of intranasal delivery route of drug administration for brain targeting. *Brain Res. Bull.*, **143**, 155–170.
15. Musumeci, T., Bonaccorso, A., Puglisi, G. (2019). Epilepsy disease and nose-to-brain delivery of polymeric nanoparticles: an overview. *Pharmaceutics*, **11**(3), E118.
16. Manda, P., Kushwaha, A. S., Kundu, S., Shivakumar, H. N., Jo, S. B., Murthy, S. N. (2016). Delivery of ziconotide to cerebrospinal fluid via intranasal pathway for the treatment of chronic pain. *J. Control. Release*, **224**, 69–76.
17. Trotta, V., Pavan, B., Ferraro, L., Beggiato, S., Traini, D., Des Reis, L. G., Scalia, S., Dalpiaz, A. (2018). Brain targeting of resveratrol by nasal administration of chitosan-coated lipid microparticles. *Eur. J. Pharm. Biopharm.*, **127**, 250–259.
18. League-Pascual, J. C., Lester-McCully, C. M., Shandilya, S., Ronner, L., Rodgers, L., Cruz, R., Peer, C. J., Figg, W. D., Warren, K. E. (2017). Plasma and cerebrospinal fluid pharmacokinetics of select chemotherapeutic agents following intranasal delivery in a non-human primate model. *J. Neurooncol.*, **132**(3), 401–407.
19. Seju, U., Kumar, A., Sawant, K. K. (2011). Development and evaluation of olanzapine-loaded PLGA nanoparticles for nose-to-brain delivery: in vitro and in vivo studies. *Acta Biomater.*, **7**(12), 4169–4176.

20. Serralheiro, A., Alves, G., Fortuna, A., Falcao, A. (2014). Intranasal administration of carbamazepine to mice: a direct delivery pathway for brain targeting. *Eur J. Pharm. Sci.*, **60**, 32–39.

21. Serralheiro, A., Alves, G., Fortuna, A., Falcao, A. (2015). Direct nose-to-brain delivery of lamotrigine following intranasal administration to mice. *Int. J. Pharm.*, **490**(1–2), 39–46.

22. Chapman, C. D., Frey, W. H., 2nd, Craft, S., Danielyan, L., Hallschmid, M., Schioth, H. B., Benedict, C. (2013). Intranasal treatment of central nervous system dysfunction in humans. *Pharm. Res.*, **30**(10), 2475–2484.

23. Dhuria, S. V., Hanson, L. R., Frey, W. H., 2nd. (2010). Intranasal delivery to the central nervous system: mechanisms and experimental considerations. *J. Pharm. Sci.*, **99**(4), 1654–1673.

24. Pardeshi, C. V., Belgamwar, V. S. (2013). Direct nose to brain drug delivery via integrated nerve pathways bypassing the blood-brain barrier: an excellent platform for brain targeting. *Expert Opin. Drug Deliv.*, **10**(7), 957–972.

25. Illum, L. (2002). Nasal drug delivery: new developments and strategies. *Drug Discov. Today*, **7**(23), 1184–1189.

26. Chow, H. S., Chen, Z., Matsuura, G. T. (1999). Direct transport of cocaine from the nasal cavity to the brain following intranasal cocaine administration in rats. *J. Pharm. Sci.*, **88**(8), 754–758.

27. Ganger, S., Schindowski, K. (2018). Tailoring formulations for intranasal nose-to-brain delivery: a review on architecture, physico-chemical characteristics and mucociliary clearance of the nasal olfactory mucosa. *Pharmaceutics*, **10**(3), E116.

28. Chauhan, M. B., Chauhan, N. B. (2015). Brain uptake of neurotherapeutics after intranasal versus intraperitoneal delivery in mice. *J. Neurol. Neurosurg.*, **2**(1), 009.

29. Mittal, D., Ali, A., Md, S., Baboota, S., Sahni, J. K., Ali, J. (2014). Insights into direct nose to brain delivery: current status and future perspective. *Drug Deliv.*, **21**(2), 75–86.

30. Wong, Y. C., Zuo, Z. (2010). Intranasal delivery--modification of drug metabolism and brain disposition. *Pharm. Res.*, **27**(7), 1208–1223.

31. Lochhead, J. J., Thorne, R. G. (2014). Intranasal drug delivery to the brain, in *Drug Delivery to the Brain: Physiological Concepts, Methodologies and Approaches*, Hammarlund-Udenaes, M., de Lange, E. C. M., Thorne, R. G., eds., Springer, pp. 401–431.

32. Thorne, R. G., Emory, C. R., Ala, T. A., Frey, W. H., 2nd (1995). Quantitative analysis of the olfactory pathway for drug delivery to the brain. *Brain Res.*, **692**(1–2), 278–282.

33. Barakat, N. S., Omar, S. A., Ahmed, A. A. (2006). Carbamazepine uptake into rat brain following intra-olfactory transport. *J. Pharm. Pharmacol.*, **58**(1), 63–72.

34. Czapp, M., Bankstahl, J. P., Zibell, G., Potschka, H. (2008). Brain penetration and anticonvulsant efficacy of intranasal phenobarbital in rats. *Epilepsia*, **49**(7), 1142–1150.

35. Banks, W. A., Morley, J. E., Niehoff, M. L., Mattern, C. (2009). Delivery of testosterone to the brain by intranasal administration: comparison to intravenous testosterone. *J. Drug Targeting*, **17**(2), 91–97.

36. Pardridge, W. M. (2011). Drug transport in brain via the cerebrospinal fluid. *Fluids Barriers CNS*, **8**(1), 7.

37. Illum, L. (2000). Transport of drugs from the nasal cavity to the central nervous system. *Eur. J. Pharm. Sci.*, **11**(1), 1–18.

38. Ross, T. M., Martinez, P. M., Renner, J. C., Thorne, R. G., Hanson, L. R., Frey, W. H., 2nd (2004). Intranasal administration of interferon beta bypasses the blood-brain barrier to target the central nervous system and cervical lymph nodes: a non-invasive treatment strategy for multiple sclerosis. *J. Neuroimmunol.*, **151**(1–2), 66–77.

39. Mistry, A., Stolnik, S., Illum, L. (2009). Nanoparticles for direct nose-to-brain delivery of drugs. *Int. J. Pharm.*, **379**(1), 146–157.

40. Thorne, R. G., Pronk, G. J., Padmanabhan, V., Frey, W. H., 2nd (2004). Delivery of insulin-like growth factor-I to the rat brain and spinal cord along olfactory and trigeminal pathways following intranasal administration. *Neuroscience*, **127**(2), 481–496.

41. Illum, L. (2004). Is nose-to-brain transport of drugs in man a reality? *J. Pharm. Pharmacol.*, **56**(1), 3–17.

42. van den Berg, M. P., Verhoef, J. C., Romeijn, S. G., Merkus, F. W. (2004). Uptake of estradiol or progesterone into the CSF following intranasal and intravenous delivery in rats. *Eur. J. Pharm. Biopharm.*, **58**(1), 131–135.

43. Wang, X., He, H., Leng, W., Tang, X. (2006). Evaluation of brain-targeting for the nasal delivery of estradiol by the microdialysis method. *Int. J. Pharm.*, **317**(1), 40–46.

44. Jayachandra Babu, R., Dayal, P. P., Pawar, K., Singh, M. (2011). Nose-to-brain transport of melatonin from polymer gel suspensions: a microdialysis study in rats. *J. Drug Targeting*, **19**(9), 731–740.

45. van den Berg, M. P., Merkus, P., Romeijn, S. G., Verhoef, J. C., Merkus, F. W. (2004). Uptake of melatonin into the cerebrospinal fluid after nasal and intravenous delivery: studies in rats and comparison with a human study. *Pharm. Res.*, **21**(5), 799–802.

46. Pires, P. C., Santos, A. O. (2018). Nanosystems in nose-to-brain drug delivery: a review of non-clinical brain targeting studies. *J. Control. Release*, **270**, 89–100.

47. Agu, R. U., Ugwoke, M. I. (2008). In situ and ex vivo nasal models for preclinical drug development studies, in *Drug Absorption Studies: In Situ, In Vitro and In Silico Models*, Ehrhardt, C., Kim, K., eds., Springer, pp. 112–134.

48. Mercier, C., Perek, N., Delavenne, X. (2018). Is RPMI 2650 a suitable in vitro nasal model for drug transport studies? *Eur. J. Drug Metab. Pharmacokinet.*, **43**(1), 13–24.

49. Goncalves, V. S. S., Matias, A. A., Poejo, J., Serra, A. T., Duarte, C. M. M. (2016). Application of RPMI 2650 as a cell model to evaluate solid formulations for intranasal delivery of drugs. *Int. J. Pharm.*, **515**(1–2), 1–10.

50. Kim, D. (2008). In vitro cellular models for nasal drug absorption studies, in *Drug Absorption Studies: In Situ, In Vitro and In Silico Models*, Ehrhardt, C., Kim, K., eds., Springer, pp. 216–234.

51. Zhang, L., Du, S. Y., Lu, Y., Liu, C., Tian, Z. H., Yang, C., Wu, H. C., Wang, Z. (2016). Puerarin transport across a Calu-3 cell monolayer - an in vitro model of nasal mucosa permeability and the influence of paeoniflorin and menthol. *Drug Des. Dev. Ther.*, **10**, 2227–2237.

52. Engelhardt, L., Rohm, M., Mavoungou, C., Schindowski, K., Schafmeister, A., Simon, U. (2016). First steps to develop and validate a CFPD model in order to support the design of nose-to-brain delivered biopharmaceuticals. *Pharm. Res.*, **33**(6), 1337–1350.

53. Pozzoli, M., Ong, H. X., Morgan, L., Sukkar, M., Traini, D., Young, P. M., Sonvico, F. (2016). Application of RPMI 2650 nasal cell model to a 3D printed apparatus for the testing of drug deposition and permeation of nasal products. *Eur. J. Pharm. Biopharm.*, **107**, 223–233.

54. Ugwoke, M. I., Verbeke, N., Kinget, R. (2001). The biopharmaceutical aspects of nasal mucoadhesive drug delivery. *J. Pharm. Pharmacol.*, **53**(1), 3–21.

55. Oliveira, P., Fortuna, A., Alves, G., Falcao, A. (2016). Drug-metabolizing enzymes and efflux transporters in nasal epithelium: influence on the bioavailability of intranasally administered drugs. *Curr. Drug Metab.*, **17**(7), 628–647.

56. Ravouru, N., Kondreddy, P., Korakanchi, D., Haritha, M. (2013). Formulation and evaluation of niosomal nasal drug delivery system of folic acid for brain targeting. *Curr. Drug Discov. Technol.*, **10**(4), 270–282.

57. Shingaki, T., Hidalgo, I. J., Furubayashi, T., Sakane, T., Katsumi, H., Yamamoto, A., Yamashita, S. (2011). Nasal delivery of P-gp substrates to the brain through the nose-brain pathway. *Drug Metab. Pharmacokinet.*, **26**(3), 248–255.

58. Hussain, A. A. (1998). Intranasal drug delivery. *Adv. Drug Deliv. Rev.*, **29**(1–2), 39–49.

59. Kozlovskaya, L., Abou-Kaoud, M., Stepensky, D. (2014). Quantitative analysis of drug delivery to the brain via nasal route. *J. Control. Release*, **189**, 133–140.

60. Smolnik, R., Perras, B., Molle, M., Fehm, H. L., Born, J. (2000). Event-related brain potentials and working memory function in healthy humans after single-dose and prolonged intranasal administration of adrenocorticotropin 4-10 and desacetyl-alpha-melanocyte stimulating hormone. *J. Clin. Psychopharmacol.*, **20**(4), 445–454.

61. Wall, A., Kagedal, M., Bergstrom, M., Jacobsson, E., Nilsson, D., Antoni, G., Frandberg, P., Gustavsson, S. A., Langstrom, B., Yates, R. (2005). Distribution of zolmitriptan into the CNS in healthy volunteers: a positron emission tomography study. *Drugs R D*, **6**(3), 139–147.

62. Yates, R., Sorensen, J., Bergstrom, M., Antoni, G., Nairn, K., Kemp, J., Langstrom, B., Dane, A. (2005). Distribution of intranasal C-zolmitriptan assessed by positron emission tomography. *Cephalalgia*, **25**(12), 1103–1109.

63. Merkus, P., Guchelaar, H. J., Bosch, D. A., Merkus, F. W. (2003). Direct access of drugs to the human brain after intranasal drug administration? *Neurology*, **60**(10), 1669–1671.

64. Born, J., Lange, T., Kern, W., McGregor, G. P., Bickel, U., Fehm, H. L. (2002). Sniffing neuropeptides: a transnasal approach to the human brain. *Nat. Neurosci.*, **5**(6), 514–516.

65. Padowski, J. M., Pollack, G. M. (2010). Examination of the ability of the nasal administration route to confer a brain exposure advantage for three chemical inhibitors of P-glycoprotein. *J. Pharm. Sci.*, **99**(7), 3226–3233.

66. Gizurarson, S. (2012). Anatomical and histological factors affecting intranasal drug and vaccine delivery. *Curr. Drug Deliv.*, **9**(6), 566–582.

67. Kaur, P., Garg, T., Vaidya, B., Prakash, A., Rath, G., Goyal, A. K. (2015). Brain delivery of intranasal in situ gel of nanoparticulated polymeric carriers containing antidepressant drug: behavioral and biochemical assessment. *J. Drug Targeting*, **23**(3), 275–286.

68. Lochhead, J. J., Thorne, R. G. (2012). Intranasal delivery of biologics to the central nervous system. *Adv. Drug Deliv. Rev.*, **64**(7), 614–628.

69. Merkus, F. W., van den Berg, M. P. (2007). Can nasal drug delivery bypass the blood-brain barrier?: questioning the direct transport theory. *Drugs R D*, **8**(3), 133–144.

70. Harkema, J. R. (2012). Nose, sinus, pharynx, and larynx, in *Comparative Anatomy and Histology: A Mouse and Human Atlas*, Treuting, P. M., Dintzis, S. M., eds., Elsevier, pp. 71–94.

71. Van den Berg, M. P., Merkus, P., Romeijn, S. G., Verhoef, J. C., Merkus, F. W. (2003). Hydroxocobalamin uptake into the cerebrospinal fluid after nasal and intravenous delivery in rats and humans. *J. Drug Targeting*, **11**(6), 325–331.

72. Djupesland, P. G. (2013). Nasal drug delivery devices: characteristics and performance in a clinical perspective: a review. *Drug Deliv. Transl. Res.*, **3**(1), 42–62.

73. Charlton, S. T., Davis, S. S., Illum, L. (2007). Nasal administration of an angiotensin antagonist in the rat model: effect of bioadhesive formulations on the distribution of drugs to the systemic and central nervous systems. *Int. J. Pharm.*, **338**(1–2), 94–103.

74. Kumar, A., Garg, T., Sarma, G. S., Rath, G., Goyal, A. K. (2015). Optimization of combinational intranasal drug delivery system for the management of migraine by using statistical design. *Eur. J. Pharm. Sci.*, **70**, 140–151.

75. Southam, D. S., Dolovich, M., O'Byrne, P. M., Inman, M. D. (2002). Distribution of intranasal instillations in mice: effects of volume, time, body position, and anesthesia. *Am. J. Physiol. Lung Cell. Mol. Physiol.*, **282**(4), L833–839.

76. Hussain, A. A., Dakkuri, A., Itoh, S. (2000). Nasal absorption of ondansetron in rats: an alternative route of drug delivery. *Cancer Chemother. Pharmacol.*, **45**(5), 432–434.

77. Ishikawa, F., Murano, M., Hiraishi, M., Yamaguchi, T., Tamai, I., Tsuji, A. (2002). Insoluble powder formulation as an effective nasal drug delivery system. *Pharm. Res.*, **19**(8), 1097–1104.

78. Raghavan, C. V., Abimon, V. D. (2001). Intranasal delivery of tenoxicam in rat. *Int. J. Pharm.*, **221**(1–2), 227–229.

79. Sinswat, P., Tengamnuay, P. (2003). Enhancing effect of chitosan on nasal absorption of salmon calcitonin in rats: comparison with hydroxypropyl- and dimethyl-beta-cyclodextrins. *Int. J. Pharm.*, **257**(1–2), 15–22.

80. Wang, Q., Chen, G., Zeng, S. (2007). Pharmacokinetics of Gastrodin in rat plasma and CSF after i.n. and i.v. *Int. J. Pharm.*, **341**(1–2), 20–25.

81. Yokogawa, K., Toshima, K., Yamoto, K., Nishioka, T., Sakura, N., Miyamoto, K. (2006). Pharmacokinetic advantage of an intranasal preparation of a novel anti-osteoporosis drug, L-Asp-hexapeptide-conjugated estradiol. *Biol. Pharm. Bull.*, **29**(6), 1229–1233.

82. Ozsoy, Y., Gungor, S. (2011). Nasal route: an alternative approach for antiemetic drug delivery. *Expert Opin. Drug Deliv.*, **8**(11), 1439–1453.

83. Bell, G. S., Sander, J. W. (2002). The epidemiology of epilepsy: the size of the problem. *Seizure*, **11**(Suppl A), 306–314; quiz 315–306.

84. Singh, R. M., Kumar, A., Pathak, K. (2013). Mucoadhesive in situ nasal gelling drug delivery systems for modulated drug delivery. *Expert Opin. Drug Deliv.*, **10**(1), 115–130.

85. Wong, Y. C., Zuo, Z. (2013). Brain disposition and catalepsy after intranasal delivery of loxapine: role of metabolism in PK/PD of intranasal CNS drugs. *Pharm. Res.*, **30**(9), 2368–2384.

86. Wu, H., Hu, K., Jiang, X. (2008). From nose to brain: understanding transport capacity and transport rate of drugs. *Expert Opin. Drug Deliv.*, **5**(10), 1159–1168.

87. Kaur, P., Kim, K. (2008). Pharmacokinetics and brain uptake of diazepam after intravenous and intranasal administration in rats and rabbits. *Int. J. Pharm.*, **364**(1), 27–35.

88. Chou, K. J., Donovan, M. D. (1997). Distribution of antihistamines into the CSF following intranasal delivery. *Biopharm. Drug Dispos.*, **18**(4), 335–346.

89. Bagger, M., Bechgaard, E. (2004). A microdialysis model to examine nasal drug delivery and olfactory absorption in rats using lidocaine hydrochloride as a model drug. *Int. J. Pharm.*, **269**(2), 311–322.

90. Bagger, M. A., Bechgaard, E. (2004). The potential of nasal application for delivery to the central brain-a microdialysis study of fluorescein in rats. *Eur. J. Pharm. Sci.*, **21**(2–3), 235–242.

91. Dahlin, M., Bjork, E. (2001). Nasal administration of a physostigmine analogue (NXX-066) for Alzheimer's disease to rats. *Int. J. Pharm.*, **212**(2), 267–274.

92. Kao, H. D., Traboulsi, A., Itoh, S., Dittert, L., Hussain, A. (2000). Enhancement of the systemic and CNS specific delivery of L-dopa by the nasal administration of its water soluble prodrugs. *Pharm. Res.*, **17**(8), 978–984.

93. Zhao, Y., Tao, T., Wu, J., Pi, J., He, N., Chai, X., Chen, Q. (2008). Pharmacokinetics of tramadol in rat plasma and cerebrospinal fluid after intranasal administration. *J. Pharm. Pharmacol.*, **60**(9), 1149–1154.

94. Bergstrom, U., Franzen, A., Eriksson, C., Lindh, C., Brittebo, E. B. (2002). Drug targeting to the brain: transfer of picolinic acid along the olfactory pathways. *J. Drug Targeting*, **10**(6), 469–478.

95. Wang, F., Jiang, X., Lu, W. (2003). Profiles of methotrexate in blood and CSF following intranasal and intravenous administration to rats. *Int. J. Pharm.*, **263**(1–2), 1–7.

96. Jogani, V. V., Shah, P. J., Mishra, P., Mishra, A. K., Misra, A. R. (2007). Nose-to-brain delivery of tacrine. *J. Pharm. Pharmacol.*, **59**(9), 1199–1205.

97. Johnson, N. J., Hanson, L. R., Frey, W. H. (2010). Trigeminal pathways deliver a low molecular weight drug from the nose to the brain and orofacial structures. *Mol. Pharm.*, **7**(3), 884–893.

98. Dufes, C., Olivier, J. C., Gaillard, F., Gaillard, A., Couet, W., Muller, J. M. (2003). Brain delivery of vasoactive intestinal peptide (VIP) following nasal administration to rats. *Int. J. Pharm.*, **255**(1–2), 87–97.

99. Erkkinen, M. G., Kim, M. O., Geschwind, M. D. (2018). Clinical neurology and epidemiology of the major neurodegenerative diseases. *Cold Spring Harb. Perspect. Biol.*, **10**(4), a033118.

100. Collins, P. Y., Insel, T. R., Chockalingam, A., Daar, A., Maddox, Y. T. (2013). Grand challenges in global mental health: integration in research, policy, and practice. *PLoS Med.*, **10**(4), e1001434.

101. Collins, P. Y., Patel, V., Joestl, S. S., March, D., Insel, T. R., Daar, A. S., Scientific Advisory, B., the Executive Committee of the Grand Challenges on Global Mental, H., Anderson, W., Dhansay, M. A., Phillips, A., Shurin, S., Walport, M., Ewart, W., Savill, S. J., Bordin, I. A., Costello, E. J., Durkin, M., Fairburn, C., Glass, R. I., Hall, W., Huang, Y., Hyman, S. E., Jamison, K., Kaaya, S., Kapur, S., Kleinman, A., Ogunniyi, A., Otero-Ojeda, A., Poo, M. M., Ravindranath, V., Sahakian, B. J., Saxena, S., Singer, P. A., Stein, D. J. (2011). Grand challenges in global mental health. *Nature*, **475**(7354), 27–30.

102. Institute for Health Metrics and Evaluation (IHME) (2018). *Findings from the Global Burden of Disease Study 2017*. IHME, Seattle, WA.

103. Van Woensel, M., Wauthoz, N., Rosière, R., Amighi, K., Mathieu, V., Lefranc, F., Van Gool, S. W., De Vleeschouwer, S. (2013). Formulations for intranasal delivery of pharmacological agents to combat brain disease: a new opportunity to tackle GBM? *Cancers*, **5**(3), 1020.

104. Gonçalves, J., Bicker, J., Gouveia, F., Liberal, J., Oliveira, R. C., Alves, G., Falcão, A., Fortuna, A. (2019). Nose-to-brain delivery of levetiracetam after intranasal administration to mice. *Int. J. Pharm.*, **564**, 329–339.

105. Shimazu, S., Minami, A., Kusumoto, H., Yoneda, F. (2005). Antidepressant-like effects of selegiline in the forced swim test. *Eur. Neuropsychopharmacol.*, **15**(5), 563–571.

106. Singh, D., Rashid, M., Hallan, S. S., Mehra, N. K., Prakash, A., Mishra, N. (2016). Pharmacological evaluation of nasal delivery of selegiline hydrochloride-loaded thiolated chitosan nanoparticles for the treatment of depression. *Artif. Cells Nanomed. Biotechnol.*, **44**(3), 865–877.

Part II

Nanomedicines

Chapter 4

Organic Nanocarriers for Brain Drug Delivery

Marlene Lúcio,[a,b] Carla M. Lopes,[c] Eduarda Fernandes,[a] Hugo Gonçalves[d] and Maria Elisabete C. D. Real Oliveira[a]
[a]*Centre of Physics of Universities of Minho and Porto (CF-UM-UP), University of Minho, Campus de Gualtar, 4710-057 Braga, Portugal*
[b]*Centre of Molecular and Environmental Biology (CBMA), University of Minho, Braga, Portugal*
[c]*Fernando Pessoa Energy, Environment and Health Research Unit/ Biomedical Research Center (FP-ENAS/CEBIMED), Faculty of Health Sciences, Fernando Pessoa University, Portugal*
[d]*Paralab SA, Rua Dr. Joaquim Manuel Costa 946 B, 4420-437 Valbom, Portugal*
mlucio@fisica.uminho.pt

Although the blood–brain barrier remains a major barrier to drug delivery, organic nanocarriers (ONCs) have been demonstrated to be effective in targeting and delivering therapeutic agents to the brain and have provided promising preclinical outcomes. Because of their favourable physicochemical properties, such as biocompatible composition, nanometric dimensions, large surface area compared to volume and easily tuneable surfaces, ONCs have

Nanoparticles for Brain Drug Delivery
Edited by Carla Vitorino, Andreia Jorge and Alberto Pais

ISBN 978-981-4877-31-2 (Hardcover), 978-1-003-11932-6 (eBook)
www.jennystanford.com

proven to be excellent transport vehicles capable of prolonging drug (or other therapeutic agents) circulation time and of addressing the challenges posed by numerous diseases affecting the brain. This chapter presents an overview of the different types of ONCs for brain delivery, including a description of their advantages and disadvantages, and a set of preclinical studies illustrating the most effective strategies for effective brain distribution. Biodegradation and bioelimination issues and future challenges for effective clinical translation are also addressed.

4.1 Introduction

Brain pathologies, the most prevalent of which are neurodegenerative diseases (e.g. Alzheimer's disease [AD], Huntington's disease [HD], amyotrophic lateral sclerosis [ALS], Parkinson's disease [PD], multiple sclerosis [MS]), vascular pathologies (e.g. cerebral ischaemia/reperfusion [CIR]) and brain cancer (BC), are very difficult to treat [1–3].

The main difficulties in the treatment of these diseases are associated with the blood–brain barrier (BBB), a selective permeability barrier which controls the entry of systemic circulating drugs and nutrients into the brain. Only small (molecular weight <400 Da), moderately lipophilic (log octanol/water partition coefficient between 0.5 and 6.0) compounds which are neutral at physiological pH and form less than 8 hydrogen bonds with water are able to pass through the BBB by passive diffusion [4]. Regrettably, most therapeutic agents (including small drugs, proteins or peptides) do not satisfy these requirements and are unable to cross the BBB [5]. Therefore, one of the most difficult and costly market niches for pharmaceutical companies is the development of new approaches to treat brain diseases. The costs of completing phase I clinical trials can go up to $100 million and around $1 billion before hitting the market during production and discovery of new drugs for brain diseases [6]. With these statistics in mind, success in the development phase of brain therapeutics is of paramount importance. In recent years, however, there are only a small number of drugs for brain on the market (3%–5%) since most of them failed to cross the BBB in vivo [6]. Thus, strategies to pass the BBB constitute the key challenge for the delivery of therapeutic agents to the brain.

Presently, progress in the field of nanomedicine has developed numerous platforms to enhance the therapeutic transport across the BBB. Among these platforms, the development of nanosystems capable of carrying drugs (also termed as 'nanocarriers' [NCs]) is rapidly moving forward as one of the most promising to improve the outcomes of current brain therapeutic delivery [2, 3, 6–11]. Compared to conventional therapeutic dosage forms, NCs offer several benefits, including (i) encapsulating one or more drugs, (ii) controlling drug release and (iii) carrying drugs and directing them to diseased locations [2, 12]. Encapsulation prevents the release of drugs before they reach their target tissues, which is particularly significant for toxicity issues usually associated with nonspecific drug distribution in off-target and target tissues [2, 12]. The ability of NCs to release drugs in a sustained or triggered manner is also an important advantage, as controlled release kinetics often affects therapeutic efficacy and toxicity. Finally, the capacity of NCs to target drugs to diseased tissues is possibly their most attractive attribute as it may reduce off-target toxic effects and favour drug accumulation at the diseased site [2, 12]. These are the general advantages presented by NCs for the delivery of drugs. However, using well-established endogenous BBB transport routes, NCs are particularly suitable for overcoming the BBB and effectively delivering drugs to the brain [2, 9]. Indeed, the rational design of the NC and its proper surface functionalisation may, at the same time, specifically direct NCs to endothelial BBB cells (promoting a local high concentration gradient between the blood and the brain which would favour a greater passive diffusion of drugs) or promote transport of NCs across the BBB [2, 7, 9].

Regarding their dimensions, NCs are nanostructured systems, generally characterised by a high surface-to-volume ratio, which should have a size range of 1–100 nm in at least one dimension [10, 11, 13]. NCs may also have submicron sizes (usually <500 nm) [11, 13] as long as there is a relationship between their dimensions and their physical, chemical and biological properties [11, 13, 14].

In terms of composition, NCs can be broadly divided into organic and inorganic nanocarriers (ONCs and INCs) (Fig. 4.1).

ONCs are composed of carbon-based nanomaterials, while INCs do not contain carbon and are composed of inorganic elements (e.g. silicon, gold and silver) [6, 10, 14]. However, there are some NCs composed of allotropes of carbon (e.g. fullerenes, carbon nanotubes, graphene-based nanosystems or graphene quantum dots) [15] for which this classification is not so clear, and they may be placed in a group aside excluded from this classification of ONCs/INCs [16] or can become hybrid materials being functionalised with several INCs or ONCs [17].

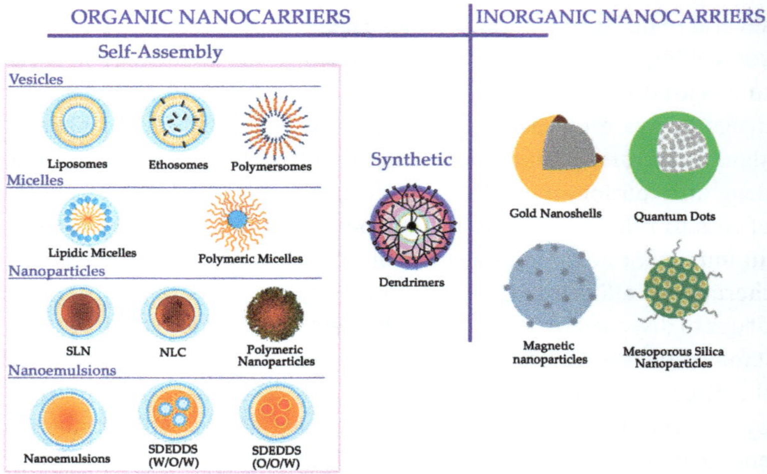

Figure 4.1 Organic and inorganic nanocarriers. SDEDDS, self-double-emulsion drug delivery systems; W, water phase; O, oil phase. Liposomes, ethosomes, lipidic micelles, solid lipid nanoparticle (SLNs), nanostructured lipid carriers (NLCs) and nanoemulsions were reprinted from Ref. [2], Copyright (2018), with permission from Elsevier.

INCs provide advantages over ONCs in terms of size and shape control and ease of preparation and functionalisation [6]. Most importantly, it is easier to track INCs through microscopy or analytical techniques. Furthermore, inorganic nanomaterials exhibit interesting mechanical, optical, physical and electrical phenomena at the nanoscale, which can be tailored through changes in material, phase, shape, size and surface characteristics. However, INCs also present disadvantages. It is often necessary to add a biocompatible surface to INCs to avoid toxicity, especially for heavy metals. Moreover, INCs may not be degraded, which imposes concerns regarding their biocompatibility and biosafety [6]. On the other hand, as carbon is a main component of our body, ONCs are generally characterised by high biocompatibility [6, 14]. In addition, ONCs allow versatile control of both morphology and chemical composition, while their colloidal stability and relatively large size make it possible to incorporate and carry a wide combination of hydrophilic/lipophilic drugs [14]. These characteristics provide protection to drugs and facilitate significant drug loading, minimising toxicity and increasing blood circulation time (increasing the possibility that the drug reaches its therapeutic target). The disadvantages of ONCs are related to their less easy preparation, which in some cases promotes less standardisation and batch-to-batch variability [6, 14]. Also, ONCs are more difficult to track than INCs. Therefore, if we could classify the different functions of NCs in a simple way, we could say that INCs are good for functionalisation and monitoring purposes [11] or for alternative treatments such as photothermal therapy [18, 19] and hyperthermia [20–22], while ONCs are more interesting for drug delivery and for their higher biocompatibility and safety [11, 12, 14]. Hybrid NCs often combine INCs and ONCs, gathering their advantages in a single carrier.

This chapter focuses on the use of ONCs for brain drug delivery. In the following sections, we provide an overview of the possible administration routes, transport mechanisms across the BBB and biodegradation/bioelimination pathways of ONCs. Additionally, the chapter describes a set of literature examples of ONCs developed for brain drug delivery.

4.2 Pathways for Nanocarrier Administration to the Brain

This section presents a brief overview of the routes used for NC administration, providing an analysis of the advantages and disadvantages of each route of administration. The routes presented are used for NC administration in general and are not just used for ONC administration, although their revision is essential for the subsequent understanding of the examples given in the literature. Some common strategies for tuning NCs to improve the efficiency of their brain delivery are also discussed. Finally, in the case of systemic administration, where NCs must cross the BBB, the transport routes commonly used by NCs are revised with a brief overview of the targeting strategies commonly applied. This section also provides a basis for understanding some of the strategies used in the revised literature examples.

4.2.1 Administration Routes

The NC administration routes can be classified into two main categories, local NC delivery and systemic administration. The benefit of local NC administration is that successful therapeutic concentrations of drugs in the brain are ensured, as well as a precise control of the concentration which is placed in the brain, guaranteeing that a drug is fully bioavailable and that any physiological obstacles to the drug, including the BBB, are prevented. However, local NC administration requires surgical procedures in order to put NCs in the brain. Additional surgeries may also be needed if multiple doses are required for the treatment. Local NC administration examples include intracerebroventricular (i.c.v.) administration using a catheter, osmotic pumps for intraventricular drug infusion or stereotaxic implantation, that is, a type of surgical intervention which uses a 3D coordinate device to position NCs in brain. Despite the advantages mentioned, local NC administration is rarely used because of the technical requirements it involves [2, 23].

The majority of NCs are systemically delivered to the brain, most likely by intravenous (i.v.) injection because of the ease of administration and avoidance of the first pass effect [2, 23]. When in blood circulation, and especially in the case of NCs with sizes greater than 200 nm [24], immune system mononuclear phagocyte cells (dendritic cells, monocytes and macrophages) may easily recognise NCs, removing them from circulation [2, 25, 26] and thereby reducing their chances to reach the target brain tissues. To avoid this early NC clearance, it is common to use stealth strategies which consist of coating the NC surface with hydrophilic chains, such as polyethylene glycol (PEG), in a process called PEGylation [2, 25, 26].

Systemic administration includes all routes which involve the passage of NCs to the blood circulation, such as classical intraperitoneal (i.p.) injections or those through the digestive tract (like oral administration), lungs or transdermal administrations [2, 23]. In such administration routes, NCs also require stealth strategies. Moreover, NCs face more off-target tissues, and if a targeted strategy is not adequate to direct NCs to the brain, they can be metabolised in the liver, thereby modifying the amount of circulating therapeutics available to the brain [23]. Furthermore, the liver, kidneys, intestine, skin, lungs and organs which separate the brain from the blood flow release enzymes which can metabolise xenobiotics and may likewise metabolise NCs [23]. Another part of the NCs can be excreted by the kidneys (especially if NC sizes are smaller than 5 nm) [24], which makes it difficult to estimate the accurate amount of the medication which finally enters the brain [2, 23].

Intranasal (i.n.) administration has recently been studied as an alternative to i.v. and other systemic administration routes as it avoids the BBB [2, 23, 27–31]. This route offers NCs a direct access into the brain through axonal transport along the olfactory nerve and can be explored as a new tool to manage chronic neurological conditions and diseases. The advantages of i.n. administration are increased bioavailability due to a lack of first-pass liver metabolism and subsequent rapid absorption, resulting in a fast therapeutic effect [2, 23, 27–31]. The disadvantages of i.n. administration are related to the limited amounts of therapeutic formulation which can be delivered into the brain because of the limited volume available for administration through the nasal cavity [23, 31]. However, if this is a disadvantage considering classical formulations, it might not be the case of NCs which can, in a small volume of formulation, concentrate higher doses of a drug loaded in the NCs. NC surface modification appears to be a key strategy to optimise drug delivery by the i.n. route because of mucociliary clearance mechanisms [32]. Mucociliary clearance is one of the physiological mechanisms which has a major impact on nasal delivery and drug transport inside the brain. This respiratory defence mechanism allows efficient and rapid removal of toxic substances, nanoparticles and microorganisms which are caught into the mucus layer [32]. Therefore, the surface electrostatic charges of NCs and their coating with mucoadhesive/mucopenetrating polymers are considered paramount to control their residence time in the nasal mucosa and their efficient delivery from the nose to the brain [32]. This is especially important in the case of ONCs (e.g. polymeric nanoparticles) since several polymers are considered to possess either mucopenetrating (e.g. PEG) or mucoadhesive properties (e.g. chitosan), and tuning the surface coating of NCs with those polymers permits enough mucoadhesion to avoid their rapid removal from the nasal mucosa, but it also confers some mucopenetrating properties so that NCs do not become entrapped on the mucus layer and can move from the nose to the brain [27, 32, 33]. Some other ONCs like lipid-based NCs may also benefit from the mucoadhesive properties of some lipids (e.g. monoolein) or the mucopenetration properties of fatty acids [32, 34, 35]. These mucopenetration properties have been attributed to the surfactant nature of fatty acids which may cause disruption of the nasal membrane and to the ability of NCs composed of fatty acids to be flexible and pass through the opening of the olfactory epithelium [32]. Lastly, positive and hydrophobic surfaces of NCs enhance the adherence of NCs to the mucus because of electrostatic attraction and hydrophobic interaction established with the negatively charged sialic acid and hydrophobic domains of mucin [32].

4.2.2 Transport Routes across the BBB

When NCs are administrated by systemic routes, and after facing all the obstacles found during blood circulation, they eventually reach their target tissue, where they face their most important barrier before entering the brain: the BBB. NCs may not cross the BBB at this point and can simply serve to deliver high concentrations of drugs to the luminal surface of BBB cells, establishing a local high concentration gradient between blood and brain which increases the passive diffusion of the drug through the BBB [7]. Alternatively, NCs may cross the BBB using certain transport routes while carrying the drug which is released in the brain [2, 7, 9].

Between the transport routes across the BBB, adsorptive-mediated transcytosis (AMT), receptor-mediated transcytosis (RMT) and carrier-mediated transcytosis (CMT) are those with the highest potential for brain uptake of NCs (Fig. 4.2) [2, 3, 7, 9].

AMT is based on electrostatic interactions established between the NC cationic surface and the anionic plasma membrane of the endothelial cells [36, 37]. Since this transport route is dependent solely on electrostatic interaction rather than on ligand–receptor binding, it is nonspecific and weaker than RMT [9, 36]. NCs must have cationic surfaces conferred either by their components or by cationic ligands attached to their surface to achieve this transport route [2, 7, 9, 36]. Typical cationic ligands used for AMT purposes are cell-penetrating peptides (CPPs). CPPs are short amphipathic or cationic peptides which usually display high BBB-crossing capacity by AMT, thus not needing transport mediated by receptors. Examples of CPPs used to functionalise the surface of NCs are TAT peptide (peptide derived from human immunodeficiency virus), antennapedia peptide (Antp), penetratin (a shorter peptide derived from Antp), transportan and poly-L-arginine [38–43].

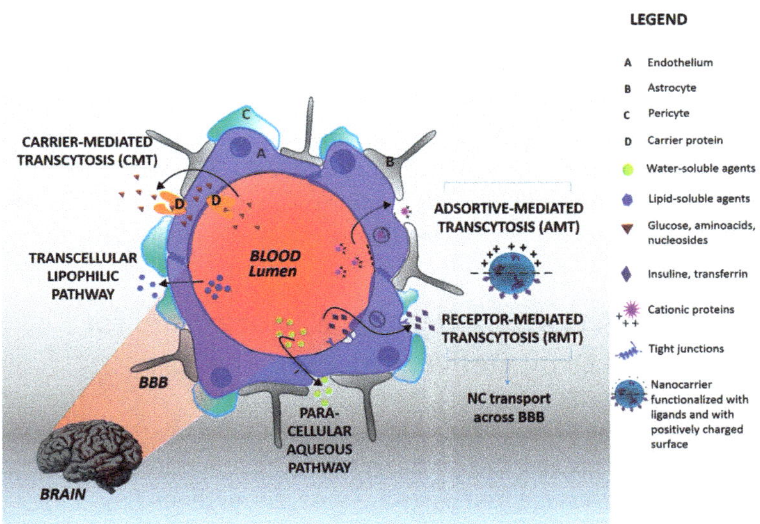

Figure 4.2 Schematic representation of transport routes across the blood–brain barrier (BBB) and types of solutes which use each route. Also highlighted are the nanocarrier (NC) preferential routes. Reprinted from Ref. [2], Copyright (2018), with permission from Elsevier.

In the physiological activities of the BBB as a transport barrier, the RMT route is used for transport of macromolecules which are necessary for brain function, such as (i) transferrin (Tf), (ii) lactoferrin (Lf), (iii) insulin (Ins), (iv) low-density lipoproteins (LDLs) and (v) leptin (Lep). The transport of these molecules is possible because of the expression of several specific receptors on the luminal side of the BBB: (i) Tf receptors (TfRs), (ii) Lf receptors (LfRs), (iii) Ins receptors (InsRs) and Ins-like growth factor receptors (IGF1R and IGF2R), (iv) LDL receptors (LDLRs), acetylated LDLR (AceLDLR), LDLR-related protein (LRP) and scavenger receptors class B type which are also receptors for LDL (SR-B) and (v) Lep receptors (LepRs) [2, 7, 9]. By conjugating the surface of the NCs with ligands which specifically bind to these receptors, it is possible to achieve an active targeting strategy which helps NCs to transpose the BBB and enter the brain [2, 7, 9].

In the brain endothelium there are many types of transporters which transport nutrients (e.g. glucose) and endogenous substances (e.g. amino acids, hormones, purine bases) to the brain by passive diffusion [3]. CMT is a substrate-selective transport system, and thus, only drugs which closely mimic these substrates can use and benefit from this route [44]. Examples of these specific transport systems include glucose receptors (GLUTs) [45–47], the neutral amino acid transporter (NAAT) [48], the cationic amino acid transporter (CAAT) [49], the anionic amino acid transporter (AAAT) [50], the beta amino acid transporter (AAT) [51], the choline transporter (ChT) [52], fatty acids (FATs) [53–55] and nucleoside transporters (NTs) [56].

4.3 Self-Assembly Organic Nanocarriers for Brain Drug Delivery

According to the preparation methods of ONCs, we may divide them into two major groups, ONCs which exploit the self-assembly process and those which come from specific synthetic methods (Fig. 4.1).

ONCs based on self-assembly processes result from basic building blocks that auto-organise in a supramolecular structure. This process is spontaneous but is conducted by noncovalent interactions like the hydrophobic effect, van der Waals interactions, hydrogen bonding, hydration and electrostatic forces, π–π staking interactions, steric and depletion interactions, coordination bonding and solvation [14, 57]. Many of the self-assembly ONCs are based on amphiphilic molecules which possess a hydrophilic portion (anionic, cationic or zwitterionic) which tends to be exposed to the surrounding aqueous solvent, while the hydrophobic portions (usually hydrocarbon chains) face each other minimising contact with the aqueous solvent [14, 57].

This section reviews different types of self-assembly ONCs for brain delivery. However, because all the self-assembly methods of preparation of these ONCs have been widely described in a number of previous review articles [58–62], we only briefly introduce each ONC without getting into details. Among the ONCs described, more attention is given to lipid-based nanosystems for their biocompatibility, which show higher chances of clinical translation. Moreover, lipid-based nanosystems, such as liposomes, SLNs, NLCs, microemulsions and nanoemulsions, have already demonstrated their capacity for enhancing brain transport, making it easier to move into the central nervous system (CNS) and enabling the administration of medicines which could support the treatment of neurological pathologies [63]. Other non-lipid-based ONCs are discussed more briefly, along with some examples of their use in CNS diseases. Focus is also placed on the presentation of a comparison between the ONCs regarding advantages and disadvantages (Table 4.1), as well as the brain delivery strategies used with these ONCs.

Table 4.1 Advantages and disadvantages of organic nanocarriers for brain delivery

Types of ONCs	Advantages	Disadvantages
Liposomes	• Encapsulation of both hydrophilic and hydrophobic compounds • Biocompatibility • Biodegradability and low toxicity • Flexibility and ease of passing through pores in human brain tissue • Versatility in terms of size, preparation method, lipid composition, charge of liposome surface • Can be composed by responsive lipids to produce a triggering drug release	• Physicochemical instability • In vivo stability problems • Limited routes of administration (preferably i.n. and i.v.) • Manufacturing methods difficult to scale
Ethosomes	• Same as liposomes • Enhanced BBB permeability	• Same as liposomes • Higher toxicity than liposomes because of increased ethanol content

(*Continued*)

Table 4.1 (*Continued*)

Types of ONCs	Advantages	Disadvantages
Polymersomes and polymeric nanoparticles	• High encapsulation of both hydrophilic and hydrophobic compounds • Higher stability and robustness compared to liposomes • Can be composed by responsive polymers to produce triggering drug release	• Release dependent on polymer degradability • Lack of reproducibility in production • Higher toxicity than lipid-based nanocarriers
Micelles	• Polymeric micelles have high drug-loading capacity. • Good biocompatibility	• Polymeric micelles exhibit higher toxicity than lipid-based nanocarriers. • Lipid micelles require concentrations above the critical micellar concentration (CMC) and can release the cargo upon dilution.
Lipid nanoparticles	• Controlled release of encapsulated compounds • Protects encapsulated compounds from degradation • Biocompatibility, biodegradability • Use of physiological lipids and generally recognised as safe (GRAS) excipients • Physical stability in the circulatory system • Natural tendency to cross the BBB by LDLR • Use of excipients which are regulatory-approved and do not induce drug alterations (e.g. protein denaturation, chemical degradation)	• Not ideal to encapsulate hydrophilic compounds • Toxicity is lower than polymeric nanocarriers but depends on the surfactant composition.

Types of ONCs	Advantages	Disadvantages
	• Ease of manufacture/scaling on an industrial scale cost-effectively with reproducibility in drug loading • Less toxic than polymeric nanocarriers	
Micro-/ Nanoemulsions	• Use of safe ingredients such as edible oils and biocompatible surfactants • Increased solubilisation of lipophilic compounds • Improved drug transport and delivery due to the large interfacial area • Easy manufacturing and scale-up • Improved stability of therapeutic agents	• Use of a large concentration of surfactants and co-surfactants necessary for stabilising the nanodroplets • Limited solubilising capacity for high melting substances • Stability influenced by environmental parameters such as temperature and pH • Nanoemulsions are also more susceptible to undergo instability phenomena over time.
Dendrimers	• Load therapeutic compounds by either covalent conjugation or electrostatic adsorption on their surface • Encapsulate different types of molecules with hydrophobic, hydrophilic and amphiphilic properties • Highly monodisperse nanostructures • Promising for gene therapy because of a positively charged surface • Amyloid β (Aβ) peptide aggregation inhibitors – important in neurodegenerative diseases	• Toxicity • Low biocompatibility • Complex synthesis

4.4 Vesicles: Liposomes, Ethosomes and Polymersomes

4.4.1 Liposomes

Liposomes are formed by amphiphiles (e.g. phospholipids) which, once dispersed in an aqueous media, self-assemble as vesicles [2, 64, 65]. These vesicles are made up of lipid bilayers, where the hydrophobic part of the amphiphiles (hydrophobic fatty acid chains) is oriented away from the aqueous polar phase, while the polar portions of the molecules (headgroup regions) are exposed to the aqueous solvent which exists in the vesicle core and also around the vesicle [2, 64, 65]. The amphiphilic nature of liposomes permits the encapsulation of a vast number of drugs with different polarities. While hydrophilic drugs are located nearby the hydrophilic headgroup region or in the aqueous core, hydrophobic drugs are loaded inside the lipid bilayer within the acyl chains region [66]. In addition to the advantages of ease of encapsulation, the lipid composition of liposomes, often resembling the phospholipid composition of biological membranes, also gives these systems advantages of biocompatibility [2, 14] (Table 4.1).

The use of liposomes as NCs for drug delivery is focused on the production of three types of liposomes (Fig. 4.3): multilamellar vesicles (MLVs), consisting of numerous concentric lipid bilayers which are polydisperse and present dimensions from 500 nm to several μm; large unilamellar vesicles (LUVs), with one lipid bilayer usually forming a monodisperse group of vesicles with defined dimensions which can range between 100 and 500 nm; and small unilamellar vesicles (SUVs), also composed of a single lipid bilayer forming monodisperse or polydisperse groups of vesicles (according to the preparation method) with dimensions smaller than 100 nm [2, 65, 66].

The route of administration of liposomes to the brain should be preferably i.v. or i.n. because of the high degradation of lipids in the gastrointestinal tract [14, 67, 68]. For brain delivery purposes, MLVs are the least interesting type of liposomes as their dimensions may not be appropriate for diffusion within the brain parenchyma. Indeed, although the dimensions of the NCs are not likely to be sought, it could be very important to take this into account in view of the fact that the NCs need to pass through the BBB and the extracellular space of the brain's parenchyma could prevent them from entering the brain [7]. Therefore, it is estimated that human brain tissue has some pores larger than 200 nm, but the majority have dimensions slightly greater than 100 nm, indicating that NCs should never exceed 200 nm [7, 24]. Nevertheless, liposomes have advantages in this context, since they are soft-matter NCs and therefore highly flexible and can pass through pores even if their sizes are larger than pore diameters [69]. The disadvantage of such a soft composition is that liposomes are more fragile than, for example, other ONCs such as polymeric nanoparticles [14]. On the other hand, liposomes can be easier to manufacture than polymeric ONCs because of the commercial availability of phospholipids and other lipid components which can be used in simple self-assembly processes [14].

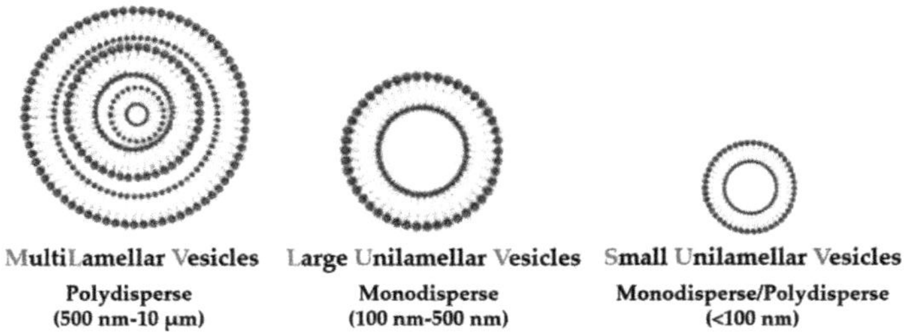

Figure 4.3 Schematic representation of three liposomal structures: MLV, LUV, and SUV.

As the flexibility of the liposomes can be detrimental in terms of stability, cholesterol (Chol) can be added to the composition of liposomes as it reduces the permeability of the bilayer and increases its stability [7]. In fact, the fluidity of liposomes, which depends on their composition and the temperature at which they are exposed, has been shown to have a significant impact on liposomal stability, drug release and cellular uptake [70, 71]. With increasing temperature, the lipid bilayer of liposomes can pass from a highly ordered gel phase to a more mobile and flexible fluid phase [70]. Accordingly, it may be interesting to produce a liposome system which is in the gel phase at the physiological temperature of healthy tissues (37°C) but which becomes fluid at higher temperatures characteristic of inflammatory conditions such as those found in brain cancer and neurodegenerative diseases [2, 72–74]. This can constitute a triggering strategy, as the liposome system is more stable while it is distributed throughout the body in off-target tissues but becomes more fluid and releases its contents into the target tissue [2, 14].

Other advantages of liposomes, as potential ONCs for brain drug delivery, are related to their very adjustable properties which may change with size, preparation method and lipid composition, which also defines the type of charge and charge density of the liposomal surface [2, 65, 66]. In terms of brain delivery, it may be beneficial to include cationic lipids, such as 1,2-dioleoyl-3-trimethylammonium-propane (DOTAP), dioctadecyldimethylammonium bromide (DODAB) or dioctadecyldimethylammonium chloride (DODAC), in the composition of the liposomes, rendering them with a positively charged surface. Cationic liposomes cross the BBB through the AMT mechanism [2, 14, 75, 76]. Moreover, cationic liposomes may also be used as transfection carriers to deliver genetic material into the cells, avoiding lysosomal digestion [77]. In this case, besides bearing cationic lipids, liposomes are also composed of neutral-charged *helper lipids*, like 1,2-dioleoyl-*sn*-glycero-3-phosphoethanolamine (DOPE) or monoolein, with fusogenic properties [77, 78]. These nucleic acid–loaded NCs, called lipoplexes, are formed by nucleic acid complexation and compaction, a process which initiates with electrostatic interaction between the cationic liposomal surface and anionic phosphate groups in nucleic acid material [77] (Fig. 4.4).

Generally, the lipoplexes formed retain a slight excess of positive charge which will allow them to still cross the BBB through AMT mechanisms [14]. In addition, the *helper* lipid fuses and destabilises the endosomal membrane, which promotes the endosomal escape of nucleic acids, thereby avoiding their enzymatic degradation and allowing their delivery in the cytosol of brain cells [14, 80, 81].

In summary, the tuneable nature of liposomes reinforces their potential for encapsulation of drugs of different lipophilicity, genetic material and other bioactive compounds [2, 65, 66], and despite presenting problems of in vivo stability which limit their route of administration and require careful selection of their composition, liposomes gather a set of attractive properties which still make them the most prevalent NCs in clinically approved therapeutic formulations [82].

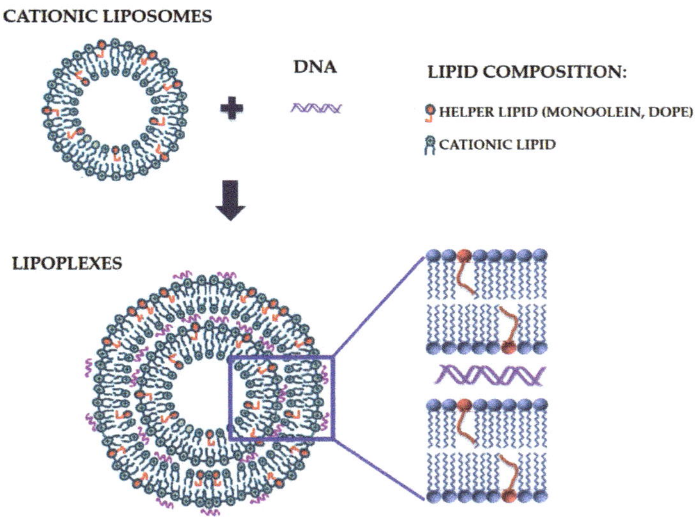

Figure 4.4 Schematic representation of cationic liposomes (top) and the correspondent DNA-lipoplexes (bottom). Reprinted from Ref. [79], Copyright (2014), with permission from Elsevier.

Liposomes are not only the most prevalent NCs in clinically approved formulations, but these ONCs are also one of the most explored in brain delivery research studies. The list of examples is endless, and there is a very good review on the subject [83]. Herein we give several examples focusing on liposomes used for different brain delivery purposes and composed exclusively of lipids. Therefore, all hybrid nanosystems produced by liposomes and polymeric coatings or other hybrid compositions have been excluded. Liposomes functionalised with different ligands, proteins or monoclonal antibodies were considered as these ligands are not part of the NC composition but are part of the targeting strategy and are adjuvants of therapeutic loads.

4.4.1.1 Liposomes in Alzheimer's disease

Two very similar liposomal formulations were developed as potential therapeutic strategies for AD [84, 85]. In these studies liposomes were composed of sphingomyelin (SM) and Chol (1:1 molar ratio), mixed with phosphatidic acid (PA) and functionalised on the surface with apolipoprotein E (ApoE)-derived peptide (mApoE) and were i.p. [85] or i.v. [84] administered to mice. ApoE is a protein involved in the metabolism of fats in the body which is also implicated in AD and cardiovascular disease [86]. Since ApoE is the main carrier of Chol in the brain, it must enter the brain. Indeed, ApoE specifically interacts with the LDLR and enters the brain through RMT [86]. mApoE is a peptide derived of human ApoE, modified with the addition of a tryptophan, glycine, and cysteine residue at the C-terminal [84, 85]. Therefore, the functionalisation of the liposome surface with apolipoproteins, such as mApoE, is a brain delivery strategy which promotes the interaction of liposomes with the LDLR, favouring the RMT BBB crossing [2]. The inclusion of PA and ApoE in the liposomes is also related to their therapeutic potential in AD. The observation of senile plaques is a hallmark of AD and is associated with the presence of amyloid β (Aβ) which undergoes aggregation from soluble oligomers to peptides aggregates which then form insoluble fibrils, ending in the deposition of the plaques between the nerve cells [2, 87]. These Aβ aggregates are neurotoxic and cause a gradual decline of neurological functions [2, 87]. It has been shown that under slightly acidic conditions (such as those encountered in inflamed AD brains), the protonation of three histidine residues in Aβ promotes the formation of β-sheet aggregates by reducing electrostatic repulsion [88]. Therefore, the destabilisation of Aβ aggregates is believed to be driven by electrostatic interactions [88], which in these studies occur between the charged Aβ residues and the charged liposomes [84, 85]. The ability of mApoE-PA liposomes to disaggregate Aβ assemblies has been confirmed in vivo by the synergistic interaction of both the negatively charged PA phosphate group and the positively charged mApoE amino acids with oppositely charged residues present on Aβ peptide at physiological pH [84, 85]. Additionally, mApoE-PA liposomes have been shown to be effective in reducing brain plaques in mice model animals, and this reduction was still observable 3 months after treatment [85]. Moreover, the neurodegeneration process seemed to slow down, as observed by the significant recovery of mice with impaired memory [85]. Finally, in vitro biocompatibility studies on different types of cells (endothelial and differentiated neuroblastoma cells) showed that mApoE-PA liposomes did not affect cell viability, BBB monolayer integrity and nitric oxide production and did not induce endoplasmic reticulum stress [84]. Taken together, the results of both studies suggest that mApoE-PA liposomes can affect the aggregation/disaggregation process of Aβ and are able to cross the BBB, thus possessing valuable potential in vivo applicability for the treatment of AD [84, 85].

In addition to controlling the aggregation and deposition of Aβ, other approaches to AD therapy include the treatment of neuroinflammation and the control of oxidative stress [2]. In this context, natural compounds (e.g. baicalein, curcumin [CRM], quercetin, sasanqua saponin, etc.) which possess anti-inflammatory and antioxidant properties and sometimes also exhibit anti-Aβ aggregation properties are emerging as prophylactic and therapeutic agents for AD control [2]. Furthermore, liposomes are also emerging as efficient NCs for these natural compounds, improving their poor pharmacokinetic profile. For example, baicalein-loaded liposomes, despite presenting fragility in simulated gastrointestinal fluids, were administered orally to rats and significantly improved (threefold more) the bioavailability of this natural compound [89]. Liposomes were also used to encapsulate another natural compound with neuroprotective effects relevant to suppression of oxidative stress, elimination of free radicals and inhibition of inflammation (sasanqua saponin) [90]. These liposomes composed of phosphatidylcholine (PC) and Chol also contained pheophorbide, an effective photosensitiser capable of generating singlet oxygen radicals while excited by 670 nm [90]. Singlet oxygen radicals break up phosphodiester bonds in phosphatidylcholine, causing liposome rupture and release of sasanqua saponin [90]. Following i.v. administration of liposomes in mice and near-infrared (NIR) irradiation, neuroprotective effects have been observed by improving locomotion activity in mice with increased expression of tyrosine hydroxylase (TH) and decreased inflammatory cytokines – tumour necrosis factor alpha (TNF-α) and interleukin 1 beta (IL-1β) – in the brain [90]. The decrease of inflammatory cytokines reflects the anti-inflammatory effect of sasanqua saponin. TH is a key enzyme in the synthesis of monoamine neurotransmitters such as dopamine and noradrenaline in neurons, and its expression is lowered in the brain tissues of patients with neurodegenerative diseases, making the observed increase in TH expression a sign of neuroprotection [90, 91]. Lazar et al. (2013) developed CRM-conjugated liposomes (CnLs) as a theranostic (therapeutic+diagnostic) for AD [92]. CnLs were composed of 1,2-dipalmitoyl-*sn*-glycerol-3-phosphatidylcholine

(DPPC), Chol and CRM–phospholipid conjugate. CnLs were nontoxic in vitro, downregulated the secretion of amyloid peptide and partially prevented Aβ-induced toxicity [92]. Intracranial stereotaxic injection of CnLs in the hippocampus and in the neocortex of mice showed that these liposomes were able to specifically stain the Aβ deposits in vivo [92]. CnLs also strongly labeled Aβ deposits in postmortem brain tissue of AD patients and mice, indicating that they could be used both as a targeting strategy for AD plaques and also as a diagnostic tool indicating the location of these plaques [92]. Finally, the natural compound quercetin was loaded into two very similar liposomal formulations (composed of PC and Chol) which were i.n. administered in rats [93, 94]. It was observed that quercetin-loaded liposomes attenuated the death of neurons and improved learning and memory deficits, probably because of the reduction of oxidative stress caused by quercetin [93, 94].

4.4.1.2 Liposomes in Parkinson's disease

PD is also a neurodegenerative disease with several aetiologies, including the death of dopamine-generating neurons in the brain area called *substantia nigra*, which causes a decrease in dopamine levels and motor symptoms such as tremor and rigidity. Currently available therapies are based on the administration of a natural precursor of dopamine (levodopa). In this regard, liposomal formulations composed by PC and Chol and loaded with levodopa were i.p. administered in mice, improving the release of dopamine in the *striatum* region [95, 96]. Moreover, these formulations by carrying levodopa to the brain avoided peripheral conversion to dopamine, which causes side effects of nausea, sleepiness and dyskinesia (involuntary movements which may occur with long-term levodopa use). Levodopa-loaded liposomes have also inhibited akinaesia (a failure to move or a much smaller version of movement) more effectively.

Glial cell–derived neurotrophic factor (GDNF) is a small protein which promotes the survival of many types of neurons [97]. Accordingly, ongoing studies have shown that GDNF can promote the growth, regeneration and survival of substantia nigra dopamine neurons, preventing the progression of PD when given at an early stage of the disease [83, 97]. In this regard, the liposomal formulation composed by 1,2-dioleoyl-*sn*-glycero-3-phosphocholine (DOPC),

Chol and stearylamine (SA) loaded with GDNF was i.n. administered in rats. GDNF demonstrated neurotrophic and neuroprotective effects of GDNF protein in the brain of rats either in GDNF not encapsulated or in GDNF encapsulated in liposomes. However, the liposomal formulation may have the advantage of a protective effect on the protein, preventing it from degrading [98].

As for AD, natural compounds which can control oxidative stress will be able to control the selective loss of PD dopaminergic nigral neurons [2, 99]. For instance, resveratrol (RSV) is a natural compound well known for its antioxidant effects. Therefore, liposomes composed of PC, Chol and dicetylphosphate (DCP) were loaded with RSV and administered orally to a rat PD model [99]. After 14 days of oral treatment with free RSV or RSV-loaded liposomes, the abnormal rotational behaviour, loss and apoptosis of nigral cells and total reactive oxygen species (ROS) decreased significantly and the overall antioxidant capacity of the nigral tissues improved significantly [99]. Furthermore, RSV-loaded liposomes showed more profound effects than free RSV, likely due to its increased bioavailability with encapsulation in liposomes [99].

4.4.1.3 Liposomes in cerebral ischaemia/reperfusion

The prevalence, impairment and mortality of CIR is high, in comparison to other neurological disorders mentioned so far [83]. CIR is characterised by a sudden decrease in brain blood flow because of cerebral vasculature obstruction, which affects the neural tissue (ischaemical penumbra zone) [83]. Unfortunately, CIR treatment is constrained by the poor ability to deliver therapeutic agents throughout the BBB [83]. Therefore, efforts have been made to recognise and improve the mechanisms of drug delivery to the brain [83]. Liposomes are considered potentially helpful to improve therapeutic effects in the treatment of CIR [83]. One of the possible treatments of CIR is citicoline, also known as cytidine diphosphate-choline (CDP-choline), the main phospholipid of the neuronal membrane which is degraded to free radicals and fatty acids throughout brain ischaemia [83]. Unfortunately, the crossing of the BBB was much lower than desired because of the polar nature of citicoline [83]. Therefore, liposomes containing CDP-choline have been found to enhance its bioavailability and its therapeutic efficacy in treating CIR [83, 100]. For example, liposomes composed of DPPC, dipalmitoylphosphatidylserine (DPPS), Chol and monosialotetrahexosylganglioside (GM1) were loaded with CDP-choline. In a similar approach to PEGylation of liposomes, the incorporation of GM1 ganglioside and anionic lipids such as DPPS into liposomes causes prolonged circulation time in vivo [100]. Thus, it is possible to obtain a stealth strategy without preparing a hybrid NC, as GM1 is a glycosphingolipid, and the resultant NC is entirely made of lipid components. After intraventricular injection in ischaemic rats, treatment with CDP-choline liposomes significantly decreased cerebral infarction compared to the equivalent dose of free CDP-choline [100]. The beneficial effects of CDP-choline liposomes in CIR may derive from a synergistic effect between the phospholipid components of liposomes and the encapsulated CDP-choline [100].

Natural compound–loaded liposomes have also proved to be beneficial in the treatment of CIR [2, 101, 102]. Liposomes containing PC, Chol and vitamin E were prepared to encapsulate luteolin and administered i.p. in rats as post-ischaemic treatment [102]. Vitamin E was used as an antioxidant agent. In general, luteolin as a neuroprotective agent acts by anti-ischaemic activity, which is likely through the re-equalisation of the pro-oxidant/antioxidant status [102]. Therefore, the liposomal formulation has substantially avoided behavioural and histologic injuries caused by CIR [102]. Furthermore, encapsulated luteolin not only lowered the increase in the level of mitochondrial ROS but also substantially upregulated the decrease in the activity of catalase and glutathione in the brain of CIR rats [102]. Liposomes composed of PC, Chol and DCP were loaded with quercetin and coated with aminophenyl-α-d-mannoside by covalent coupling to the surface [101]. The resulting mannosylated liposomes were administered i.v. in rats as preischaemic therapy [101]. Mannosylated liposomes were demonstrated to be nontoxic, non-immunogenic, noncarcinogenic, nonthrombogenic and biodegradable [101]. Moreover, because of the presence of mannose receptors in the brain, mannosylated liposomes are effective as an active RMT targeting strategy for the delivery of quercetin to brain tissue [101]. In summary, it has been shown that mannosylated liposomes loaded with quercetin not only prevented the development of CIR-induced lipid peroxidation and cerebral oedema but also protected the endogenous cerebral antioxidant defence in young and old rat brains [101].

4.4.1.4 Liposomes in brain tumours

The brain and CNS include more than 100 types of tumours. Our focus in this chapter is the use of ONCs in glioma, which includes all glial cell tumours such as astrocytomas, oligodendrogliomas, ependypomas and glioblastoma multiforme [83]. The treatment of glioma is very limited by the inadequate ability to deliver therapeutic agents over two specific brain barriers: the BBB and the blood–brain tumour barrier (BBTB). As a result, the enhanced permeability and retention (EPR) effect in the case of glioma is not as effective in NC accumulation in the brain as in the case of other cancers [83]. Therefore, efforts have been made to identify and enhance brain drug delivery systems. In this sense, liposomes are described as a possible valuable system for better treatment of gliomas, since several targeting strategies show their ability to reach the brain and target the tumour [83]. Most of the targeting strategies involve the coating of liposomes with polymers which act as spacers to bind the ligands which are recognised by the overexpressed receptors in the BBB [83]. Hybrid liposomes made of lipids and polymeric coatings are therefore the vast majority of NCs used in glioma [83]. However, since this chapter does not cover hybrid NCs, we present examples of liposomes which are entirely made up of lipids which still use targeting strategies or which use triggering strategies (e.g. ultrasounds) or other combination therapies (e.g. genetic therapy) which can be applied as therapeutic approaches for glioma. For example, Chen et al. (2010) used a cholesterol derivative – cholest-5-en-3-ol-(3β)-[2-[[4-[(carboxymethyl)dithio]-1-iminobutyl] amino] ethyl] carbamate (CHETA) – and PC to prepare procationic liposomes (pcl) [103]. The ligand Lf, which was positively charged at physiological pH, was adsorbed onto the surface of the pcl (negatively charged) via electrostatic interaction, forming lactoferrin-coated procationic liposomes (Lf-pcl) [103]. Lf-pcl combined two targeting strategies: AMT and RMT. First, the AMT strategy was used, as under physiological pH conditions, the positively charged Lf will adsorb to the negatively charged BBB membrane. Second, the pcl were neutral or negatively charged in a physiological environment, but when Lf-pcl reached brain capillary endothelial cells, the disulphide bond inside CHETA was cleaved by protein disulphide isomerase or thioredoxin reductase (TrxR) on the cellular membrane, changing the surface charge of pcl to positively charged liposomes which can once more take advantage of AMT [103]. Furthermore, since LfRs are highly expressed in endothelial cells of the BBB, Lf-pcl were specifically bound to these receptors and internalised by RMT [103]. As a result, Lf-pcl had an improved uptake profile in the brain capillary endothelial cells, increased ability to cross the BBB in vitro, increased in vivo brain accumulation and lower cell toxicity compared to conventional and cationic liposomes [103]. Thus, although this liposomal system has not been tested for a specific type of drug, it appears to be promising to deliver drugs to the brain, particularly in the case of glioma because of a dual targeting strategy. The AMT strategy was also explored by Joshi et al. (2015) [104]. These authors compared the performance of cationic, anionic and neutral liposomes. Cationic liposomes were composed of dimyristoylphosphatidylcholine (DMPC), DOTAP and Chol. Neutral liposomes were composed of DMPC and Chol. Anionic liposomes were composed of dimyristoylphosphatidylglycerol (DMPG) and Chol [104]. The three types of liposomes were loaded with a dialkyl carbocyanine membrane label (DiD), a dye which can be quantified by light absorbance and fluorescence methods. The three types of liposomes were separately injected via the internal carotid artery of healthy rats during transient cerebral hypoperfusion. Rats bearing gliomas were injected with cationic liposomes [104]. Following intra-arterial injection, a strong uptake of cationic as opposed to anionic and neutral liposomes in the brain parenchyma was observed. Postmortem multispectral fluorescence imaging showed that the cationic liposomal charge was related to more effective brain delivery indicating an AMT-targeting mechanism [104]. This study demonstrates that highly cationic liposomes, administered directly to the brain via an intracarotid route, can be an effective method for drug delivery to glioma. Two research studies have used focused ultrasound (FU) waves as a triggering strategy for delivery of the anticancer drug doxorubicin (DOX) from liposomes [105, 106]. Besides triggering DOX release, FU can induce a transient permeabilisation of the BBTB without effects on normal tissues [105, 106]. One of these studies complemented this strategy with the use of cationic liposomes composed of PC, DOPE, Chol, DODAB and cetyltrimethylammonium bromide (CTAB) [106]. Combining the advantages of the BBB and BBTB reversible opening by FU and glioma-targeted binding through AMT, these cationic liposomes could achieve glioma-targeted delivery, which could be established as a possible strategy for future brain tumour treatment [106]. Cationic liposomes (composed of DOTAP and DOPE) were also developed to produce lipoplexes carrying nucleic acids used for genetic therapy as a strategy for glioma treatment [107]. Lipoplexes were formed from the compaction of cationic liposomes with a recombinant plasmid encoding for the protein of the matrix of vesicular stomatitis virus, a protein which can inhibit rat glioma growth either in vitro or in situ. Lipoplexes loaded with protein of the matrix (LPM) were i.v. injected in rats bearing gliomas [107]. In vivo experiments confirmed the uptake of lipoplexes by glioma cells and the effects of LPM in those cells, as a smaller tumour volume and prolonged survival time was found in the LPM-treated group [107].

4.4.2 Ethosomes

While classic liposomes are excellent candidates to deliver drugs and other bioactives, ethosomes (Fig. 4.1) – made up of phospholipids, high quantities of ethanol (20%–45%) and water – enhance permeation via gastrointestinal epithelia and skin, improving oral and transdermal delivery [2, 108].

The increase in permeability observed with ethosomes is based on the interaction of ethanol with lipid molecules located in the polar headgroup region, which increases the fluidity of the lipid membrane. Ethanol, known as an effective enhancer of permeability, can provide soft flexible properties to the vesicles [2, 108], making it possible to penetrate deeper layers of the skin or of the gastrointestinal epithelia [2, 109, 110]. The same reasoning can be applied to brain delivery as the characteristics of ethosomes may enhance BBB permeability and delivery of drugs or bioactives to the brain [2].

Accordingly, ethosomes loaded with catechin and orally administered in rats were successful in increasing plasma concentrations of this natural compound compared to the free compound in solution [111]. Consequently, ethosomes delivered a high concentration of catechin to different regions of the brain (thalamus, hippocampus, cortex and striatum) [111] and can be promising as protectors against age-related neurodegenerative diseases, given the beneficial effects of catechin as a natural antioxidant which ameliorates the progression of AD and PD [110, 111]. Ethosomes were also investigated for the transdermal administration in rats of ligustrazine – a natural antioxidant for the treatment of AD [109]. Both the penetration ability and the deposition in skin were significantly higher when ligustrazine was carried in the ethosomes in comparison to administration of free ligustrazine [109]. Ligustrazine-loaded ethosomes were also able to recover the activities of the antioxidant enzymes and the levels of lipid peroxidation in the brain of amnesic rats to the similar state of normal rats, which was also indirectly reflected by the improvement in the behavioural performance [109]. In conclusion, ligustrazine-loaded ethosomes might offer a potential therapeutic alternative for AD with the advantage of using transdermal delivery as a patient-friendly administration route [109].

4.4.3 Polymersomes

Polymers are chemical compounds composed of many repeated monomers and may exist as chains or in branched form and can be from natural origin, like chitosan, alginate and other polysaccharides, or can be synthetic like poly(caprolactone) (PCL), polylactide (PLA), poly(methyl methacrylate) (PMMA), polydimethylsiloxane (PDMS), poly(2-methyl-2-oxazoline) (PMOXA), poly(*N*-vinylpyrrolidone) (PVP), poly(vinyl alcohol) (PVA) and PEG [112, 113]. Block copolymers are macromolecules which contain multiple adjacent blocks of chemical monomers with different structures or distributed in different sequences [112, 113]. A block copolymer, consisting of two types of monomers is called a diblock copolymer and has amphiphilic properties [112, 113]. Triblock copolymers composed of an inner hydrophobic block attached to outer hydrophilic blocks are also amphiphilic. In aqueous solution, amphiphilic block copolymers, either diblock or triblock, can self-assemble into various supramolecular polymeric structures such as micelles, rods, nanoparticles, or polymersomes (POs) [112, 113]. The final structure of the self-assembly aggregates depends on several parameters such as concentration, molecular weight, geometry of the amphiphilic block copolymers or the ratio of the different blocks [112, 113]. POs are self-assembled vesicles of amphiphilic block copolymers

[112–116]. The most common polymer arrangement used in PO formation are diblock (AB) or triblock copolymers (ABA or rarely ABC, where A and C are the hydrophilic blocks and B the hydrophobic block) (Fig. 4.5) [114].

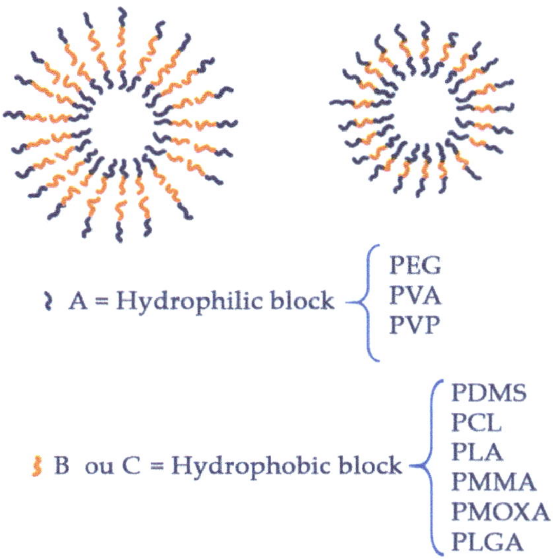

Figure 4.5 Schematic representation of polymersomes and diblock or triblock copolymers.

Structurally, POs are very similar to liposomes, that is, they present an aqueous core where hydrophilic therapeutic agents can be encapsulated, and surrounding the aqueous core there is a polymeric hydrophobic membrane where lipophilic therapeutic agents can be loaded. However, the polymeric membrane of POs is thicker (5–30 nm) than the lipid membrane of liposomes (3–5 nm), conferring to POs more stability and robustness [114] (Table 4.1). These properties may be useful for drug delivery purposes to ensure that the drug is not released before reaching the target tissues [112, 113, 115, 116]. Because of their increased stability, POs are emerging as promising vesicles to replace liposomal formulations [115]. Nevertheless, POs also have some drawbacks relative to liposomes. One drawback comes from POs' superior stability, which could hinder or prolong the release of the drug over time [115]. In this regard, stimulus-responsive polymers, which may be degraded with changes in pH or temperature, have been used extensively to control drug release and increase the bioavailability of the drug at the target site [115]. Another inconvenience is the lack of reproducibility in the production of POs (Table 4.1). In fact, as opposed to lipids, block copolymers are polydisperse, and the use of different batches of the same polymers affects the self-assembly and originates different final PO structures [114]. Finally, PO constitution and durability are still causing some caution with regard to their long-term use, and therefore these ONCs remain interesting in academic studies but are still not translatable to the same extent as liposomes in the clinical context [115].

Despite these drawbacks of POs, the appealing tuneable properties and improved stability of these ONCs make them good candidates for drug delivery purposes and their exploitation as brain delivery systems is also increasing. A few examples illustrative of the use of POs for brain drug delivery in neurodegenerative diseases and glioma are presented in Table 4.2.

4.5 Micelles: Polymeric and Lipidic

Micelles are self-assembly aggregates with 5–50 nm of amphiphilic agents (lipidic or polymeric) which occur above a well-defined concentration which is called the critical micelle concentration (CMC). Unlike liposomes or POs which are vesicles containing an aqueous core, micelles possess hydrophilic portions turned towards aqueous surroundings and a hydrophobic core made of the hydrophobic portions of the amphiphilic agents (Fig. 4.1) [2]. As described before, although using the same type of amphiphilic constituents, whether an amphiphile is assembled in a micelle or in a vesicle, it depends on several parameters, such as concentration, molecular weight, geometry of the amphiphilic block copolymers or amphiphilic lipids or the ratio of the different blocks.

Like vesicles, micellar drug carriers have also been particularly attractive in studies of BBB penetration and brain drug delivery for their tuneable self-assembly, high drug-loading capacity, good biocompatibility, increased brain drug accumulation and extended circulation half-life. Moreover, their surface can also be decorated with targeting ligands which will actively direct the ONCs to the corresponding BBB endothelial cell receptors and facilitate transcytosis of drug across the BBB [117]. Some illustrative examples of the use of micelles for brain drug delivery in different CNS diseases and glioma are presented in Table 4.2.

4.6 Nanoparticles: Lipid Nanoparticles and Polymeric Nanoparticles

4.6.1 Lipid Nanoparticles

Another important lipid-based ONC is lipid nanoparticles which are colloidal dispersions containing a solid lipid matrix in which hydrophobic therapeutic agents can be effectively carried. These ONCs present a size distribution ranging from 10 to 1000 nm. The term 'lipid nanoparticles' includes two types of nanoparticles which differ in their inner lipidic structure because of the composition and organisation of the lipids in the solid matrix: solid lipid nanoparticles (SLNs) and nanostructured lipid carriers (NLCs) [118] (Fig. 4.1). SLNs are an alternative of submicron-sized oil-in-water (o/w) emulsions, where the liquid lipid (oil) is replaced by a solid lipid (e.g. glyceryl behenate, tripalmitin, stearic acid, glyceryl monostearate [GMS], cetyl palmitate, tristearin, tripalmitate [TP], glyceryl palmitostearate, glyceril trimyristate), which remains in the solid state at room temperature. In contrast, the lipid matrix of NLCs is composed of a mixture of liquid and solid lipids, that is, a solid matrix which entraps liquid lipid nanocompartments, and is also solid at room temperature [58]. Some examples of liquid lipids include octyldodecanol, Miglyol® 812 (caprylic/capric triglycerides), oleic acid and propylene glycol monocaprylate. Although NLCs contain a liquid lipid, these nanoparticles remain in the solid state at room temperature by setting the proportion of liquid lipids in the formulation [58]. The use of functional lipids in ONCs can enhance the dissolution and bioavailability of poorly water-soluble drugs, while the solid matrix allows the controlled release of encapsulated molecules and protects them from degradation, thus increasing the long-term stability of the system [119].

To enhance brain uptake of therapeutic agents, lipid nanoparticles are considered highly attractive colloidal systems because of their general properties [120–126]:

- Biocompatibility, biodegradability generating natural degradation by-products
- Non-immunogenicity, nonthrombogenicity and non-inflammatory because of the use of physiological lipids and generally recognised as safe (GRAS) excipients
- Physical stability in the circulatory system
- Natural tendency to cross the BBB by endocytosis or by transcytosis mechanism of endothelial cells [120] lining blood capillaries in the brain or permeate the tight junctions between cells because of their lipophilic nature and small size
- Possibility of surface functionalisation to target the BBB
- Use of excipients which are regulatory-approved and do not induce drug alterations (e.g. protein denaturation, chemical degradation)
- Ease of manufacturing/scaling up at an industrial scale cost-effectively with reproducibility in drug loading
- Capacity to encapsulate a wide variety of biologically active compounds

Despite the development of lipid matrices being described several decades ago, nowadays lipid nanoparticles are gaining a special interest for therapeutic brain delivery because of the increasing availability of lipophilic excipients with well-known safety profiles which offer the possibility of modulating release profiles [127, 128]. In vitro studies have shown that lipid nanoparticles are less toxic than polymeric ones [129]. In addition, these nanosystems can present high physicochemical stability; for example, Blasi et al. [130] demonstrated that SLNs composed of cetyl palmitate are stable when stored at 4°C for four years. These authors reinforced the potential of lipid nanoparticles as ONCs for brain drug delivery based on long-term physicochemical stability and the in vivo safety profile.

The use of both lipid nanoparticles (i.e. SLNs and NLCs) has been widely investigated to mediate targeting of therapeutic agents for different brain pathologies (e.g. neurodegenerative, psychotic disorders or tumours) and overcome the constraints on the transport of therapeutics across the BBB. These ONCs have already demonstrated their high value in improving the delivery of therapeutics to the brain, crossing the BBB more easily. Some examples of these studies are explored in the next sections.

4.6.1.1 Solid lipid nanoparticles

As mentioned before, the presence of physiological barriers, particularly the BBB, restricts the accessibility of many therapeutic agents to the brain, which may compromise the therapeutic efficacy in brain diseases. In accordance with Pardridge [131], more than 98% of potentially therapeutic agents for brain-associated diseases fail in vivo since they cannot passively cross the BBB and reach therapeutic levels. Therefore, SLNs can be used as drug carriers because of their lipophilic properties which lead them to the CNS by an endocytosis mechanism, overcoming the BBB. On the basis of these considerations, Bondi et al. [132] developed SLNs composed of biocompatible solid lipid (glyceryl behenate – Compritol 888® ATO) and phosphatidylcholine and taurocholate sodium salt as a surfactant and co-surfactant agents, respectively, for brain delivery of riluzole. Riluzole, a glutamate release inhibitor, is a potent neuroprotective agent which is useful for the treatment of neurodegenerative diseases. This compound represents the first approved disease-modifying treatment for ALS [133], and its clinical use is linked to limited efficacy due to the abnormal hepatic function history in patients. The SLNs containing riluzole had an average diameter of approximately 88 nm; a highly charged surface, as indicated by the zeta potential of approximately −46 mV; and excellent loading capacity; and the release profile of riluzole was pH-dependent [132]. After i.p. administration to rats, biodistribution studies indicated that the entrapped riluzole crossed the BBB with greater facility than free non-encapsulated riluzole, reaching a significantly higher concentration in the CNS, which resulted in more efficacy in delaying damage clinical signs (i.e. damage of neurons and axons in myelin basic protein of an animal model) using induced experimental allergic encephalomyelitis (EAE) in Sprague–Dawley rats. Additionally, a low biodistribution of riluzole in other organs – liver, spleen, heart, kidneys and lungs – was verified when the drug was loaded in SLNs, which could imply less systemic toxicity. This was proved by the fact that the rats treated with the SLNs developed clinical signs of EAE later than those treated with free riluzole. Moreover, SLNs can be used not only to improve the drug targeting to the brain but also to enhance drug bioavailability. For example, Misra et al. [134] proposed the development of galantamine hydrobromide (GH)-loaded SLNs formulated with biodegradable and biocompatible components (solid lipid was glyceryl behenate) to overcome some shortcomings of GH, particularly its poor brain penetration which results in low bioavailability to the target site, requiring repeated dosing. Additionally, the cholinergic side effects of GH are also another obstacle to the optimal use of this agent. GH is a reversible and competitive acetylcholinesterase (AchE) inhibitor which has been shown to improve attention and has beneficial effects on cognitive and functional outcomes for AD [135, 136] because of its neuroprotective effects [137, 138]. The mean size of SLNs was lower than 100 nm (i.e. ideal for brain-targeted therapeutic delivery), and the maximum drug entrapment was 83.42 ± 0.63%. SLN were able to modulate both the in vitro GH release profile and the in vivo time course of the drug. After oral administration, the group of rats to which the SLNs were administered showed an increase in bioavailability of approximately twofold and a significant improvement of cognitive impairment in the AD-like preclinical protocol using rats in comparison with the free drug. Similarly, Natarajan et al. [139] developed SLNs to improve the bioavailability of olanzapine (OLZ), an antipsychotic drug, in the brain by embedding the minimum dose of the drug into SLNs, thereby reducing the side effects of the drug. Despite the high clinical value of OLZ in the treatment of schizophrenia, it has some limitations such as poor bioavailability (57%) due to extensive hepatic first-pass metabolism, requiring the administration of high doses to reach therapeutic levels in the brain and, thus, increasing the likelihood of adverse effects associated with antipsychotic agents, such as extrapyramidal symptoms (EPS) like rigidity, bradykinaesia, tremor, akathisia, and dyskinaesia. OLZ-loaded SLNs were formulated using tripalmitate (TP-SLN) or glyceryl monostearate (GMS-SLN) as a solid lipid and Tween® 80 as a surfactant and SA as a positive charge inducer. Generally, the optimal size range for SLNs in brain targeting ranges from 50 to 300 nm. The mean particle size and zeta potential of GMS-SLNs and TP-SLNs were 165.1 ± 2.2 nm and 110.5 ± 0.5 nm, respectively, and +35.29 ± 1.2 and +66.50 ± 0.7 mV, respectively (i.e. ideal for brain targeting by the AMT route). SLNs revealed a sustained drug release profile. Pharmacokinetics studies were conducted in male Wistar rats through i.v. administration. SLNs enhanced the relative bioavailability of OLZ in the brain up to 23-fold and reduced the clearance compared to pure OLZ suspension. The authors suggest that this may be because of the transport of intact OLZ-loaded SLNs across the BBB via the endocytosis mechanism. These results are promising at reducing the OLZ dose required, which could reduce the EPS.

An additional approach to increase the amount of therapeutic agent which reaches the brain is through active targeting by binding specific ligands to the surface of ONCs which interact with surface proteins expressed constitutively in the BBB (i.e. receptors involved in the RMT pathway). This modification has been proven to enhance the selectivity uptake of therapeutics via RMT [140]. Kuo and Wang explored this strategy using a monoclonal melanotransferrin antibody (mMAb) [141], since human brain microvascular endothelial cells (HBMECs) expressed a large quantity of membrane-bound melanotransferrin [142]. In addition to mMAb, the authors also conjugated tamoxifen (TX), a modulator of selective oestrogen receptor, on etoposide (ETP – chemotherapeutic agent)-loaded SLNs (ETP-SLNs) to target the BBB and glioblastoma multiforme (GBM) [141]. Several chemotherapeutic agents are substrates of the active efflux transporters (e.g. P-glycoprotein [P-gp] and multidrug resistance–related proteins [MRPs]) at the BBB and so the agents do not achieve therapeutic levels [143, 144]. Therefore, TX was used to prolong the ETP residence in the brain parenchyma because of its potential ability to suppress the activity of MRPs which limited the efficacy of chemotherapeutic agents [145]. The mMAb- and TX-conjugated ETP-SLNs (mMAb-TX-ETP-SLNs) were used to penetrate the BBB composed of a monolayer of human astrocyte–regulated HBMECs and to inhibit the growth of malignant U87MG cells (Uppsala 87 Malignant Glioma [U87MG]) [141]. After treating with mMAb-TX-ETP-SLNs, a high viability of HBMECs proved acceptable cytotoxicity for the integrity of the BBB, suggesting high biocompatibility of the developed formulation. Both TX-grafted and mMAb-grafted SLNs significantly increased the BBB permeability coefficient for ETP. mMAb-TX-ETP-SLNs have also been demonstrated to be more effective in both BBB permeability and coupling melanotransferrin in GBM than ETP-SLNs. Moreover, the efficiency in antiproliferation against U87MG cells was in the order of mMAb-TX-ETP-SLNs > TX-ETP-SLNs > ETP-SLNs > SLNs. Cationic bovine serum albumin (CBSA) is another example of a targeting ligand which has been investigated to bypass the BBB, maintaining the integrity of the BBB tight junction [146, 147]. On the basis of this consideration, Agarwal et al. prepared DOX-loaded SLNs containing tristearin, soya lecithin and stearic acid as a lipid phase stabilised with a Poloxamer 188 (surfactant agent) aqueous phase and conjugated with CBSA [148]. Stearic acid was added for the conjugation of CBSA to the SLNs. CBSA uses the AMT pathway to bypass the BBB, which involves electrostatic interaction between the positively charged protein (CBSA) and negatively charged membrane cells at the BBB [149, 150]. The results demonstrated that CBSA-conjugated SLNs allow sustained and brain-targeted delivery [148]. SLN-DOX and CBSA-SLN-DOX had a mean size of 80.9 ± 1.7 nm (polydispersity index [PDI] of 0.082 ± 0.008) and 95.1 ± 1.8 nm (PDI of 0.073 ± 0.011), respectively. The zeta potential of SLN-DOX was −13.5 ± 0.5 mV and increased to +14.1 ± 0.7 mV upon ligand conjugation. Cellular studies using HNGC-1 cell lines revealed that the targeting ligand enhanced the cellular uptake of SLNs, almost six times, and was more cytotoxic as compared to DOX solution or nonconjugated SLNs. CBSA-anchored SLNs also demonstrated the maximum transcytosis ability across brain capillary endothelial cells. In vivo studies were carried out in mice and confirmed the more efficient delivery of DOX to brain tissues and the least immunogenic effect with a CBSA-conjugated formulation.

In another active brain-targeting study related to AD, Yusuf et al. [151] assessed the efficacy of brain-targeted piperine (PIP)-loaded SLNs (PIP-SLNs) in an experimentally induced AD model at a low dose of 2 mg/kg. PIP has beneficial effects in AD, including a strong antioxidant effect, inhibits the enzyme AchE and improves the cholinergic system in the brain. The delivery of PIP to the brain is complicated since this molecule undergoes intense first-pass metabolism, pH-mediated metabolism and photo-isomerisation [152, 153]. Therefore, the authors proposed the development of SLNs containing glycerol monostearate as a solid lipid and Epikuron™ 200 (purified phosphatidylcholine) and Tween® 80 or polysorbate-80 (PS-80) as surfactants [151]. The prepared

PIP-SLNs were overcoated with PS-80 to produce PS-80-PIP-SLNs, since PS-80-coated nanoparticles penetrate the BBB by endocytosis (transcytosis) through specific adsorption of ApoE – a lipoprotein fragment of LDL – on its surface, and the nanoparticles mimic the natural LDL particles which could interact with the LDL receptors located in the BMEC, followed by nanoparticle endocytic uptake into the brain [154, 155]. Thus, the coating of nanoparticles with polysorbates can improve the targeting of therapeutics to the brain and, additionally, inhibit P-gp activity, minimising the efflux of the drug [156, 157]. The PS-80-PIP-SLN formulation was administered to animals (albino rats) via the i.p. route [151]. Although the size of PS-80-PIP-SLNs was 312.0 ± 5.1 nm, there was a high concentration of PIP in brain tissues, which can be explained by transcytosis, as previously reported in other studies [158, 159]. The PIP in SLNs demonstrated positive therapeutic results in the AD model via acting on the oxidative cascade (i) by decreasing the superoxide dismutase values by 504 ± 44.24 m units ($p < 0.05$), (ii) on the cholinergic system by enhancing AchE values by 29.24 ± 4.29 μg/mg ($p < 0.01$) and (iii) reducing the amyloidal plaque and tangle contents in the brain tissues which were proved by histopathology studies. On the basis of the significant antitumoural activity exhibited by PS-80 nanoparticles in the glioma animal model [160, 161], the coating of cetyl palmitate-based SLNs with PS-80 and PS-60 was also a strategy investigated by Martins et al. [162] to deliver cytotoxic camptothecin (CPT) into the brain parenchyma by crossing the BBB after i.v. administration. Both polysorbates (i.e. PS-60 and PS-80) are reported to be promising surfactant agents for enhancing drug brain delivery [154]. Although CPT has already revealed antitumour activity in glioblastomas models [163], its instability in physiological conditions, the limited aqueous solubility and its several toxic effects limit its therapeutic value [164, 165]. The CPT-loaded SLNs had a mean size below 200 nm, a low PDI (<0.25), a negative surface charge (–20 mV) and high encapsulation efficiency (>94%) [162]. Cytotoxicity studies against human glioma cell lines (A172, U251, U373, U87) revealed higher antitumour activity when CPT was encapsulated into SLNs compared to free CPT in solution/suspension or in a physical mixture with SLNs. In vivo biodistribution studies in rats demonstrated superior brain accumulation and lower deposition of CPT in peripheral organs with CPT-loaded SLNs, revealing the positive role of SLNs on brain targeting and, thus, the potential reduction of CPT toxic side effects. Estella-Hermoso de Mendoza et al. [166] obtained similar results after oral administration of anticancer edelfosin loaded in Compritol® and Precirol® lipid nanoparticles on a xenograft mouse glioma model [166]. The results demonstrated that the high edelfosin accumulation in the brain with lipid nanoparticles is attributed to the inhibition of P-gp by Tween® 80, which was verified using a P-gp drug interaction assay. The authors also proved that after 14 days of treatment, drug-loaded lipid nanoparticles in mice bearing a C6 glioma xenograft tumour exhibited a highly significant decrease in tumour growth after 14 days from the beginning of treatment [166].

To improve the access of drugs to the brain, the rational use of alternative routes of administration has been triggered, with the i.n. route (non-invasive technique) being an important focus for the transport of neurotherapeutic agents, since the molecules bypass the BBB and directly access the brain through the olfactory region of the nasal mucosa, without previous absorption to the blood circulation [167–169]. Moreover, i.n. administration improves the bioavailability of compounds since it avoids gastrointestinal and first-pass hepatic metabolic processes. In conclusion, the development of nose-to-brain ONCs represents a promising approach for neurotherapeutic agents which have a short circulation half-life ($t_{1/2}$), a rapid degradation rate, or poor ability to pass through the BBB because of their unsuitable molecular weight, lipophilicity or surface charge. Taking these considerations into account, and to overcome some shortcomings related to risperidone (RSP), Patel et al. [170] encapsulated this drug in SLNs (solid lipid: glyceryl behenate; surfactant: Pluronic F-127) and explored the brain-targeting efficiency through nose-to-brain delivery. RSP is an antipsychotic agent which has been approved for the management of psychotic disorders. This compound has advantages over conventional antipsychotic agents because of a lower EPS; however, this benefit depends on the dose of the drug, requiring a low-dose therapy. In addition, RSP has some drawbacks which limit its clinical use, such as poor aqueous solubility, poor oral bioavailability since it undergoes extensive first-pass hepatic metabolism and P-gp efflux [171]. SLNs presented an RSP encapsulating efficiency (EE) of 59.65% ± 1.18%, a mean particle size of 148.05 ± 0.85 nm, a PDI of 0.148 ± 0.028 (i.e. a monodisperse stable system) and a zeta potential of −25.35 ± 0.45 mV. SLNs demonstrated a sustained release of RSP [170]. Both pharmacodynamic and pharmacokinetic studies carried out in mice demonstrated that RSP-loaded SLNs (RSLNs) administrated by the i.n. route effectively reach the brain. In vivo biodistribution and gamma scintigraphy imaging studies showed that i.n. administration of RSLN provides higher RSP levels in the brain (with a brain/blood ratio 1 h postadministration of 1.36 ± 0.06) than i.v. administration of the free drug (with a brain/blood ratio of 0.17 ± 0.05) and i.v. administration of RSLN (with a brain/blood ratio of 0.78 ± 0.07), that is, nearly 10- and 5-fold higher, respectively.

4.6.1.2 Nanostructured lipid carriers

NLCs represent an enhanced generation of lipid nanoparticles and theoretically present some advantages over SLNs, namely high capacity to accommodate a greater quantity of therapeutics, while avoiding drug expulsion during storage [172]. NLCs have shown potential as ONCs to improve the bioavailability of drugs with the aim to reach therapeutic concentrations in the brain. For example, Kumar et al. [173] investigated the use of NLCs composed of Compritol 888® ATO (solid lipid) and tocopherol acetate (liquid lipid) and PC (surfactant) to encapsulate quercetin for brain delivery after oral administration [173]. As previously referred, quercetin is a natural compound which shows protective effects against neuronal cell damage and thus may play an important role in the prevention or therapy of AD and PD. However, despite possessing many advantages, its administration also presents various challenges, like poor oral bioavailability (<2%), extensive first-pass metabolism, poor brain permeability, a hydrophobic nature and physiological pH instability, which hinder its proper usage [174]. NLCs offered better loading of quercetin and controlled drug release with appreciable stability [173]. In vitro antioxidant performance of quercetin was improved after encapsulation in NLCs, and these nanoparticles were substantially uptaken by Caco-2 cells [173]. In vivo, NLCs substantially enhanced quercetin bioavailability (approx. sixfold), enhanced biological residence (2.5 times) and appreciably retarded quercetin clearance (approx. sixfold) [173]. On the other hand, NLCs were able to substantially deliver quercetin to the brain. NLCs were observed to enhance the brain drug permeability in a noticeable manner [173]. In conclusion, NLCs can significantly improve brain delivery of quercetin [173].

NLCs have also been widely exploited as ONCs in order to improve the penetration of therapeutic agents to the brain using the i.n.

administration strategy. Some studies reported that drugs loaded in NLCs provide significant differences in the pharmacokinetic profile and distribution after i.n. administration. For example, Eskandari et al. [175] developed valproic acid (VPA)-loaded NLCs with the aim of reducing the dose of the drug and maintaining therapeutic levels in the brain for a prolonged period. VPA, an anticonvulsant agent, is used in the treatment of epilepsy, bipolar disorders, migraine and cancer [176]. Generally, this therapeutic agent requires high doses to achieve effective clinical effects, since its delivery and distribution into the brain are limited. Additionally, Scism et al. [177] assessed the VPA efflux clearance at the BBB and proved that it was 2.7-fold superior than the influx clearance compared to control animals. The developed NLCs contained cetyl palmitate and octyldodecanol as solid and liquid lipids, respectively, and were stabilised with soy lecithin S 100 and Poloxamer 188 (i.e. surfactants) [175]. The mean size of NLCs was 154 ± 16 nm with drug loading of 47% ± 0.8% and drug release of 75% ± 1.9% after 21 days. In vivo pharmacodynamics studies were performed using rats which received VPA-loaded NLCs by i.p. or i.n. administration. The results revealed that VPA-NLCs provide a superior protective effect than a solution of VPA ($p < 0.05$) after treatment via the i.n. route. A similar protective effect to systemic administration was achieved with much lower doses when rats were treated with VPA-NLCs by the i.n. route ($p > 0.05$). The results proved that i.n. administration of NLCs maintains the protective effect of VPA with a much higher (about 20 times) brain:plasma concentration ratio compared to i.p. administration (i.e. positive control group), requiring lower doses of VPA. Alam et al. [178] also explored the efficacy of i.n. NLC administration – using GMS as a solid lipid, oleic acid as a liquid lipid and Tween® 80 and Poloxamer 188 as surfactants – to improve the brain targeting of lamotrigine (LMT), an antiepileptic agent [178]. The brain access of LMT is limited by overexpression of P-gp in the BBB [179], requiring the administration of high doses to achieve a therapeutic concentration; however, this challenge enhances its blood concentration and, consequently, the adverse effects of LMT. Therefore, the i.n. route was evaluated in order to improve clinical utility and therapeutic efficacy of LMT. NLCs had an average size of 151.6 ± 7.6 nm, a PDI of 0.249 ± 0.035, an average zeta potential of +11.75 ± 2.96 mV and an EE of 96.64% ± 4.27%. NLCs exhibited a sustained drug concentration (24 h) after i.n. administration. Scintigraphy studies evidenced that i.n. administration of NLCs provides higher accumulation of LMT in rats' brains and a higher protective effect (even with lower doses – that is, one-fifth of the oral dose) than i.n. and oral administration of the drug solution. Likewise, duloxetine hydrochloride (DLX)-loaded NLCs for i.n. administration were developed and their efficacy against depression was investigated in a rat model [180]. DLX is a potent and balanced dual reuptake inhibitor of both serotonin and norepinephrine which is used in the treatment of major depressive disorder (MDD). This therapeutic agent has also all the properties required to be loaded into NLCs and delivered by the i.n route [181, 182]: it undergoes hepatic first-pass metabolism, presents poor oral bioavailability (~50%), has chemical instability in gastric pH and has low cerebrospinal fluid (CSF) concentration on oral administration. The lipid matrix of NLCs included Capryol™ propylene glycol monocaprylate (PGMC) and GMS, which was stabilised in a surfactant aqueous solution of Poloxamer (Pluronic F68) and bile salt (sodium taurocholate) [180]. Lyophilised DLX-NLCs had an average particle size of 137.2 ± 2.88 nm with a PDI of 0.639 ± 0.355, a zeta potential of +31.53 ± 11.21 mV and an EE of 79.15 ± 4.17%. In vivo studies conducted in rats demonstrated that i.n. DLX-NLC treatment significantly improves behaviour analysis (i.e. the total swimming, climbing time and locomotor activity), as well as revealed a higher concentration of drug in brain when compared with DLX solution.

In addition to the antioxidant effects useful in the treatment of AD, CRM is also a promising agent for cancer treatment because of its potent antiproliferative effects, although it is also associated with pharmacokinetic problems such as poor aqueous solubility, chemical instability in alkaline medium, rapid metabolism and poor absorption from the gastrointestinal tract. With the perspective to solubilise CRM in a physiologic stable medium and maybe to improve its brain targeting, Madane and Mahajan [183] also proposed its encapsulation into NLCs (solid lipid: Precirol® ATO; liquid lipid: Capmul™ MCM – mixture of monoacylglycerols; surfactant and stabiliser: Tween® 80 and soy lecithin) for i.n. delivery to the CNS. The CRM-loaded NLCs (CRM-NLCs) had a mean size of 146.8 nm, a PDI of 0.18, an EE of 90.86% and a zeta potential of –21.4 mV. CRM-NLCs presented higher cytotoxicity against astrocytoma–glioblastoma cells (U373MG) than free CRM. Biodistribution studies in rats demonstrated that CRM-NLCs after i.n. administration enhance the concentration of CRM in brain and its nasal bioavailability.

Cryptococcus neoformans–mediated meningoencephalitis is a severe infection of the human CNS. The poor penetration of therapeutic agents across the BBB limits the efficiency of available treatments. Therefore, Du et al. [184] evaluated the potential of NLCs as nose-to-brain carriers for treating meningoencephalitis [184]. The authors used Miglyol® 812 (caprylic/capric triglycerides) as a liquid lipid, glyceryl behenate as a solid lipid and Tween® 80 and Solutol HS 15 (a permeability enhancer) as surfactant agents. Firstly, fluorescent-dye-loaded NLCs were prepared to investigate their uptake into the cytoplasm of *C. neoformans* cells. The results suggested that NLCs present excellent penetration ability into the thick capsule structure of *C. neoformans*. The authors also prepared ketoconazole (keto)-loaded NLCs with the following properties: average particle size of 102.1 ± 0.44 nm; PDI of 0.195 ± 0.005, indicating a homogeneous particle size distribution; average zeta potential of –2.1 ± 0.18 mV; EE of 70.4% ± 3.4%; and good stability over two weeks. In vitro studies revealed that keto-loaded NLCs had higher antifungal activity, with a cell inhibition rate fourfold higher than the free drug, even at low concentrations. Animal imaging analysis demonstrated that NLCs can enter brain tissues via the olfactory bulbs after i.n. administration, bypassing the BBB, as well as that the NLCs remained in tissue for longer periods. Moreover, i.n.-administrated keto-NLCs significantly inhibited cerebral *C. neoformans* colonisation and proliferation in mouse brain tissue when compared to free keto.

Despite i.n. administration being a useful tool for rapid transport of drugs to the brain, the low residence time in the nasal cavity because of mucocilliary clearance represents a constraint, resulting in incomplete drug absorption [185]. To prolong ONCs in the nasal cavity and improve drug absorption by the nasal mucosa, some authors proposed the development of mucoadhesive systems [186]. The mucoadhesive nanoparticles can perturb the microstructure of mucus, which increases the pore size of mucus up to 380–470 nm; thus larger-size particles can easily pass by the mucous membrane. Mucoadhesive nanoparticles can be achieved by coating the nanoparticles with mucoadhesive polymers or by using a composition which renders its surface with positive charges which will electrostatically bind to mucin negative charges. Herein we restrict our examples to lipid nanoparticles which are positively charged, as the polymeric coating of lipid nanoparticles produces hybrid polymeric lipid nanoparticles which are not a focus of this chapter. On the basis of these considerations, Gabal et al. [187] encapsulated the anti-Parkinson agent ropirinole in NLCs, with the aim to overpass the limitations in the uptake of this hydrophilic compound, and studied the influence of NLC surface charge on brain delivery through the i.n. route. The authors used Compritol 888® ATO as a solid lipid and Labrafac lipophile WL1394 (caprylic/capric triglycerides) as a liquid lipid. As mentioned before, the electrostatic attraction between cationic nanoparticles and negatively charged brain endothelial cells can increase their contact time and thus enhances the penetration of nanoparticles to the brain via AMT [188]. Previous studies also reported that in addition to cationic nanoparticles, anionic nanoparticles can also cross the BBB [189, 190]. Anionic and cationic NLCs with similar sizes (175 nm and 160 nm, respectively) and an absolute surface charge of +34 mV were successfully prepared [187]. In vivo toxicity assessment was performed on the nasal mucosa of rats and demonstrated that cationic NLCs caused severe injury and destruction of the lining epithelium, whereas mild inflammation, including inflammatory cell infiltration, was reported for anionic NLCs. However, the incorporation of aqueous dispersions of NLCs in Poloxamer 188 in situ gels resulted in no histopathological alterations in the treated animals, eliminating the adverse effects previously reported. Both anionic and cationic NLC gels increased ropirinole's absolute bioavailability (44% and 77.3%, respectively) compared to i.n. drug solution (7.4%). In addition, a higher accumulation in the brain was observed for the cationic NLCs. Likewise, Wavikar and Vavia [191] explored the potential of NLCs for nose-to-brain delivery of rivastigmine (RV), used in the treatment of AD, which was additionally enhanced by their incorporation into an in situ gelling system of gellan gum, extending the retention period in the nasal cavity. RV is a hydrophilic compound and is thus unable to overcome the BBB. NLCs were prepared using GMS (solid lipid), Capmul™ MCM (liquid lipid), lecithin and Tween® 80 (surfactants and stabilisers). NLCs had an average size of 123.2 ± 2.3 nm with an EE of 68.34% ± 3.4%. The in situ gel presented physical properties in terms of elasticity, rheology and mucoadhesion which allow its adhesion to the upper nasal mucosa, thus increasing the residence time in this region. In situ gelling RV-NLCs demonstrated a twofold enhancement in nasal permeation of the drug and superior enzyme inhibition efficacy (threefold increase) when compared to RV solution.

4.6.2 Polymeric Nanoparticles

Polymeric nanoparticles (Fig. 4.1) are solid colloidal particles with diameters ranging usually from 60 to 200 nm which are composed of a polymeric core matrix in which drugs can be embedded [7, 192]. Most popular polymers used in the composition of polymeric nanoparticles are synthetic or semisynthetic polymers, like PLA, poly(lactic-*co*-glycolic acid) (PLGA), polyanhydrides, polycyanoacrylates and PCL, and natural polymers, like chitosan [7]. In the case of polymeric nanoparticles, reports are also available describing enhanced drug delivery to the brain mediated by these ONCs. Table 4.2 shows a few examples of these reports.

Among these polymer nanoparticles, Kreuter et al. worked extensively on the use of polycyanoacrylate nanoparticles for BBB crossing [155, 193, 194]. However, these works have not been included in this chapter since their composition involves other components (e.g. non-ionic surfactants, phospholipids) other than polymeric compositions and should therefore be considered as hybrid nanoparticles.

4.7 Micro- and Nanoemulsions

Micro- and nanoemulsions are colloidal dispersion heterogeneous systems consisting of immiscible liquid phases, generally containing an aqueous phase and an oil phase, with one dispersed as droplets in the other, stabilised by surfactant agent(s). These systems can be considered as ONCs and can be classified into water-in-oil (w/o) or o/w, each designating the composition of the dispersed phase (droplets) within the continuous phase or bicontinuous systems depending on the concentration, nature and arrangement of the constituents [195]. Although in the literature, the terms 'nanoemulsion' and 'microemulsion' are often used indistinctly because of the similarity of the size range of droplets dispersed, these colloidal systems present differences related to their physical and physicochemical properties [195–197]. Microemulsions are defined as thermodynamically stable dispersions which are spontaneously (i.e. self-assembly) formed by mixing water and oil and stabilised by a surfactant(s) or a mixture of surfactant and co-surfactant agents.

The droplet sizes of microemulsions generally range from 10 to 100 nm, resulting in optically transparent (or translucent) dispersions [195, 196, 198]. Although these systems are formed by self-assembly at optimal component ratios and temperature, the application of an external low energy (e.g. heating or stirring) is frequently needed because of kinetic energy barriers or mass transport limitations [195, 198]. Nanoemulsions are also composed of an emulsified oil phase (e.g. triglycerides and soybean oil; vitamin E), an aqueous phase and adequate surface-active agents (surfactant and possibly co-surfactant) as stabilisation agents (e.g. egg phosphatidylcholine, lecithin and Tween® 80), wherein the inner phase (i.e. droplets dispersed) has a size in the nanometer scale [199] which can range from 20 to 500 nm [195, 200–202], taking into consideration optical properties and, often, the intended application [200]. Although nano- and microemulsions have similar components in their composition, a higher ratio of the surfactant-to-oil phase is usually needed to form a microemulsion. The main difference between a microemulsion and a nanoemulsion is based on thermodynamic stability [195]. Even though nanoemulsions are kinetically stable isotropic systems, these ONCs are non-equilibrium, thermodynamically unstable systems because of the positive free energy created in the interface between oil and aqueous phases, which requires a higher external energy input to generate a colloidal dispersion when compared to microemulsions [195, 203]. Nanoemulsions can be produced using diverse methods which can be broadly classified as either high-energy (e.g. high-pressure homogenisation, microfluidisation and ultrasonication) or low-energy (e.g. spontaneous emulsification, solvent displacement/diffusion and phase inversion temperature/point) emulsification approaches [202, 204]. Nanoemulsions are also more susceptible to undergo instability phenomena over time, such as coalescence, flocculation, Ostwald ripening and gravitational separation [195, 203]. The droplet size of a nanoemulsion can be controlled by both the preparation method and the formulation components (i.e. type of surfactants and oils, as well as concentration of surfactants). Figure 4.1 shows examples of o/w nanoemulsions and the self-double-emulsion drug delivery systems (SDEDDS), which can be w/o/w or o/o/w [2].

Nanoemulsions are used as promising ONCs to achieve brain targeting because of their outstanding properties, including [199, 205–207]:

- Use of safe ingredients such as edible oils and biocompatible surfactants (e.g. egg phosphatidylcholine, lecithin)
- Ability to increase solubilisation of lipophilic therapeutic agents
- Ability to improve drug transport and delivery due to the large interfacial area; ability to functionalise the surface for targeting delivery
- Easy manufacture and scale-up
- Improved stability of therapeutic agents, protecting them from degradation

As mentioned before, the i.n. route is being studied as a non-invasive, practical and effective route for administration of therapeutic agents directly into the brain, bypassing the BBB, which can be important to achieve therapeutic concentrations in the brain [208–210]. For example, Yadav et al. [210] proposed i.n. administration of cationic nanoemulsions carrying small interference RNA (siRNA) which silences the expression of TNF-α to protect against neuroinflammation, which is frequent in neurodegenerative conditions. TNF-α is a potent pro-inflammatory/pro-apoptotic tumoural cytokine which plays a crucial role in neuroinflammation cell death [211, 212]. The authors used the cationic lipid DOTAP, which is important for precondensing the negatively charged oligonucleotide and include it in the oil phase of the nanoemulsion. The nanoemulsion was formulated with flaxseed oil and an aqueous phase containing Lipoid® E80 and Tween® 80 as surfactants using the sonication method. The cationic nanoemulsions had sizes less than 400 nm. Qualitative and quantitative intracellular uptake studies revealed superior siRNA transfection of the nanoemulsion compared to Lipofectamine® (a commercially available cationic lipid transfection reagent). The optimised nanoemulsion caused the reduction of TNF-α levels in lipopolysaccharide (LPS)-stimulated macrophages. The i.n. administration in rats provided a higher brain uptake (almost 5 times) compared to non-encapsulated siRNA. In addition, the developed nanoemulsion significantly lowered the upregulated TNF-α levels in an LPS-induced animal model of neuroinflammation.

Many therapeutic agents are not effective to treat CNS diseases because of their low lipid solubility for BBB penetration. Docetaxel

(DTX), an inhibitor of microtubule depolymerisation, has been used for the treatment of many malignancies, including brain cancer [213]. DTX presents restricted clinical use which is explained by its poor aqueous solubility and nonspecific in vivo distribution, resulting in toxic effects [214, 215]. To overcome these limitations, Gaoe et al. [206] proposed the use of nanoemulsions to encapsulate DTX. The authors prepared nanoemulsions by the high-energy homogenisation method using soybean oil and egg lecithin and poloxamer 188 as surfactant agents. The mean droplet size of the nanoemulsion was 72.3 nm with a PDI of 0.19, the average zeta potential was −6.38 mV and the EE was 93.1%. In vitro toxicity tests demonstrated that the nanoemulsion had comparable antiproliferative effects in both U87MG cells and bEnd.3 cells. In vivo toxicity studies in healthy mice resulted in a slight change in the liver cells for the DTX-loaded nanoemulsion-treated group, whereas the administration of Taxotere® (commercial formulation) induced hydropic degeneration of liver cells. The main adjuvant used in Taxotere® is PS-80 which is associated with adverse effects such as peripheral neuropathy and acute hypersensitivity reaction [216]. In addition, nanoemulsions, i.v.-administered in mice, have been distributed to the brain, have accumulated at the glioma site and have been effective at targeting glioma sites and extending the median survival time of glioma mice.

Although the BBB prevents most substances from entering the brain, it presents special entry mechanisms, such as RMT, which can be used to target drug delivery [217]. A nanosystem coating with polysorbate, such as Tween® 80, has shown high potential to cross the BBB [218–220]. Prabhakar et al. [221] reported that the use of Tween® 80, a hydrophilic non-ionic surfactant, enhanced the uptake of nanoemulsions into the brain via the LDLR of brain endothelial cells. Furthermore, this surfactant inhibits the P-gp function, which promotes the drug to efflux from the CNS. Therefore, Harum et al. [222] proposed the use of nanoemulsions encapsulating cefuroxime (a cephalosporin antibiotic), aiming to enhance the permeation of the drug into the brain via passive diffusion after i.p. administration. Nanoemulsions were composed of an oil mixture (soybean oil, sunflower seed oil), Tween® 80 and lecithin as surfactants and were formulated using a high-pressure homogenisation technique. D-α-tocopherol (vitamin E) (1%) was used in the nanoemulsion composition to prevent the oxidation of the drug in the oil phase. To comply with the requirement of osmolarity for i.p. administration, glycerol (2.3%) was included. The nanoemulsion presented compatible parameters for i.p. administration with a droplet size of 100.32 ± 0.75 nm, a PDI of 0.18 ± 0.01, a zeta potential of −46.9 ± 1.39 mV, viscosity of 1.24 ± 0.34 cps and osmolality of 285.33 ± 0.58 mOsm/kg. These physicochemical parameters remained stable when the formulation was stored at 4°C for 6 months. On the basis of the EE value (~100%), the authors concluded that cefuroxime is completely encapsulated in the oil phase of the nanoemulsion. The nanoemulsion promoted sustained release of cefuroxime and improved the in vivo pharmacokinetic profile (i.e. enhanced the maximum concentration, prolonged $t_{1/2}$ and reduced clearance from both plasma and brain), demonstrating higher biodistribution of cefuroxime in the brain of the rats treated with the cefuroxime-loaded nanoemulsion when compared to cefuroxime-free-solution-treated rats.

As previously explained in Section 4.2.2, Lf, a single-chain mammalian cationic iron-binding glycoprotein, also has specific receptors at the BBB level (in the brain endothelial capillary cells, cerebral microvasculature and glial cells [223]), and the use of this ligand at the ONC surface makes them able to cross the BBB through RMT [224]. Therefore, Lf has been used as a targeting agent for enhanced brain penetration [225–227]. Indinavir (IDV), an antiretroviral protease inhibitor useful for controlling human immunodeficiency virus (HIV) infection, is a poorly aqueous-soluble compound and has restricted access to the brain because of efflux by P-gp frequently expressed at the BBB. Taking into consideration these facts, together with the potential of o/w nanoemulsions as ONCs for therapeutic agent delivery into the brain, Karami et al. [228] formulated IDV-loaded nanoemulsions using the high-speed homogenisation method and functionalised their surface with Lf to improve the IDV concentration in the brain. The nanoemulsion contained olive oil as the oil phase, oleic acid as a negative charge inducer, α-tocopherol as antioxidant agent, glycerol as an isotonicity agent and a mixture of surfactants (span 8 and PS-80). IDV-loaded nanoemulsions had spherical droplets with a size of 112 ± 3.5 nm, a PDI of 0.20 ± 0.02, a zeta potential of −33.2 ± 2.6 mV, a high EE (95.70% ± 3.6%), a viscosity of 3.392 ± 0.04 mPa·s and osmolality of 317.85 ± 1.91 mOsm/kg. The in vivo neuropharmacokinetic study performed in rats after i.p. administration demonstrated that the free IDV presents limited brain entry probably because of the effective function of P-gp. In addition, the concentration of IDV in the brain was higher (~fivefold) in the Lf-nanoemulsion-treated group compared to the free drug–treated group. The area under the curve of the brain concentration–time profile of the Lf-coated nanoemulsions group was superior (4.1-fold) than the free drug, and the brain uptake was much higher than the free drug. The authors explained these achievements by the effective targeting of Lf to the BBB, which has directed the drug to the brain and kept the drug inside the brain for a longer time.

4.8 Synthetic Organic Nanocarriers for Brain Drug Delivery

4.8.1 Dendrimers

Dendrimers are hyperbranched globular polymeric structures which resemble the structure of a tree [14, 229, 230]. In general, dendrimers are composed of a centric core (single atom or group of atoms), repeat structural units attached to the core and known as generations and surface functional groups which may have positive, negative or neutral charges (Fig. 4.1) [14, 229, 230].

Dendrimers are obtained by specific synthetic methods based on reaction sequences which enable precise control of molecular design parameters, resulting in highly monodisperse nanostructures, as opposed to the self-assembly systems described previously [14]. In addition, the structure of dendrimers confers flexibility to these ONCs for the loading of therapeutic compounds by either covalent conjugation or electrostatic adsorption on their surface. Furthermore, there are spaces ('cavities') in the branch-like dendrimer structures which can be used to store different types of molecules with hydrophobic, hydrophilic or amphiphilic properties [14, 230]. Despite these advantages of dendrimers as ONCs for drug delivery purposes, dendrimers also have limitations in their use which are related with their toxicity (Table 4.1). Toxicity of dendrimers depends on the generation of the dendrimer and the functional groups on the surface [14, 230]. For example, dendrimers with positively charged functional groups on their surface usually cause destabilisation of the anionic cell membrane or even cell lysis, resulting in low biocompatibility, while neutral or anionic dendrimers exhibit relatively less haemolysis [14, 230]. The same stealth strategy as for other ONCs is thus required to reduce the toxicity of dendrimers, that is, to coat their surface with biosafe polymers, such as PEG [14, 230].

Several types of dendrimers can be devised according to their composition: polyamidoamine (PAMAM) dendrimers; polypropyleneimine (PPI) dendrimers and poly-l-lysine (PLL) dendrimers (also called dendri-grafted poly-l-lysine, or DGL) [230]. Other dendrimer compositions are being developed for drug delivery, like phosphorus (PPH) dendrimers and carbosilane dendrimers [230], but because of their hybrid nature are out of this chapter's focus.

In terms of the delivery of drugs to the brain, dendrimers have several advantages. First, their synthesis is finely tuned, and their surface can be functionalised with a myriad of ligands which favour the BBB crossing [229, 230]. Then their hyperbranched nature provides a very good coverage of these ligands on the dendrimer surface, optimising cellular recognition. Also, their small size and monodisperse nature allow for better control of brain uptake. In addition, their cationic surface groups can be explored for conjugation with nucleic acids which turn dendrimers into promising ONCs for gene therapy [14]. Finally, the composition of dendrimers is also favourable in some brain diseases such as AD. For example, PAMAM dendrimers have been shown to be Aβ aggregation inhibitors by binding to Aβ peptides and have been able to remove existing toxic forms of aggregated proteins by accelerating the dissolution of fibrils [229]. At the same time, it was observed that the Aβ aggregation process can be modulated by PPI dendrimers if the sugar groups are attached to the surface [229].

A few examples illustrative of the use of dendrimers for brain drug delivery in different CNS diseases and gliomas are presented in Table 4.2.

Disease or application	Formulation designation	ONC composition	Targeting ligand (type of BBB transport)	Drug or therapeutic agent	Administration route and animal model	Main outcomes	Refs.
				Polymersomes			
Brain delivery	Tf-PO	PEG-PCL (AB)	Tf (RMT)	C6 (model compound)	i.v. in rats	• Tf-POs cellular uptake occurred mainly by clathrin-mediated energy-dependent endocytosis. • Tf-POs increased 2.8-fold BBB PS and 2.3-fold %ID/g brain as compared with those for POs without Tf.	[231]
AD	Tf/Tet-1-PO	PEG-PLGA (AB)	Tf Tet-1 (RMT)	Curcumin	i.v. in rats with cognitive dysfunction induced with Aβ	• Tf/Tet-1-POs had significant transportation properties and possessed affinity for neurons. • Tf/Tet-1-PO BBB PS was 0.28 mL/h/g and %ID/g was 0.08, significantly higher than controls. • Tf/Tet-1-POs provided neuroprotection and ameliorated cognitive dysfunction.	[232]

(*Continued*)

Table 4.2 (*Continued*)

Disease or application	Formulation designation	ONC composition	Targeting ligand (type of BBB transport)	Drug or therapeutic agent	Administration route and animal model	Main outcomes	Refs.
Neurodegenerative diseases (PD, AD)	Lf-PO	PEG-PLGA (AB)	Lf (RMT)	• C-6 (model compound) • S14G	i.v. in rats with cognitive dysfunction induced with Aβ	• Lf-POs were effectively transferred into the brain. • Lf-POs obtained the greatest BBB PS and %ID/g compared with Tf-POs and albumin-modified POs. • Lf-POs showed a neuroprotective effect against (i) learning and memory impairment induced by Aβ and (ii) overexpression of apoptotic proteins exhibiting neurofibrillary tangle pathology in neurons.	[233]

Disease or application	Formulation designation	ONC composition	Targeting ligand (type of BBB transport)	Drug or therapeutic agent	Administration route and animal model	Main outcomes	Refs.
Glioblastoma	ApoE-PO	PEG-P(TMC-DTC)-SP (ABC) PEG-P(TMC-DTC) (AB)	ApoE (RMT)	RGS	i.v. in mice xenografted with brain tumours	• ApoE-POs loaded with RGS markedly enhanced the G2/M cell cycle arrest and inhibitory effect in glioblastoma cells compared with the nontargeted PO-RGS and free RGS. • ApoE-POs inhibited tumour growth, prolonged survival time and depleted adverse effects.	[234]
Micelles							
Brain drug delivery	PM	PEG-PLA (AB)	Angiopep (RMT)	No drug	i.v. in mice	• PM showed high brain accumulation for up to 24 h.	[235]

(*Continued*)

Table 4.2 (*Continued*)

Disease or application	Formulation designation	ONC composition	Targeting ligand (type of BBB transport)	Drug or therapeutic agent	Administration route and animal model	Main outcomes	Refs.
Brain drug delivery	Tat-PM	PEG-PCL (AB)	Tat (AMT)	C-6 (model compound)	i.n. in mice xenografted with brain tumours	• Tat-PEG-PCL has shown higher C-6 brain distribution than PEG-PCL. • Tat-PEG-PCL has shown higher C-6 brain distribution by i.n. than i.v. • Tat-PEG-PCL has shown smaller of target distribution than C-6.	[236]
Brain gene delivery	TGN-PM/DNA Polyplexes	PEG-PDMAEMA (AB)	TGN (AMT)	pDNA	i.v. in mice	• TGN-PM/DNA polyplexes showed widespread brain expression of pDNA and higher transfection efficiency than PM/DNA polyplexes.	[237]

Disease or application	Formulation designation	ONC composition	Targeting ligand (type of BBB transport)	Drug or therapeutic agent	Administration route and animal model	Main outcomes	Refs.
Premature ejaculation	PM	PEG–PLGA (AB)	No ligand	DPX	Oral administration in rats	• PM loaded with DPX showed higher bioavailability and efficacy to cross the BBB and distribute in the brain compared with commercial DPX tablets.	[238]
Glioma	CD-PM	PEG-DOX* (AB)	CD (RMT)	DOX	i.v. in mice xenografted with brain tumours	• CD-PM induced the most significant antitumour activity with the longest media survival time in mice. • Biodistribution of CD-PM was 2.37-fold higher than that of the PM-treated group and was 24-fold higher than that of the nonloaded DOX-treated group.	[239]

(*Continued*)

Table 4.2 (*Continued*)

Disease or application	Formulation designation	ONC composition	Targeting ligand (type of BBB transport)	Drug or therapeutic agent	Administration route and animal model	Main outcomes	Refs.
Glioma Neuropro-tection	LM	GM1-DOX**	No ligand	DOX	i.v. in mice xenografted with brain tumours intracardiac injection in zebrafish	• LMs accumulated and distributed centrally in the brain as confirmed by zebrafish experiments. • LMs significantly prolonged the median survival of rats bearing glioma and had simultaneously a neuroprotective effect.	[240]
Polymeric Nanoparticles							
AD	PNP	PEGCA-HDCA (AB)	mAb anti-Aβ (RMT)	No drug	i.v. in AD-like transgenic mice	• PNP led to (i) complete correction of the memory defect, (ii) significant reduction of the Aβ-soluble peptide and its oligomer level in the brain and (iii) significant increase of the plasma Aβ levels.	[241]

Disease or application	Formulation designation	ONC composition	Targeting ligand (type of BBB transport)	Drug or therapeutic agent	Administration route and animal model	Main outcomes	Refs.
PD	Lf-PNP	PEG-PLGA (AB)	Lf (RMT)	Dopamine	i.n. in PD-induced rats	• i.n. administration of Lf-PNPs effectively alleviated the 6-hydroxydopamine-induced striatum lesion in rats. • In vivo distribution of Lf-PNPs in rat brain was significantly higher than that of PNPs.	[242]
LSD	PNP	PVA-PLGA (AB)	g7 (AMT)	Albumin (model for enzymes to be delivered for LSD therapy)	i.v. in MPS mice models	• PNPs crossed the BBB and delivered albumin into the brain of all injected mice, underlying the ability of NPs to deliver high-MW enzymes to the brain.	[243]

(*Continued*)

Table 4.2 (*Continued*)

Disease or application	Formulation designation	ONC composition	Targeting ligand (type of BBB transport)	Drug or therapeutic agent	Administration route and animal model	Main outcomes	Refs.
GBM	PNP	PVA-PLGA (AB)	No ligand	Bevacizumab	i.n. in mice xenografted with GBM	• PNPs demonstrated a reduction in tumour growth accompanied by a higher antiangiogenic effect compared to free bevacizumab. • Only PNPs (and not free bevacizumab) were found in the brain of mice after 14 days of formulation administration, with no systemic off-target toxicity.	[244]

Disease or application	Formulation designation	ONC composition	Targeting ligand (type of BBB transport)	Drug or therapeutic agent	Administration route and animal model	Main outcomes	Refs.
Dendrimers							
Brain delivery	Angiopep-Dd/DNA	G5 PAMAM-PEG	Angiopep (RMT)	pEGFP (reporter gene as model for gene therapy)	i.v. in mice	• Angiopep-Dd/DNA showed higher efficiency in crossing the BBB than unmodified Dd and was more accumulated in the brain, indicating that LRP1-mediated endocytosis may be the main mechanism of cellular internalisation of angiopep-Dd/DNA. • Angiopep-Dd/DNA also showed higher efficiency in gene expression in the brain than unmodified Dd.	[245]

(*Continued*)

Table 4.2 (*Continued*)

Disease or application	Formulation designation	ONC composition	Targeting ligand (type of BBB transport)	Drug or therapeutic agent	Administration route and animal model	Main outcomes	Refs.
PD	Angiopep-Dd/DNA	G3 DGL-PEG	Angiopep (RMT)	pDNA encoding hGDNF	i.v. in rats with induced lesions in nigrostriatal systems	• Angiopep-Dd/DNA exhibited higher cellular uptake and gene expression in brain cells compared to unmodified Dd. • The pharmacodynamic results showed that rats in the group with five injections of angiopep-Dd/DNA obtained best-improved locomotor activity and apparent recovery of dopaminergic neurons compared to those in other groups.	[246]

Disease or application	Formulation designation	ONC composition	Targeting ligand (type of BBB transport)	Drug or therapeutic agent	Administration route and animal model	Main outcomes	Refs.
CIR	Dd/siRNA	G4 PAMAM	No ligand	siRNA to silence the gene encoding for HMGB1	i.n. in post-ischaemic rats	• Dd/siRNA significantly knocked out the target gene in many brain regions, including the prefrontal cortex and *striatum*. • Dd/siRNA markedly suppressed infarct volume in the post-ischaemic rat brain (maximal reduction to 42.8% ± 5.6% 48 h after 60 min middle cerebral artery occlusion, and this protective effect was manifested by recoveries from neurological and behavioural deficits	[247]

(*Continued*)

Table 4.2 (*Continued*)

Disease or application	Formulation designation	ONC composition	Targeting ligand (type of BBB transport)	Drug or therapeutic agent	Administration route and animal model	Main outcomes	Refs.
Glioma	FA-BO-Dd	G5 PAMAM	FA (RMT) BO	DOX	i.v. in mice xenografted with brain tumours	• BO-Dd reduced the cytotoxicity of Dd, while efficiently boosting BBB permeability by twofold compared to naked Dd, while FA-BO-Dd improved BBB permeability by threefold. • FA-BO-Dd improved DOX accumulation in the brain tumour. The survival time and tumour growth inhibition were significantly increased compared to free DOX or other controls.	[248]

* and ** These formulations were not considered hybrid as they are solely constituted by polymeric (*) or glicolipidic (**) monomers, but the hydrophobic portion of the micelle is the drug encapsulated.

AB, diblock copolymer with hydrophilic (A) and hydrophobic (B) polymeric monomers; ABC, triblock copolymer with hydrophilic (A) and hydrophobic (B) and hydrophilic (C) polymeric monomers; Aβ, amyloid β peptide; AD, Alzheimer's disease; angiopep, 19-amino-acid peptide derived from the Kunitz domain which possesses a brain penetration capability by low-density lipoprotein receptor and its related protein (LRP-1), a receptor expressed in the central nervous system and overexpressed in glioblastomas; ApoE, apolipoprotein E; BBB, blood–brain barrier; BBB PS, blood–brain barrier permeability surface area product; BO, borneol, a drug from traditional Chinese medicine which facilitates BBB permeability and reduces the toxicity of naked cationic dendrimers; CD, choline derivate with dual BBB and glioma transporter affinities; Dd, dendrimer; DGL, dendri-grafted poly-l-lysine; DOX, doxorubicin; DPX, dapoxetine, a drug of choice for the specific treatment of premature ejaculation; FA, folic acid; G3, generation 3; G4, generation 4; G5, generation 5; g7, 7-amino-acid glycopeptide which uses clathrin and endocytic pathways to cross the BBB and reach neuronal cells; GBM, glioblastoma multiforme GM1, monosialoganglioside which can play neuroprotective and neurorestorative roles in neuronal injury; HDCA, hexadecyl cyanoacrylate; hGDNF, human glial cell line-derived neurotrophic factor; HMGB1, high-mobility group box 1 is a protein which is released by necrotic cells in acute damaging processes like post-ischaemic brain, inducing inflammation, microglia activation and apoptotic neuronal death; ID/g (%), brain percentage of injected dose per gram of brain; i.v., intravenous; Lf, lactoferrin; LMs, lipid micelles; LSD, lysosomal storage disorders, a group of about 50 metabolic diseases, mostly due to the deficit of lysosomal enzymes which generally cause a neurological impairment; mAb anti-Aβ, monoclonal antibodies against Aβ peptide; MPS, mucopolysaccharidoses, a subgroup of lysosomal storage disorders; MW, molecular weight; PAMAM, polyamidoamine; PCL, poly(caprolactone); PD, Parkinson's disease; PDMAEMA, poly(2-(dimethylamino) ethyl methacrylate; pDNA, DNA plasmide; PEG, polyethylene glycol; PEGCA, polyethylene glycol cyanoacrylate; pEGFP, DNA plasmide used as a reporter gene to express enhanced green fluorescent protein; PLA, polylactic acid; PLGA, poly(lactic-*co*-glycolic acid); PMs, polymeric micelles; PNPs, polymeric nanoparticles; POs, polymersomes; P(TMC-DTC), poly(trimethylene carbonate-co-dithiolane trimethylene carbonate; PVA, polyvinyl alcohol; RGS, rigosertib, a small-molecule inhibitor of the interactions of oncogene *RAS* and effector proteins. RGS actions lead to apoptosis of cancer cells; S14G is a variant shorter peptide of humanin (neuroprotective peptide), but its efficacy is 1000-fold greater than humanin; SP, spermine; Tat, 11-amino-acid peptide synthesised from human immunodeficiency virus Tat protein, functioning as a cell-penetrating peptide; Tet-1, 12-amino-acid peptide which possesses a high affinity for GT1B receptor on neurons; Tf, transferrin.

4.9 Biodegradation/Bioelimination of Organic Nanocarriers from the Brain

Although several types of INCs have been more thoroughly studied for their potential toxicity [249, 250], fewer studies have been conducted with ONCs, as these are considered to be composed of elements (carbon, hydrogen, oxygen) which are part of the chemical compounds existent in the body and therefore are regarded as biocompatible and possibly risk-free. Among the ONCs, less attention is paid to the toxicity issues which lipid-based ONCs may possess. This more relaxed view of the toxicity assessment is based on the argument that lipid-based formulations have been used for a long time. Lipid-based parenteral nutrition, for example, has been used clinically since the early 1960s. Moreover, liposomal formulations have dominated the clinical use of nanotherapy. In addition, all lipid ONC components for human use are GRAS [251].

It is true from a general point of view that lipid ONCs can be considered to have higher acceptability than INCs and other ONCs made of polymeric materials. It is also important to stress, however, that in addition to the well-tolerated lipid constituents, other components are often used in lipid-based ONC formulations. For example, SLNs and NLCs are composed of surfactants which must also be regarded as safe so that the entire system is considered to be biodegradable [251]. Another example of the influence of surfactants in biodegradation is when triglycerides with long-chain fatty acids and/or sterically impeding surfactants such as Poloxamer 407 or Poloxamine 908 are part of the SLN composition, biodegradation has shown to be slower. In contrast, lipid nanoparticles composed of short-chain fatty acid triglycerides and/or surfactants such as bile salts (e.g. cholic acid sodium salt) were degraded faster [252]. In addition, lipid-based ONC degradation products, like free fatty acids, should not be considered safe hazardous metabolites, especially in the brain. Indeed, neurons in specific brain regions (e.g. hypothalamus, hippocampus or striatum) are responsive to free fatty acids which can affect nervous activity [253]. It is therefore not hard to assume that local lipid ONC hydrolysis can also be involved in brain lipid sensing because of its free fatty acids which could act then in the sensitive neurons. Phospholipids can also be the products of lipid ONC degradation and exercise their function as precursors of inflammation which may cause neuronal damage [254]. In addition, lipid ONC degradation products, that is, free fatty acids and phospholipids, can both undergo further degradation pathways like lipid oxidation, resulting in increased levels of oxidative stress products which can lead to inflammation and neuron injury [255, 256]. In conclusion, despite lipids being considered GRAS components, the biodegradation of lipid ONCs and lipid by-products of such degradation must be cautiously investigated as they might be involved in inflammation or neuron modulation.

As a matter of fact, the biocompatibility of the components of ONCs is not a guarantee of lack of toxicity, as there are other factors besides composition which may cause toxic effects in ONCs, of which we are not aware. Such toxic effects depend not only on the composition of the ONC and its biodegradation and biocompatibility, but also on the size, shape, structure, solubility and aggregation of the ONC [7, 11]. Considering that the dimensions of ONCs are close to dimensions of the cells, it is understandable that unpredictable interactions may occur between ONCs and living cells and tissues [257]. Therefore, when determining the potential neurotoxicity of the ONC, it should be noted that beyond its core structure and composition, its size and surface functionality should also be regarded as being able to significantly alter the biological response and cause neurotoxicity of the otherwise safe ONC [7]. Another factor to be considered is the route of administration, since various risks are to be weighed. For instance, in i.v. administration of ONCs, their compatibility with blood cells, blood coagulation and platelet function should be evaluated [11]. Furthermore, it is worth mentioning that most of effective brain delivery ONC formulations still significantly accumulate in other major organs, such as the spleen, liver and kidneys, prior to elimination [6, 9]. Therefore, in addition to systemic toxicity, the potential neurotoxicity of off-targeted ONCs in healthy brains is a legitimate concern [6, 9]. Through any route of exposure, after crossing the BBB, ONCs tend to accumulate in specific brain regions, where they can access the neural cells, including neurons, astrocytes and microglia [257].

There ONCs can cause a direct change to the structure or activity of the neural system or can cause glial activations and glial–neuronal interactions with resultant neurotoxicity [257]. Many ONCs are therefore not readily removed by clearance mechanisms and may cause brain bioaccumulation leading to additional cytotoxicity, which makes it important to determine the biological fate of any ONCs developed for brain delivery purposes [258].

These recommendations are even more important in the context of ONCs for which the toxicity concerns are higher than those of lipid-based ONCs. Polymeric-based ONCs are one of such examples. Although authors claim that polymers like PLGA are biocompatible and biodegraded in organic acids (e.g. lactic and glycolic acids) with minimal toxicity, we can speculate the effect of these acidic by-products in the already acidic inflamed brain tissue. The long-term stability of polymeric ONCs also raises questions about their possible accumulation. Finally, some solvents used in some preparation processes as well as catalysts used in click chemistry functionalisation should be also evaluated regarding their toxicity, especially in a long-term administration context [112, 115, 116]. Dendrimers also raise significant toxicity concerns, which is why long-term safety issues and unforeseen drug release kinetics associated with dendrimers place restrictions on their use in the delivery of brain drugs [230]. Interplay between the surface cationic charge of dendritic molecules and the negative charge of erythrocyte membranes, known as haemolytic toxicity, has also been observed [230]. The systemic clearance of dendrimers, in addition to their possible neurotoxicity, restricts their use in drug delivery. Due to their tiny size, smaller dendrimers (G2–G4) can be removed quickly through renal filtration. On the other hand, the reticuloendothelial system is inclined to identify and eliminate larger dendrimers [230]. Although certain biodegradable dendrimers show significant superiority, most biodegradable dendrimers are polyester dendrimers, which may lead to the production of acid by-products which cause local inflammation [230]. Therefore, it is necessary to explore the synthesis and application of new biosafe dendrimers which should be preferably processed into nontoxic compounds which may be consumed by the biological system or excreted after therapeutic tasks have been completed [230].

Overall, it can be assumed that several factors have an impact on the biodegradation of ONCs, the rate of which depends on several factors, such as composition, particle size and surface decoration. New and more detailed studies dealing with the neurotoxic effects of several ONC classes on the function of the CNS are therefore mandatory.

4.10 Conclusions and Future Perspectives

ONCs offer great opportunities to deliver drugs and other therapeutic compounds to the brain. Besides providing a carrier system which can resolve most of the pharmacokinetic problems of drugs (e.g. low solubility and permeability), ONCs present better properties than their inorganic counterparts to match the physicochemical conditions encountered in the biological environment, thus constituting the best example of biocompatible NCs. Moreover, ONCs can achieve optimised BBB penetration and brain accumulation because of their stealth, targeting and triggering strategies. Accordingly, the benefits of ONCs in the brain delivery of drugs and other therapeutic agents have been clearly demonstrated by the impressive growth of research and novel applications. In this chapter we have attempted to cover a wide range of these applications, even though most of the advances and breakthroughs in ONC-based therapy have been dedicated to the treatment of glioma. The development of ONCs as an effective therapeutic strategy for AD, PD and CIR still requires further exploration to improve the pharmacokinetic and toxicological aspects so that clinical trials are carried out, as most of the investigations are currently conducted only in preclinical studies.

The lack of clinical trials and low academic-to-clinical translation is due to the many challenges which the development of ONCs still faces. One important challenge relates to the difficulty of fully describing the complex structural and dynamic processes which occur during the interaction of ONCs with biological interfaces. In this regard, a systematic study of the effect of very important parameters, such as surface density and chemistry and/or ONC size and topology, should be part of the development process. A thorough characterisation of these key factors in the design of ONCs is mostly overlooked, and ONCs are produced and almost immediately tested in vivo in animal models without first fully understanding the reasons for their unpredictable biological interactions and off-target accumulation. Related to this off-target distribution, another important challenge which merits further investment is the development of ONCs which can target specific brain cells, such as dopaminergic neurons (PD targets), microglia (neuroinflammation targets) or neural stem cells (neuronal repair targets). Investment in specific brain targets could increase the potential therapeutic value of ONCs. Additionally, there is also a challenge arising from the limitations imposed by animal models used to test the ONCs, which cannot fully mimic human disease. What is not toxic to animals can be toxic to humans, and vice versa. Another limitation is the time required to determine the neurotoxicity, clearance mechanism and long-term side effects of ONCs. A full assessment of ONC toxicity may take decades in humans. Finally, other challenges which need to be addressed are those related to the scalability of the ONC production processes as well as the reproducibility of those processes, which are often practical problems which may delay their clinical translation.

Despite the current scientific and regulatory challenges which ONCs still face before being applied to clinical brain delivery, the potential of these NCs with high BBB-crossing capacity is very promising in a medical field where an effective treatment spectrum is urgently needed. It is therefore anticipated that it will only be a matter of time until the ONCs developed in the preclinical studies described herein become a clinical reality to improve the quality of life of patients with brain diseases.

Acknowledgements

The authors acknowledge Fundação para a Ciência e Tecnologia (FCT) in the framework of the Strategic Funding [UIDB/04650/2020], and in the ambit of the project CONCERT [POCI-01-0145-FEDER-032651 and PTDC/NAN-MAT/326512017], co-financed by the European Regional Development Fund (ERDF), through COMPETE 2020, under Portugal 2020, and FCT I.P. M Lúcio thanks FCT and ERDF for a doctoral position [CTTI-150/18-CF (1)] in the ambit of the project CONCERT. Eduarda Fernandes is thankful for a doctoral grant (SFRH/BD/147938/2019).

References

1. Durães, F., Pinto, M., Sousa, E. (2018). Old drugs as new treatments for neurodegenerative diseases. *Pharmaceuticals (Basel)*, **11**(2), 44.
2. Soares, T. B., et al. (2018). Lipid nanocarriers loaded with natural compounds: potential new therapies for age related neurodegenerative diseases? *Prog. Neurobiol.*, **168**, 21–41.
3. Mendes, M., et al. (2018). Targeted theranostic nanoparticles for brain tumor treatment. *Pharmaceutics*, **10**(4), 181.
4. Pasha, S., Gupta, K. (2010). Various drug delivery approaches to the central nervous system. *Expert Opin. Drug Deliv.*, **7**(1), 113–135.
5. Reinhard, G. (2009). Blood-brain barrier transport of drugs for the treatment of brain diseases. *CNS Neurol. Disord. Drug Targets*, **8**(3), 195–204.
6. Saraiva, C., et al. (2016). Nanoparticle-mediated brain drug delivery: overcoming blood–brain barrier to treat neurodegenerative diseases. *J. Control. Release*, **235**, 34–47.
7. Masserini, M. (2013). Nanoparticles for brain drug delivery. *ISRN Biochem.*, **2013**, 18.
8. Saeedi, M., et al. (2019). Applications of nanotechnology in drug delivery to the central nervous system. *Biomed. Pharmacother.*, **111**, 666–675.
9. Tang, W., et al. (2019). Emerging blood–brain-barrier-crossing nanotechnology for brain cancer theranostics. *Chem. Soc. Rev.*, **48**(11), 2967–3014.
10. Teleanu, D. M., et al. (2018). Blood-brain delivery methods using nanotechnology. *Pharmaceutics*, **10**(4), 269.
11. Zottel, A., Videtič Paska, A., Jovčevska, I. (2019). Nanotechnology meets oncology: nanomaterials in brain cancer research, diagnosis and therapy. *Materials*, **12**(10), 1588.
12. Mitragotri, S., Stayton, P. (2014). Organic nanoparticles for drug delivery and imaging. *MRS Bull.*, **39**(3), 219–223.
13. D'Mello, S. R., et al. (2017). The evolving landscape of drug products containing nanomaterials in the United States. *Nat. Nanotechnol.*, **12**(6), 523–529.
14. Lombardo, D., Kiselev, M. A., Caccamo, M. T. (2019). Smart nanoparticles for drug delivery application: development of versatile nanocarrier platforms in biotechnology and nanomedicine. *J. Nanomater.*, **2019**, 26.

15. Viseu, T., et al. (2018). A systematic review and critical analysis of the role of graphene-based nanomaterials in cancer theranostics. *Pharmaceutics*, **10**(4), 282.

16. Pirzada, M., Altintas, Z. (2019). Nanomaterials for healthcare biosensing applications. *Sensors*, **19**(23), 5311.

17. Tian, P., et al. (2018). Graphene quantum dots from chemistry to applications. *Mater. Today Chem.*, **10**, 221–258.

18. Cherukula, K., et al. (2016). Multifunctional inorganic nanoparticles: recent progress in thermal therapy and imaging. *Nanomaterials (Basel)*, **6**(4), 76.

19. Colombeau, L., et al. (2016). Inorganic nanoparticles for photodynamic therapy, in *Light-Responsive Nanostructured Systems for Applications in Nanomedicine*, Sortino, S., ed., Springer International, Cham, pp. 113–134.

20. del Pino, P., Pelaz, B. (2012). Hyperthermia using inorganic nanoparticles, in *Frontiers of Nanoscience*, de la Fuente, J. M., Grazu, V., eds., Elsevier, pp. 309–335.

21. Kaur, P., et al. (2016). Hyperthermia using nanoparticles--promises and pitfalls. *Int. J. Hyperthermia*, **32**(1), 76–88.

22. Chang, D., et al. (2018). Biologically targeted magnetic hyperthermia: potential and limitations. *Front. Pharmacol.*, **9**(831).

23. Kreuter, J., Alyautdin, R. (2000). *Using Nanoparticles to Target Drugs to the Central Nervous System to the CNS*, Madcel Dekker.

24. Jo, D. H., et al. (2015). Size, surface charge, and shape determine therapeutic effects of nanoparticles on brain and retinal diseases. *Nanomedicine*, **11**(7), 1603–1611.

25. Kabanov, A. V., Gendelman, H. E. (2007). Nanomedicine in the diagnosis and therapy of neurodegenerative disorders. *Prog. Polym. Sci.*, **32**(8–9), 1054–1082.

26. Suk, J. S., et al. (2016). PEGylation as a strategy for improving nanoparticle-based drug and gene delivery. *Adv. Drug Deliv. Rev.*, **99**(Pt A), 28–51.

27. Wang, Z., et al. (2019). Nose-to-brain delivery. *J. Pharmacol. Exp. Ther.*, **370**(3), 593–601.

28. Hong, S.-S., et al. (2019). Liposomal formulations for nose-to-brain delivery: recent advances and future perspectives. *Pharmaceutics*, **11**(10), 540.

29. Pardeshi, C., Belgamwar, V. (2013). Direct nose to brain drug delivery via integrated nerve pathways bypassing the blood-brain barrier: an excellent platform for brain targeting. *Expert Opin. Drug Deliv.*, **10**, 957–972.

30. Kunjan, P., et al. (2016). Nanosized drug delivery systems for direct nose to brain targeting: a review. *Recent Pat. Drug Deliv. Formul.*, **10**(2), 156–164.

31. Dong, X. (2018). Current strategies for brain drug delivery. *Theranostics*, **8**(6), 1481–1493.

32. Sonvico, F., et al. (2018). Surface-modified nanocarriers for nose-to-brain delivery: from bioadhesion to targeting. *Pharmaceutics*, **10**(1), 34.

33. Erdő, F., et al. (2018). Evaluation of intranasal delivery route of drug administration for brain targeting. *Brain Res. Bull.*, **143**, 155–170.

34. Ganem, A., Quintanar, D., Buri, P. (2000). Monoolein: a review of the pharmaceutical applications. *Drug Dev. Ind. Pharm.*, **26**, 809–20.

35. Kararli, T. T., et al. (1992). Enhancement of nasal delivery of a renin inhibitor in the rat using emulsion formulations. *Pharm. Res.*, **9**(8), 1024–1028.

36. Hervé, F., Ghinea, N., Scherrmann, J.-M. (2008). CNS delivery via adsorptive transcytosis. *AAPS J.*, **10**(3), 455–472.

37. Kumagai, A. K., Eisenberg, J. B., Pardridge, W. M. (1987). Absorptive-mediated endocytosis of cationized albumin and a beta-endorphin-cationized albumin chimeric peptide by isolated brain capillaries. Model system of blood-brain barrier transport. *J. Biol. Chem.*, **262**(31), 15214–15219.

38. El-Andaloussi, S., Holm, T., Langel, U. (2005). Cell-penetrating peptides: mechanisms and applications. *Curr. Pharm. Des.*, **11**(28), 3597–3611.

39. Tripathi, P. P., et al. (2018). Cell penetrating peptides in preclinical and clinical cancer diagnosis and therapy. *Oncotarget*, **9**(98), 37252–37267.

40. Pooga, M., et al. (1998). Cell penetration by transportan. *FASEB J.*, **12**(1), 67–77.

41. Vivès, E., Brodin, P., Lebleu, B. (1997). A truncated HIV-1 tat protein basic domain rapidly translocates through the plasma membrane and accumulates in the cell nucleus. *J. Biol. Chem.*, **272**(25), 16010–16017.

42. Mäe, M., Langel, Ü. (2006). Cell-penetrating peptides as vectors for peptide, protein and oligonucleotide delivery. *Curr. Opin. Pharmacol.*, **6**(5), 509–514.

43. Xia, H., et al. (2012). Penetratin-functionalized PEG–PLA nanoparticles for brain drug delivery. *Int. J. Pharm.*, **436**(1), 840–850.

44. Boer, A. G. D., Gaillard, P. J. (2007). Drug targeting to the brain. *Annu. Rev. Pharmacol. Toxicol.*, **47**(1), 323–355.

45. Umezawa, F., Eto, Y. (1998). Liposome targeting to mouse brain: mannose as a recognition marker. Biochem. *Biophys. Res. Commun.*, **153**(3), 1038–1044.

46. Qin, Y., et al. (2010). In vitro and in vivo investigation of glucose-mediated brain-targeting liposomes. *J. Drug Targeting*, **18**(7), 536–549.

47. Du, D., et al. (2014). The role of glucose transporters in the distribution of p-aminophenyl-α-d-mannopyranoside modified liposomes within mice brain. *J. Control. Release*, **182**, 99–110.

48. Kobayashi, K., et al. (2008). Enhanced tumor growth elicited by L-type amino acid transporter 1 in human malignant glioma cells. *Neurosurgery*, **62**(2), 493–504.

49. Barar, J., et al. (2016). Blood-brain barrier transport machineries and targeted therapy of brain diseases. *BioImpacts*, **6**(4), 225–248.

50. Smith, Q. R. (2000). Transport of glutamate and other amino acids at the blood-brain barrier. *J. Nutr.*, **130**(4), 1016S–1022S.

51. Hawkins, R. A., et al. (2006). Structure of the blood–brain barrier and its role in the transport of amino acids. *J. Nutr.*, **136**(1), 218S–226S.

52. Fenart, L., et al. (1999). Evaluation of effect of charge and lipid coating on ability of 60-nm nanoparticles to cross an in vitro model of the blood-brain barrier. *J. Pharmacol. Exp. Ther.*, **291**(3), 1017–1022.

53. Romano, A., et al. (2017). Fats for thoughts: an update on brain fatty acid metabolism. *Int. J. Biochem. Cell Biol.*, **84**, 40–45.

54. Strickland, M., Stoll, E. A. (2017). Metabolic reprogramming in glioma. *Front. Cell Dev. Biol.*, **5**, 43–43.

55. Guo, D., Bell, E. H., Chakravarti, A. (2013). Lipid metabolism emerges as a promising target for malignant glioma therapy. *CNS Oncol.*, **2**(3), 289–299.

56. Miriam, M.-A., Casado, F. J., Marcal, P.-A. (2009). Nucleoside transporter proteins. *Curr. Vasc. Pharmacol.*, **7**(4), 426–434.

57. Lombardo, D., et al. (2015). Amphiphiles self-assembly: basic concepts and future perspectives of supramolecular approaches. *Adv. Condens. Matter Phys.*, **2015**, 22.

58. Ganesan, P., Narayanasamy, D. (2017). Lipid nanoparticles: different preparation techniques, characterization, hurdles, and strategies for the production of solid lipid nanoparticles and nanostructured lipid carriers for oral drug delivery. *Sustainable Chem. Pharm.*, **6**, 37–56.

59. Patravale, V. B., Upadhaya, P. G., Jain, R. D. (2019). Preparation and characterization of micelles, in *Pharmaceutical Nanotechnology: Basic Protocols*, Weissig, V., Elbayoumi, T., eds., Springer New York, New York, pp. 19–29.

60. Akbarzadeh, A., et al. (2013). Liposome: classification, preparation, and applications. *Nanoscale Res. Lett.*, **8**(1), 102–102.

61. Rao, J. P., Geckeler, K. E. (2011). Polymer nanoparticles: preparation techniques and size-control parameters. *Prog. Polym. Sci.*, **36**(7), 887–913.

62. Has, C., Sunthar, P. (2019). A comprehensive review on recent preparation techniques of liposomes. *J. Liposome Res.*, 1–30.

63. Teixeira, I., et al. (2020). Current insights on lipid nanocarrier-assisted drug delivery in the treatment of neurodegenerative diseases. *Eur. J. Pharm. Biopharm.*, **149**, 192–217.

64. Lopes, C. M., et al. (2018). Lipid-based colloidal carriers for topical application of antiviral drugs, in *Design of Nanostructures for Versatile Therapeutic Applications*, Grumezescu, A. M., ed., William Andrew Publishing, pp. 565–622.

65. Lucio, M., Lima, J. L., Reis, S. (2010). Drug-membrane interactions: significance for medicinal chemistry. *Curr. Med. Chem.*, **17**(17), 1795–809.

66. Allen, T. M., Cullis, P. R. (2013). Liposomal drug delivery systems: from concept to clinical applications. *Adv. Drug Deliv. Rev.*, **65**(1), 36–48.

67. Parmentier, J., et al. (2012). Exploring the fate of liposomes in the intestine by dynamic in vitro lipolysis. *Int. J. Pharm.*, **437**(1), 253–263.

68. He, H., et al. (2019). Adapting liposomes for oral drug delivery. *Acta Pharm. Sin. B*, **9**(1), 36–48.

69. Liu, R. R., Cannon, J. B., Paspal, S. Y. L. (2018). Liposomes in solubilization, in *Water-Insoluble Drug Formulation*, Liu, R., ed., CRC Press, Boca Raton, USA.

70. Nagle, J. F., Tristram-Nagle, S. (2000). Structure of lipid bilayers. *Biochim. Biophys. Acta*, **1469**(3), 159–195.

71. Hafez, I. M., Cullis, P. R. (2001). Roles of lipid polymorphism in intracellular delivery. *Adv. Drug Deliv. Rev.*, **47**(2), 139–148.

72. Wang, H., et al. (2014). Brain temperature and its fundamental properties: a review for clinical neuroscientists. *Front. Neurosci.*, **8**, 307.

73. Thrall, D. E., et al. (1986). Temperature measurements in normal and tumor tissue of dogs undergoing whole body hyperthermia. *Cancer Res.*, **46**(12 Part 1), 6229–6235.

74. Sowers, J. L., et al. (2014). The role of inflammation in brain cancer, in *Inflammation and Cancer*, Aggarwal, B. B., Sung, B., Gupta, S. C., eds., Springer Basel, Basel. pp. 75–105.

75. Joshi, S., et al. (2014). Transient cerebral hypoperfusion assisted intraarterial cationic liposome delivery to brain tissue. *J. Neuro-Oncol.*, **118**(1), 73–82.

76. Joshi, S., et al. (2014). Cationic surface charge enhances early regional deposition of liposomes after intracarotid injection. *J. Neuro-Oncol.*, **120**(3), 489–497.

77. Ana, C. N. O., et al. (2019). Lipid-based nanocarriers for siRNA delivery: challenges, strategies and the lessons learned from the DODAX: MO liposomal system. *Curr. Drug Targets*, **20**(1), 29–50.

78. Oliveira, A. C. N., et al. (2016). Role of counter-ion and helper lipid content in the design and properties of nanocarrier systems: a biophysical study in 2D and 3D lipid assemblies. *RSC Adv.*, **6**(53), 47730–47740.

79. Silva, J. P. N., et al. (2014). Structural dynamics and physicochemical properties of pDNA/DODAB:MO lipoplexes: effect of pH and anionic lipids in inverted non-lamellar phases versus lamellar phases. *Biochim. Biophys. Acta, Biomembr.*, **1838**(10), 2555–2567.

80. Girão da Cruz, M. T., Simões, S., Pedroso de Lima, M. C. (2004). Improving lipoplex-mediated gene transfer into C6 glioma cells and primary neurons. *Exp. Neurol.*, **187**(1), 65–75.

81. Yang, L., Rongqin, H., Chen, J. (2011). Non-viral gene delivery and therapeutics targeting to brain. *Curr. Nanosci.*, **7**(1), 55–70.

82. Bulbake, U., et al. (2017). Liposomal formulations in clinical use: an updated review. *Pharmaceutics*, **9**(2), 12.

83. Vieira, D. B., Gamarra, L. F. (2016). Getting into the brain: liposome-based strategies for effective drug delivery across the blood-brain barrier. *Int. J. Nanomed.*, **11**, 5381–5414.

84. Bana, L., et al. (2014). Liposomes bi-functionalized with phosphatidic acid and an ApoE-derived peptide affect Aβ aggregation features and

cross the blood–brain-barrier: implications for therapy of Alzheimer disease. *Nanomed. Nanotechnol. Biol. Med.*, **10**(7), 1583–1590.

85. Balducci, C., et al. (2014). Multifunctional liposomes reduce brain β-amyloid burden and ameliorate memory impairment in Alzheimer's disease mouse models. *J. Neurosci.*, **34**(42), 14022–14031.

86. Puglielli, L., Tanzi, R. E., Kovacs, D. M. (2003). Alzheimer's disease: the cholesterol connection. *Nat. Neurosci.*, **6**(4), 345–351.

87. Palop, J. J., Mucke, L. (2010). Amyloid-β–induced neuronal dysfunction in Alzheimer's disease: from synapses toward neural networks. *Nat. Neurosci.*, **13**(7), 812–818.

88. Olubiyi, O., Strodel, B. (2012). Structures of the amyloid beta-peptides A beta(1-40) and A beta(1-42) as influenced by pH and a D-peptide. *J. Phys. Chem. B*, **116**, 3280–3291.

89. Wei, Y., et al. (2014). Preparation, pharmacokinetics and biodistribution of baicalin-loaded liposomes. *Int. J. Nanomed.*, **9**, 3623–3630.

90. Ye, Y., Xing, H., Li, Y. (2014). Nanoencapsulation of the sasanquasaponin from Camellia oleifera, its photo responsiveness and neuroprotective effects. *Int. J. Nanomed.*, **9**, 4475–4484.

91. Kastner, A., et al. (1993). Tyrosine hydroxylase protein and messenger RNA in the dopaminergic nigral neurons of patients with Parkinson's disease. *Brain Res.*, **606**(2), 341–345.

92. Lazar, A. N., et al. (2013). Curcumin-conjugated nanoliposomes with high affinity for Aβ deposits: possible applications to Alzheimer disease. *Nanomed. Nanotechnol. Biol. Med.*, **9**(5), 712–721.

93. Phachonpai, W. (2010). Neuroprotective effect of quercetin encapsulated liposomes: a novel therapeutic strategy against Alzheimer's disease. *Am. J. Appl. Sci.*, **7**, 480–485.

94. Tong-Un, T., et al. (2010). Nasal administration of quercetin liposomes modulate cognitive impairment and inhibit acetylcholinesterase activity in hippocampus. *Neurosci. Int.*, **1**(1), 21–27.

95. Yurasov, V. V., et al. (1996). Effects ofl-dopa-carrying liposomes on striatal concentration of dopamine and its metabolites and phospholipid metabolism in experimental Parkinson's syndrome. *Bull. Exp. Biol. Med.*, **122**(6), 1180–1183.

96. Yurasov, V. V., et al. (1997). Effect of long-term parenteral administration of empty and L-Dopa-loaded liposomes on the turnover of dopamine and its metabolites in the striatum of mice with experimental Parkinson's syndrome. *Bull. Exp. Biol. Med.*, **123**(2), 126–129.

97. Oo, T. F., Kholodilov, N., Burke, R. E. (2003). Regulation of natural cell death in dopaminergic neurons of the substantia nigra by striatal glial cell line-derived neurotrophic factor in vivo. *J. Neurosci.*, **23**(12), 5141–5148.

98. Migliore, M. M., et al. (2014). Neurotrophic and neuroprotective efficacy of intranasal GDNF in a rat model of Parkinson's disease. *Neuroscience*, **274**, 11–23.

99. Wang, Y., et al. (2011). Protective effect of resveratrol derived from Polygonum cuspidatum and its liposomal form on nigral cells in Parkinsonian rats. *J. Neurol. Sci.*, **304**(1), 29–34.

100. Adibhatla, R. M., Hatcher, J. F., Tureyen, K. (2005). CDP-choline liposomes provide significant reduction in infarction over free CDP-choline in stroke. *Brain Res.*, **1058**(1–2), 193–197.

101. Sarkar, S., Das, N. (2006). Mannosylated liposomal flavonoid in combating age-related ischemia–reperfusion induced oxidative damage in rat brain. *Mech. Ageing Dev.*, **127**(4), 391–397.

102. Zhao, G., et al. (2011). Postischemic administration of liposome-encapsulated luteolin prevents against ischemia-reperfusion injury in a rat middle cerebral artery occlusion model. *J. Nutr. Biochem.*, **22**(10), 929–936.

103. Chen, H., et al. (2010). Lactoferrin-modified procationic liposomes as a novel drug carrier for brain delivery. *Eur. J. Pharm. Sci.*, **40**(2), 94–102.

104. Joshi, S., et al. (2015). Cerebral hypoperfusion-assisted intra-arterial deposition of liposomes in normal and glioma-bearing rats. *Neurosurgery*, **76**(1), 92–100.

105. Aryal, M., et al. (2015). Enhancement in blood-tumor barrier permeability and delivery of liposomal doxorubicin using focused ultrasound and microbubbles: evaluation during tumor progression in a rat glioma model. *Phys. Med. Biol.*, **60**(6), 2511–2527.

106. Lin, Q., et al. (2016). Brain tumor-targeted delivery and therapy by focused ultrasound introduced doxorubicin-loaded cationic liposomes. *Cancer Chemother. Pharmacol.*, **77**(2), 269–280.

107. Zhang, H., et al. (2007). Plasmid encoding matrix protein of vesicular stomatitis viruses as an antitumor agent inhibiting rat glioma growth in situ. *Exp. Oncol.*, **29**, 85–93.

108. Abdulbaqi, I. M., et al. (2016). Ethosomal nanocarriers: the impact of constituents and formulation techniques on ethosomal properties, in vivo studies, and clinical trials. *Int. J. Nanomed.*, **11**, 2279–2304.

109. Shi, J., Wang, Y., Luo, G. (2012). Ligustrazine phosphate ethosomes for treatment of Alzheimer's disease, in vitro and in animal model studies. *AAPS PharmSciTech*, **13**(2), 485–492.

110. Walker, J. M., et al. (2015). Beneficial effects of dietary EGCG and voluntary exercise on behavior in an Alzheimer's disease mouse model. *J. Alzheimers Dis.*, **44**(2), 561–572.

111. Huang, Y.-B., et al. (2011). Elastic liposomes as carriers for oral delivery and the brain distribution of (+)-catechin. *J. Drug Targeting*, **19**(8), 709–718.

112. Zhang, X.-y., Zhang, P.-y. (2017). Polymersomes in nanomedicine: a review. *Curr. Med. Chem.*, **13**(2), 124–129.

113. Jay Prakash, J., Wubeante Yenet, A., Neeraj, K. (2011). Self assembling polymers as polymersomes for drug delivery. *Curr. Pharm. Des.*, **17**(1), 65–79.

114. Rideau, E., et al. (2018). Liposomes and polymersomes: a comparative review towards cell mimicking. *Chem. Soc. Rev.*, **47**(23), 8572–8610.

115. Anajafi, T., Mallik, S. (2015). Polymersome-based drug-delivery strategies for cancer therapeutics. *Ther. Deliv.*, **6**(4), 521–534.

116. Pawar, P. V., et al. (2013). Functionalized polymersomes for biomedical applications. *Polym. Chem.*, **4**(11), 3160–3176.

117. Costantino, L., Boraschi, D. (2012). Is there a clinical future for polymeric nanoparticles as brain-targeting drug delivery agents? *Drug Discov. Today*, **17**(7–8), 367–378.

118. Müller, R. H., Radtke, M., Wissing, S. A. (2002). Solid lipid nanoparticles (SLN) and nanostructured lipid carriers (NLC) in cosmetic and dermatological preparations. *Adv. Drug Deliv. Rev.*, **54**, S131–S155.

119. Shen, H., et al. (2015). Coating solid lipid nanoparticles with hyaluronic acid enhances antitumor activity against melanoma stem-like cells. *Theranostics*, **5**(7), 755–771.

120. Teleanu, D. M., et al. (2019). Neuronanomedicine: an up-to-date overview. *Pharmaceutics*, **11**(3), 101.

121. Patel, M., Souto, E. B., Singh, K. K. (2013). Advances in brain drug targeting and delivery: limitations and challenges of solid lipid nanoparticles. *Expert Opin. Drug Deliv.*, **10**(7), 889–905.

122. Lockman, P. R., et al. (2003). Brain uptake of thiamine-coated nanoparticles. *J. Control. Release*, **93**(3), 271–282.

123. Wang, J.-X., Sun, X., Zhang, Z.-R. (2002). Enhanced brain targeting by synthesis of 3′,5′-dioctanoyl-5-fluoro-2′-deoxyuridine and

incorporation into solid lipid nanoparticles. *Eur. J. Pharm. Biopharm.*, **54**(3), 285–290.

124. Kreuter, J. (2001). Nanoparticulate systems for brain delivery of drugs. *Adv. Drug Deliv. Rev.*, **47**(1), 65–81.

125. Kaur, I. P., et al. (2008). Potential of solid lipid nanoparticles in brain targeting. *J. Control. Release*, **127**(2), 97–109.

126. Tapeinos, C., Battaglini, M., Ciofani, G. (2017). Advances in the design of solid lipid nanoparticles and nanostructured lipid carriers for targeting brain diseases. *J. Control. Release*, **264**, 306–332.

127. Shrestha, H., Bala, R., Arora, S. (2014). Lipid-based drug delivery systems. *J. Pharm. (Cairo)*, **2014**, 801820.

128. Mittal, R., et al. (2018). Recent advancements in nanoparticle based drug delivery for gastrointestinal disorders. *Expert Opin. Drug Deliv.*, **15**(3), 301–318.

129. Müller, R., et al. (1996). Phagocytic uptake and cytotoxicity of solid lipid nanoparticles (SLN) sterically stabilized with poloxamine 908 and poloxamer 407. *J. Drug Targeting*, **4**(3), 161–170.

130. Blasi, P., et al. (2013). Lipid nanoparticles for brain targeting III. Long-term stability and in vivo toxicity. *Int. J. Pharm.*, **454**(1), 316–323.

131. Pardridge, W. M. (2009). Alzheimer's disease drug development and the problem of the blood-brain barrier. *Alzheimers Dement.*, **5**(5), 427–432.

132. Bondì, M. L., et al. (2010). Brain-targeted solid lipid nanoparticles containing riluzole: preparation, characterization and biodistribution. *Nanomedicine (London)*, **5**(1), 25–32.

133. Miller, R. G., Mitchell, J. D., Moore, D. H. (2012). Riluzole for amyotrophic lateral sclerosis (ALS)/motor neuron disease (MND). *Cochrane Database Syst. Rev.*, (3), CD001447.

134. Misra, S., et al. (2016). Galantamine-loaded solid-lipid nanoparticles for enhanced brain delivery: preparation, characterization, in vitro and in vivo evaluations. *Drug Deliv.*, **23**(4), 1434–1443.

135. Wilcock, G. K., Lilienfeld, S., Gaens, E. (2000). Efficacy and safety of galantamine in patients with mild to moderate Alzheimer's disease: multicentre randomised controlled trial. Galantamine International-1 Study Group. *BMJ*, **321**(7274), 1445–1449.

136. Raskind, M. A., et al. (2000). Galantamine in AD: a 6-month randomized, placebo-controlled trial with a 6-month extension. The Galantamine USA-1 Study Group. *Neurology*, **54**(12), 2261–2268.

137. Yanagida, T., et al. (2008). Synergistic effect of galantamine on nicotine-induced neuroprotection in hemiparkinsonian rat model. *Neurosci. Res.*, **62**(4), 254–261.

138. Hernandez, C. M., et al. (2010). Loss of α7 nicotinic receptors enhances β-amyloid oligomer accumulation, exacerbating early-stage cognitive decline and septohippocampal pathology in a mouse model of Alzheimer's disease. *J. Neurosci.*, **30**(7), 2442–2453.

139. Natarajan, J., et al. (2017). Enhanced brain targeting efficacy of Olanzapine through solid lipid nanoparticles. *Artif. Cells Nanomed. Biotechnol.*, **45**(2), 364–371.

140. Yu, X., et al. (2016). Design of nanoparticle-based carriers for targeted drug delivery. *J. Nanomater.*, **2016**, 1087250.

141. Kuo, Y.-C., Wang, I. H. (2016). Enhanced delivery of etoposide across the blood-brain barrier to restrain brain tumor growth using melanotransferrin antibody- and tamoxifen-conjugated solid lipid nanoparticles. *J. Drug Targeting*, **24**(7), 645–654.

142. Rothenberger, S., et al. (1996). Coincident expression and distribution of melanotransferrin and transferrin receptor in human brain capillary endothelium. *Brain Res.*, **712**(1), 117–121.

143. Choi, Y. K., Kim, K. W. (2008). Blood-neural barrier: its diversity and coordinated cell-to-cell communication. *BMB Rep.*, **41**(5), 345–352.

144. Wong, H. L., et al. (2010). Nanotechnology applications for improved delivery of antiretroviral drugs to the brain. *Adv. Drug Deliv. Rev.*, **62**(4), 503–517.

145. Kayyali, R., Marriott, C., Wiseman, H. (1994). Tamoxifen decreases drug efflux from liposomes: relevance to its ability to reverse multidrug resistance in cancer cells? *FEBS Lett.*, **344**(2), 221–224.

146. Thöle, M., et al. (2002). Uptake of cationzied albumin coupled liposomes by cultured porcine brain microvessel endothelial cells and intact brain capillaries. *J. Drug Targeting*, **10**(4), 337–344.

147. Xie, Y.-L., Lu, W., Jiang, X.-G. (2006). Improvement of cationic albumin conjugated pegylated nanoparticles holding NC-1900, a vasopressin fragment analog, in memory deficits induced by scopolamine in mice. *Behav. Brain Res.*, **173**(1), 76–84.

148. Agarwal, A., et al. (2011). Cationic ligand appended nanoconstructs: a prospective strategy for brain targeting. *Int. J. Pharm.*, **421**(1), 189–201.

149. Lu, W., et al. (2005). Cationic albumin conjugated pegylated nanoparticle with its transcytosis ability and little toxicity against blood–brain barrier. *Int. J. Pharm.*, **295**(1), 247–260.

150. Lu, W., et al. (2006). Cationic albumin-conjugated pegylated nanoparticles allow gene delivery into brain tumors via intravenous administration. *Cancer Res.*, **66**(24), 11878–11887.

151. Yusuf, M., et al. (2013). Preparation, characterization, in vivo and biochemical evaluation of brain targeted Piperine solid lipid nanoparticles in an experimentally induced Alzheimer's disease model. *J. Drug Targeting*, **21**(3), 300–311.

152. Bhat, B. G., Chandrasekhara, N. (1986). Studies on the metabolism of piperine: absorption, tissue distribution and excretion of urinary conjugates in rats. *Toxicology*, **40**(1), 83–92.

153. Hashimoto, K., et al. (1996). Photochemical isomerization of piperine, a pungent constituent in pepper. *Food Sci. Technol. Int.*, **2**(1), 24–29.

154. Kreuter, J. (2004). Influence of the surface properties on nanoparticle-mediated transport of drugs to the brain. *J. Nanosci. Nanotechnol.*, **4**(5), 484–488.

155. Kreuter, J., et al. (2002). Apolipoprotein-mediated transport of nanoparticle-bound drugs across the blood-brain barrier. *J. Drug Targeting*, **10**(4), 317–325.

156. Cornaire, G., et al. (2004). Impact of excipients on the absorption of P-glycoprotein substrates in vitro and in vivo. *Int. J. Pharm.*, **278**(1), 119–131.

157. Hanke, U., et al. (2010). Commonly used nonionic surfactants interact differently with the human efflux transporters ABCB1 (p-glycoprotein) and ABCC2 (MRP2). *Eur. J. Pharm. Biopharm.*, **76**(2), 260–268.

158. Wagner, S., et al. (2012). Uptake mechanism of ApoE-modified nanoparticles on brain capillary endothelial cells as a blood-brain barrier model. *PLoS One*, **7**(3), e32568.

159. Gao, K., Jiang, X. (2006). Influence of particle size on transport of methotrexate across blood brain barrier by polysorbate 80-coated polybutylcyanoacrylate nanoparticles. *Int. J. Pharm.*, **310**(1), 213–219.

160. Wang, C.-X., et al. (2009). Antitumor effects of polysorbate-80 coated gemcitabine polybutylcyanoacrylate nanoparticles in vitro and its pharmacodynamics in vivo on C6 glioma cells of a brain tumor model. *Brain Res.*, **1261**, 91–99.

161. Tian, X.-H., et al. (2011). Enhanced brain targeting of temozolomide in polysorbate-80 coated polybutylcyanoacrylate nanoparticles. *Int. J. Nanomed.*, **6**, 445–452.

162. Martins, S. M., et al. (2013). Brain targeting effect of camptothecin-loaded solid lipid nanoparticles in rat after intravenous administration. *Eur. J. Pharm. Biopharm.*, **85**(3, Part A), 488–502.

163. Çırpanlı, Y., et al. (2011). Antitumoral activity of camptothecin-loaded nanoparticles in 9L rat glioma model. *Int. J. Pharm.*, **403**(1), 201–206.

164. Rivory, L. P., Robert, J. (1995). Molecular, cellular, and clinical aspects of the pharmacology of 20(S)camptothecin and its derivatives. *Pharmacol. Ther.*, **68**(2), 269–296.

165. Giovanella, B. C., et al. (2000). Dependence of anticancer activity of camptothecins on maintaining their lactone function. *Ann. N. Y. Acad. Sci.*, **922**(1), 27–35.

166. Estella-Hermoso de Mendoza, A., et al. (2011). In vitro and in vivo efficacy of edelfosine-loaded lipid nanoparticles against glioma. *J. Control. Release*, **156**(3), 421–426.

167. Dhuria, S. V., Hanson, L. R., Frey, W. H. (2010). Intranasal delivery to the central nervous system: mechanisms and experimental considerations. *J. Pharm. Sci.*, **99**(4), 1654–1673.

168. Garcia-Garcia, E., et al. (2005). Colloidal carriers and blood–brain barrier (BBB) translocation: a way to deliver drugs to the brain? *Int. J. Pharm.*, **298**(2), 274–292.

169. Illum, L. (2000). Transport of drugs from the nasal cavity to the central nervous system. *Eur. J. Pharm. Sci.*, **11**(1), 1–18.

170. Patel, S., et al. (2011). Brain targeting of risperidone-loaded solid lipid nanoparticles by intranasal route. *J. Drug Targeting*, **19**(6), 468–474.

171. Wang, J.-S., et al. (2004). The brain entry of risperidone and 9-hydroxyrisperidone is greatly limited by P-glycoprotein. *Int. J. Neuropsychopharmacol.*, **7**(4), 415–419.

172. Müller, R. H., Radtke, M., Wissing, S. A. (2002). Nanostructured lipid matrices for improved microencapsulation of drugs. *Int. J. Pharm.*, **242**(1), 121–128.

173. Kumar, P., et al. (2016). Promises of a biocompatible nanocarrier in improved brain delivery of quercetin: biochemical, pharmacokinetic and biodistribution evidences. *Int. J. Pharm.*, **515**(1), 307–314.

174. Manach, C., et al. (1997). Bioavailability of rutin and quercetin in rats. *FEBS Lett.*, **409**(1), 12–16.

175. Eskandari, S., et al. (2011). Brain delivery of valproic acid via intranasal administration of nanostructured lipid carriers: in vivo pharmacodynamic studies using rat electroshock model. *Int. J. Nanomed.*, **6**, 363–371.

176. Stapleton, S. L., et al. (2008). Plasma and cerebrospinal fluid pharmacokinetics of valproic acid after oral administration in non-human primates. *Cancer Chemother. Pharmacol.*, **61**(4), 647–652.

177. Scism, J. L., et al. (2000). Probenecid-inhibitable efflux transport of valproic acid in the brain parenchymal cells of rabbits: a microdialysis study. *Brain Res.*, **884**(1), 77–86.

178. Alam, T., et al. (2015). Optimization of nanostructured lipid carriers of lamotrigine for brain delivery: in vitro characterization and in vivo efficacy in epilepsy. *Expert Opin. Drug Deliv.*, **12**(2), 181–194.

179. Potschka, H., Fedrowitz, M., Löscher, W. (2002). P-Glycoprotein-mediated efflux of phenobarbital, lamotrigine, and felbamate at the blood–brain barrier: evidence from microdialysis experiments in rats. *Neurosci. Lett.*, **327**(3), 173–176.

180. Alam, M. I., et al. (2012). Intranasal administration of nanostructured lipid carriers containing CNS acting drug: pharmacodynamic studies and estimation in blood and brain. *J. Psychiatr. Res.*, **46**(9), 1133–1138.

181. Paulzen, M., Hiemke, C., Gründer, G. (2009). Plasma levels and cerebrospinal fluid penetration by duloxetine in a patient with a non-fatal overdose during a suicide attempt. *Int. J. Neuropsychopharmacol.*, **12**(10), 1431–1432.

182. Lantz, R. J., et al. (2003). Metabolism, excretion, and pharmacokinetics of duloxetine in healthy human subjects. *Drug Metab. Dispos.*, **31**(9), 1142–1150.

183. Madane, R. G., Mahajan, H. S. (2016). Curcumin-loaded nanostructured lipid carriers (NLCs) for nasal administration: design, characterization, and in vivo study. *Drug Deliv.*, **23**(4), 1326–1334.

184. Du, W., et al. (2019). Development of nose-to-brain delivery of ketoconazole by nanostructured lipid carriers against cryptococcal meningoencephalitis in mice. *Colloids Surf., B*, **183**, 110446.

185. Vyas, T. K., et al. (2005). Intranasal drug delivery for brain targeting. *Curr. Drug Deliv.*, **2**(2), 165–175.

186. Ugwoke, M. I., et al. (2005). Nasal mucoadhesive drug delivery: background, applications, trends and future perspectives. *Adv. Drug Deliv. Rev.*, **57**(11), 1640–1665.

187. Gabal, Y. M., et al. (2014). Effect of surface charge on the brain delivery of nanostructured lipid carriers in situ gels via the nasal route. *Int. J. Pharm.*, **473**(1), 442–457.

188. Drin, G., et al. (2003). Studies on the internalization mechanism of cationic cell-penetrating peptides. *J. Biol. Chem.*, **278**(33), 31192–31201.

189. Lockman, P. R., et al. (2004). Nanoparticle surface charges alter blood–brain barrier integrity and permeability. *J. Drug Targeting*, **12**(9–10), 635–641.

190. Tosi, G., et al. (2008). Polymeric nanoparticles for the drug delivery to the central nervous system. *Expert Opin. Drug Deliv.*, **5**(2), 155–174.

191. Wavikar, P. R., Vavia, P. R. (2015). Rivastigmine-loaded in situ gelling nanostructured lipid carriers for nose to brain delivery. *J. Liposome Res.*, **25**(2), 141–149.

192. Bolhassani, A., et al. (2014). Polymeric nanoparticles: potent vectors for vaccine delivery targeting cancer and infectious diseases. *Hum. Vaccin. Immunother.*, **10**(2), 321–332.

193. Zybina, A., et al. (2018). Nanoparticle-based delivery of carbamazepine: a promising approach for the treatment of refractory epilepsy. *Int. J. Pharm.*, **547**(1), 10–23.

194. Wohlfart, S., et al. (2011). Efficient chemotherapy of rat glioblastoma using doxorubicin-loaded PLGA nanoparticles with different stabilizers. *PLoS One*, **6**(5), e19121.

195. McClements, D. J. (2012). Nanoemulsions versus microemulsions: terminology, differences, and similarities. *Soft Matter*, **8**(6), 1719–1729.

196. Anton, N., Vandamme, T. F. (2011). Nano-emulsions and micro-emulsions: clarifications of the critical differences. *Pharm. Res.*, **28**(5), 978–985.

197. Mason, T. G., et al. (2006). Nanoemulsions: formation, structure, and physical properties. *J. Phys.: Condens. Matter*, **18**(41), R635–R666.

198. Nastiti, C., et al. (2017). Topical nano and microemulsions for skin delivery. *Pharmaceutics*, **9**(4), 37.

199. Li, X., et al. (2017). Nano carriers for drug transport across the blood-brain barrier. *J. Drug Targeting*, **25**(1), 17–28.

200. Solans, C., Solé, I. (2012). Nano-emulsions: formation by low-energy methods. *Curr. Opin. Colloid Interface Sci.*, **17**(5), 246–254.

201. Rao, J., McClements, D. J. (2010). Stabilization of phase inversion temperature nanoemulsions by surfactant displacement. *J. Agric. Food. Chem.*, **58**(11), 7059–7066.

202. Anton, N., Benoit, J.-P., Saulnier, P. (2008). Design and production of nanoparticles formulated from nano-emulsion templates: a review. *J. Control. Release*, **128**(3), 185–199.

203. McClements, D. J. (2011). Edible nanoemulsions: fabrication, properties, and functional performance. *Soft Matter*, **7**(6), 2297–2316.

204. Jasmina, H., et al. (2017). Preparation of nanoemulsions by high-energy and low energy emulsification methods, in *CMBEBIH 2017*, Springer Singapore, Singapore.

205. Fonseca-Santos, B., Gremiao, M. P., Chorilli, M. (2015). Nanotechnology-based drug delivery systems for the treatment of Alzheimer's disease. *Int. J. Nanomed.*, **10**, 4981–5003.

206. Gaoe, H., et al. (2012). Anti-glioma effect and safety of docetaxel-loaded nanoemulsion. *Arch. Pharmacal Res.*, **35**(2), 333–341.

207. Đorđević, S. M., et al. (2017). Parenteral nanoemulsions of risperidone for enhanced brain delivery in acute psychosis: physicochemical and in vivo performances. *Int. J. Pharm.*, **533**(2), 421–430.

208. Mittal, D., et al. (2014). Insights into direct nose to brain delivery: current status and future perspective. *Drug Deliv.*, **21**(2), 75–86.

209. Pangeni, R., et al. (2014). Vitamin E loaded resveratrol nanoemulsion for brain targeting for the treatment of Parkinson's disease by reducing oxidative stress. *Nanotechnology*, **25**(48), 485102–485102.

210. Yadav, S., et al. (2016). Intranasal brain delivery of cationic nanoemulsion-encapsulated TNFα siRNA in prevention of experimental neuroinflammation. *Nanomed. Nanotechnol. Biol. Med.*, **12**(4), 987–1002.

211. Álvarez, A., et al. (2007). Serum TNF-alpha levels are increased and correlate negatively with free IGF-I in Alzheimer disease. *Neurobiol. Aging*, **28**(4), 533–536.

212. Fillit, H., et al. (1991). Elevated circulating tumor necrosis factor levels in Alzheimer's disease. *Neurosci. Lett.*, **129**(2), 318–320.

213. Sampath, P., et al. (2006). Interstitial docetaxel (taxotere), carmustine and combined interstitial therapy: a novel treatment for experimental malignant glioma. *J. Neurooncol.*, **80**(1), 9–17.

214. Upadhyay, K. K., et al. (2010). In vitro and in vivo evaluation of docetaxel loaded biodegradable polymersomes. *Macromol. Biosci.*, **10**(5), 503–512.

215. ten Tije, A. J., et al. (2003). Pharmacological effects of formulation vehicles: implications for cancer chemotherapy. *Clin. Pharmacokinet.*, **42**(7), 665–685.

216. Zhao, M., et al. (2010). Evaluation of docetaxel-loaded intravenous lipid emulsion: pharmacokinetics, tissue distribution, antitumor activity, safety and toxicity. *Pharm. Res.*, **27**(8), 1687–1702.

217. Gabathuler, R. (2010). Approaches to transport therapeutic drugs across the blood-brain barrier to treat brain diseases. *Neurobiol. Dis.*, **37**(1), 48–57.

218. Koffie, R. M., et al. (2011). Nanoparticles enhance brain delivery of blood–brain barrier-impermeable probes for in vivo optical and magnetic resonance imaging. *Proc. Natl. Acad. Sci.*, **108**(46), 18837–18842.

219. Weiss, C. K., et al. (2008). The first step into the brain: uptake of NIO-PBCA nanoparticles by endothelial cells in vitro and in vivo, and direct evidence for their blood–brain barrier permeation. *ChemMedChem*, **3**(9), 1395–1403.

220. Wilson, B., et al. (2008). Targeted delivery of tacrine into the brain with polysorbate 80-coated poly(n-butylcyanoacrylate) nanoparticles. *Eur. J. Pharm. Biopharm.*, **70**(1), 75–84.

221. Prabhakar, K., et al. (2013). Tween 80 containing lipid nanoemulsions for delivery of indinavir to brain. *Acta Pharm. Sin. B*, **3**(5), 345–353.

222. Harun, S. N., et al. (2018). Development of nanoemulsion for efficient brain parenteral delivery of cefuroxime: designs, characterizations, and pharmacokinetics. *Int. J. Nanomed.*, **13**, 2571–2584.

223. Legrand, D., et al. (2008). Lactoferrin structure and functions, in *Bioactive Components of Milk*, Bösze, Z., ed., Springer New York, New York, pp. 163–194.

224. Fillebeen, C., et al. (1999). Receptor-mediated transcytosis of lactoferrin through the blood-brain barrier. *J. Biol. Chem.*, **274**(11), 7011–7017.

225. Somani, S., et al. (2015). Enhanced gene expression in the brain following intravenous administration of lactoferrin-bearing polypropylenimine dendriplex. *J. Control. Release*, **217**, 235–242.

226. Liu, Z., et al. (2013). Lactoferrin-modified PEG-co-PCL nanoparticles for enhanced brain delivery of NAP peptide following intranasal administration. *Biomaterials*, **34**(15), 3870–3881.

227. Huang, R., et al. (2008). The use of lactoferrin as a ligand for targeting the polyamidoamine-based gene delivery system to the brain. *Biomaterials*, **29**(2), 238–246.

228. Karami, Z., et al. (2019). Neuropharmacokinetic evaluation of lactoferrin-treated indinavir-loaded nanoemulsions: remarkable brain delivery enhancement. *Drug Dev. Ind. Pharm.*, **45**(5), 736–744.

229. Aliev, G., et al. (2019). Alzheimer's disease - future therapy based on dendrimers. *Curr. Neuropharmacol.*, **17**(3), 288–294.

230. Zhu, Y., Liu, C., Pang, Z. (2019). Dendrimer-based drug delivery systems for brain targeting. *Biomolecules*, **9**(12), 790.

231. Pang, Z., et al. (2011). Brain delivery and cellular internalization mechanisms for transferrin conjugated biodegradable polymersomes. *Int. J. Pharm.*, **415**(1), 284–292.

232. Jia, T., et al. (2016). A dual brain-targeting curcumin-loaded polymersomes ameliorated cognitive dysfunction in intrahippocampal amyloid-β1-42-injected mice. *Int. J. Nanomed.*, **11**, 3765–3775.

233. Yu, Y., et al. (2014). The proton permeability of self-assembled polymersomes and their neuroprotection by enhancing a neuroprotective peptide across the blood–brain barrier after modification with lactoferrin. *Nanoscale*, **6**(6), 3250–3258.

234. Qin, H., et al. (2019). Oncoprotein inhibitor rigosertib loaded in apoE-targeted smart polymersomes reveals high safety and potency against human glioblastoma in mice. *Mol. Pharm.*, **16**(8), 3711–3719.

235. Shen, J., et al. (2011). Poly(ethylene glycol)-block-poly(d,l-lactide acid) micelles anchored with angiopep-2 for brain-targeting delivery. *J. Drug Targeting*, **19**(3), 197–203.

236. Kanazawa, T., et al. (2011). Cell-penetrating peptide-modified block copolymer micelles promote direct brain delivery via intranasal administration. *Pharm. Res.*, **28**(9), 2130–2139.

237. Qian, Y., et al. (2013). PEGylated poly(2-(dimethylamino) ethyl methacrylate)/DNA polyplex micelles decorated with phage-displayed TGN peptide for brain-targeted gene delivery. *Biomaterials*, **34**(8), 2117–2129.

238. Abourehab, M. A., et al. (2018). Self-assembled biodegradable polymeric micelles to improve dapoxetine delivery across the blood-brain barrier. *Int. J. Nanomed.*, **13**, 3679–3687.

239. Li, J., et al. (2015). Choline derivate-modified doxorubicin loaded micelle for glioma therapy. *ACS Appl. Mater. Interfaces*, **7**(38), 21589–21601.

240. Zou, D., et al. (2017). Penetration of blood-brain barrier and antitumor activity and nerve repair in glioma by doxorubicin-loaded monosialoganglioside micelles system. *Int. J. Nanomed.*, **12**, 4879–4889.

241. Carradori, D., et al. (2018). Antibody-functionalized polymer nanoparticle leading to memory recovery in Alzheimer's disease-like transgenic mouse model. *Nanomed. Nanotechnol. Biol. Med.*, **14**(2), 609–618.

242. Tang, S., et al. (2019). Brain-targeted intranasal delivery of dopamine with borneol and lactoferrin co-modified nanoparticles for treating Parkinson's disease. *Drug Deliv.*, **26**(1), 700–707.

243. Salvalaio, M., et al. (2016). Targeted polymeric nanoparticles for brain delivery of high molecular weight molecules in lysosomal storage disorders. *PLoS One*, **11**(5), e0156452–e0156452.

244. Sousa, F., et al. (2019). Enhanced anti-angiogenic effects of bevacizumab in glioblastoma treatment upon intranasal administration in polymeric nanoparticles. *J. Control. Release*, **309**, 37–47.

245. Ke, W., et al. (2009). Gene delivery targeted to the brain using an Angiopep-conjugated polyethyleneglycol-modified polyamidoamine dendrimer. *Biomaterials*, **30**(36), 6976–6985.

246. Huang, R., et al. (2013). Angiopep-conjugated nanoparticles for targeted long-term gene therapy of Parkinson's disease. *Pharm. Res.*, **30**(10), 2549–2559.

247. Kim, I.-D., et al. (2012). Intranasal delivery of HMGB1 siRNA confers target gene knockdown and robust neuroprotection in the postischemic brain. *Mol. Ther.*, **20**(4), 829–839.

248. Xu, X., et al. (2016). A novel doxorubicin loaded folic acid conjugated PAMAM modified with borneol, a nature dual-functional product of reducing PAMAM toxicity and boosting BBB penetration. *Eur. J. Pharm. Sci.*, **88**, 178–190.

249. Hu, Y.-L., Gao, J.-Q. (2010). Potential neurotoxicity of nanoparticles. *Int. J. Pharm.*, **394**(1), 115–121.

250. Costa, P. M., et al. (2016). Functionalised carbon nanotubes: from intracellular uptake and cell-related toxicity to systemic brain delivery. *J. Control. Release*, **241**, 200–219.

251. Blasi, P., et al. (2007). Solid lipid nanoparticles to improve brain drug delivery, in *Nanotechnologies for the Life Sciences*. Wiley-VCH Verlag GmbH & Co. KGaA, pp. 365–393.

252. Olbrich, C., Kayser, O., Müller, R. H. (2002). Lipase degradation of Dynasan 114 and 116 solid lipid nanoparticles (SLN)—effect of surfactants, storage time and crystallinity. *Int. J. Pharm.*, **237**(1), 119–128.

253. Cruciani-Guglielmacci, C., Magnan, C. (2017). Brain lipoprotein lipase as a regulator of energy balance. *Biochimie*, **143**, 51–55.

254. Adibhatla, R. M., Hatcher, J. F. (2008). Altered lipid metabolism in brain injury and disorders. *Subcell. Biochem.*, **49**, 241–268.

255. Foradada, M., et al. (2000). Chemical degradation of liposomes by serum components detected by NMR. *Chem. Phys. Lipids*, **104**(2), 133–148.

256. Bruce, K. D., Zsombok, A., Eckel, R. H. (2017). Lipid processing in the brain: a key regulator of systemic metabolism. *Front. Endocrinol.*, **8**, 60.

257. Teleanu, D. M., et al. (2018). Impact of nanoparticles on brain health: an up to date overview. *J. Clin. Med.*, **7**(12), 490.

258. Medina, C., et al. (2007). Nanoparticles: pharmacological and toxicological significance. *Br. J. Pharmacol.*, **150**(5), 552–558.

Chapter 5

Magnetic and Plasmonic Nanoparticles for Brain Drug Delivery

Ana Luísa Daniel-da-Silva
CICECO-Aveiro Institute of Materials, Chemistry Department, University of Aveiro, Campus Universitário de Santiago, 3810-193 Aveiro, Portugal
ana.luisa@ua.pt

The last decade has witnessed an increasing interest in the use of magnetic and plasmonic nanoparticles for brain drug delivery. Reasons behind this interest are their magnetic and optical characteristics which endow them with additional potentially useful properties. This chapter presents an overview of the magnetic iron oxide- and gold-based nanocarriers which have been developed for brain drug delivery. Most relevant properties of these nanoparticles interacting with an external magnetic field and light are highlighted. A special focus has been laid on the chemical approaches for the synthesis of gold and magnetic iron oxides with desirable size and shapes, and adequate surface decoration to improve the transport efficacy across the blood–brain barrier. Selected examples of nanosystems with potential as delivery platforms are discussed.

Nanoparticles for Brain Drug Delivery
Edited by Carla Vitorino, Andreia Jorge and Alberto Pais

ISBN 978-981-4877-31-2 (Hardcover), 978-1-003-11932-6 (eBook)
www.jennystanford.com

5.1 Introduction

The efficient delivery of drugs to the brain remains a challenge because of the extremely low permeability and selective nature of the blood–brain barrier (BBB). Overcoming the BBB and properly delivering the drug cargo are therefore the first requirements for the development of effective treatments of brain-related diseases. In an attempt to circumvent the limitations imposed by the BBB, a broad range of nanoparticles with different sizes, architectures and surface properties have been engineered for brain drug delivery [1–3]. Nanoparticles are colloidal carriers which can have a natural or synthetic origin. Nanoparticles' features, such as tuneable size, large surface-area-to-volume ratio and flexibility to undergo versatile surface modifications, make them good candidates as carriers for delivering cargoes across the BBB. Examples of colloidal carriers which have been extensively studied for drug delivery to the brain include liposomes [4], polymeric nanoparticles [2] and inorganic nanoparticles [5–10]. Inorganic nanoparticles offer advantages over polymeric nanoparticles in terms of control over size and shape and simplicity of preparation and functionalisation. Most importantly, several inorganic nanoparticles possess magnetic and optical features which endow them with additional potentially useful properties for clinical applications [11]. Magnetic nanoparticles (MNPs) can be guided magnetically to the target, facilitating uptake by brain cells, and are well established as contrast agents in magnetic resonance imaging (MRI) [12]. Meanwhile, thermal energy released by magnetic iron oxide nanoparticles under the influence of an external applied field can modulate BBB integrity, increasing its permeability [13]. This thermal energy can be also explored in cancer treatment by magnetic hyperthermia [14]. In turn, gold nanoparticles (Au NPs), apart from the applications in drug delivery, can be used in phothermal therapy and brain imaging [15].

This chapter aims to provide a critical overview of the most recent developments on magnetic and plasmonic nanoparticles for brain drug delivery. The main synthetic routes to prepare magnetic and Au NPs with adequate size and morphology are briefly described. The most suitable approaches for the surface decoration of inorganic nanoparticles aiming enhanced transport across the BBB are outlined. Finally, selected examples of nanosystems with potential as delivery platforms are presented and discussed.

5.2 Relevant Properties of Inorganic Nanoparticles for Brain Drug Delivery

5.2.1 Gold Nanoparticles

Au NPs present high chemical stability; easy and reproducible preparation and surface modification methods, shape and size controllability; and low toxicity, properties which have attracted substantial attention for several biological applications, including as carriers for delivery across the BBB [9, 16, 17]. A very important feature is the large surface-area-to-volume ratio available, which results in a high number of active sites for interacting with different chemical species, in terms of either drug loading or chemical functionalisation of the surfaces to enhance permeability through the BBB. The size of Au NPs influences their ability to permeate through the BBB [18, 19]. It has been demonstrated for spherical Au NPs that the smallest core size combined with short-chain-length polyethylene glycol (PEG) surface functionalisation favours the permeation of Au NPs in a BBB model system [19]. Spheroidal Au NPs are the most commonly Au NPs used for BBB permeation [9, 17, 20] because the synthesis of the nanoparticles uses simple methods. However, Au NPs are available in different shapes, some of them absorbing near-infrared (NIR) light, which is an advantage as the same Au NPs can be used for drug delivery, photothermal therapy and bioimaging [16, 21]. This is the case of multibranched Au NPs, also known as Au nanoflowers or Au nanostars. Multibranched Au nanoparticles are a more attractive brain-penetrating nanovehicle platform than spherical Au NPs as they have a larger surface-area-to-volume ratio than spherical Au NPs of identical size, besides absorbing NIR light [22]. The influence of the Au NPs' shape on the integrity of the BBB was assessed in an in vitro model setup [23]. The study was focused on the effect of peptide-functionalised hollow gold nanospheres and gold nanorods, which selectively bind to amyloidogenic β-amyloid structures. It was found that varying the Au NPs' morphology had no influence on BBB integrity.

Au NPs may be of potential use for diagnosis and therapy of neurodegenerative diseases and brain tumours because of their plasmonic properties, namely the noticeable band in the optical spectrum, known as the localised surface plasmon resonance (LSPR)

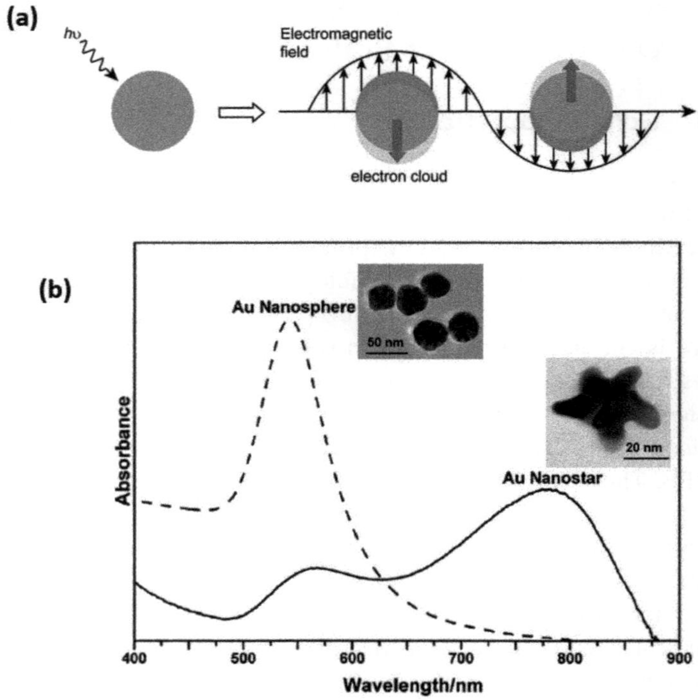

Figure 5.1 (a) Schematic illustration of the localised surface plasmon resonance effect. Conduction electrons oscillate across the metal nanoparticle because of the electromagnetic field of the incident light. Republished with permission of Royal Society of Chemistry, from Ref. [27], copyright (2012); permission conveyed through Copyright Clearance Center, Inc. (b) Visible-NIR spectra of Au nanospheres and Au nanostars and respective transmission electron microscopy (TEM) images (inset). Adapted with permission from Ref. [28]. Copyright (2018) John Wiley and Sons.

band [24]. This band arises because of the scattering and absorption of photons as a result of the resonant coherent collective oscillation of the surface electrons in Au NPs, along with the oscillating electromagnetic field of the incident light with a specific frequency (Fig. 5.1a) [25]. The wavelength of the LSPR band varies with the particle size, morphology and nature of the surrounding medium [26]. Spherical Au NPs show the LSPR in the visible (Fig. 5.1b). For biomedical purposes it is convenient to shift the LSPR band of Au NPs into the NIR window, where absorption of light by body tissues is minimal. Hence, the highest penetration depth of light into the tissues can be achieved in this spectral region. By controlling the morphology and size of Au NPs the LSPR wavelength can be shifted to the NIR region. Examples of Au NP morphologies which can absorb on the NIR region include nanorods, hollow nanospheres, nanocages, nanotriangles and multibranched Au NPs [21].

A further advantage of Au NPs is their ability to absorb light of a certain wavelength and to convert and dissipate it locally as heat through a process known as the photothermal effect [16, 29]. This effect produces a localised temperature increase which can be used to provoke tumour cells death due to a process known as hyperthermia [30–32].

5.2.2 Magnetic Nanoparticles

Iron oxide nanoparticles, more specifically magnetite (Fe_3O_4) and maghemite (γ-Fe_2O_3), are by far the most extensively investigated MNPs for targeted drug delivery due to their adequate magnetic properties, biodegradability and low toxicity [5, 33–35]. In addition, they have been extensively studied for their magnetic heating abilities for magnetic hyperthermia [14], and they are used in the clinic as contrast enhancement agents in MRI [12, 36]. More recent applications include their use as transducers in advanced neuromodulation [37]. The easy synthesis, coating or surface functionalisation provides huge versatility to these materials. Magnetite comprises both ferric (Fe^{3+}) and ferrous (Fe^{2+}) ions in its structure. Maghemite results from the topotactic oxidation of magnetite.

Magnetite nanoparticles exhibit unique size-dependent magnetic properties (Fig. 5.2) [38]. Bulk magnetite is a ferrimagnetic material composed of multiple magnetic domains. Due to magnetic domains, bulk magnetite exhibits a hysteresis curve when magnetisation (**M**) is plotted against the magnetic field (**H**) and a permanent magnetisation in absence of a magnetic field is observed. The external magnetic field necessary to bring this remanent magnetisation to zero is designated by coercivity. The decrease of the particle size from bulk to the nanoscale brings consequences in terms of magnetic properties. Below a critical particle size (~25 nm for Fe_3O_4), it is energetically more favourable for magnetite particles to be composed of single magnetic domains and therefore exhibit superparamagnetism. The magnetisation curve of superparamagnetic nanoparticles does not exhibit a hysteresis loop, which means that in the absence of an external magnetic field these particles have zero magnetisation and no coercivity. In this way the risk of aggregation of superparamagnetic iron oxide nanoparticles (SPIONs) is reduced, which is a key feature for in vivo applications. Unfortunately, superparamagnetic properties can be lost when SPIONs aggregate into clusters [39]. Thus, colloidal stability of SPIONs is of paramount importance [40].

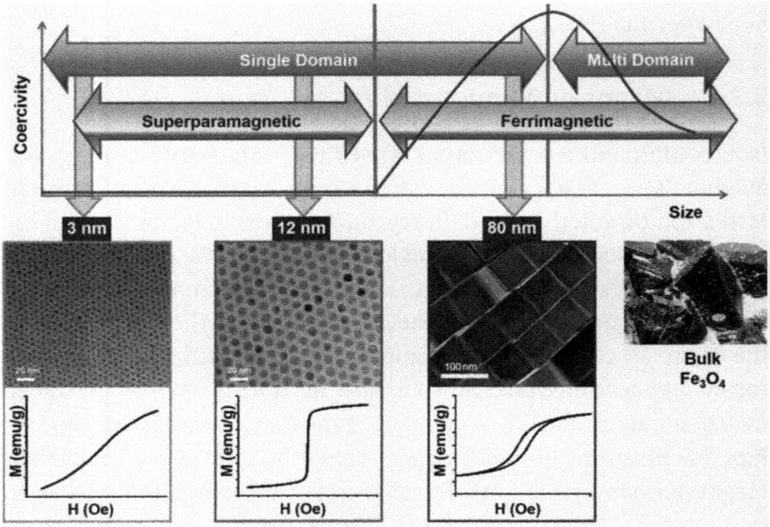

Figure 5.2 Size-dependent magnetic properties of iron oxide nanoparticles. Inset: TEM images and magnetisation curves of MNPs. Bulk magnetite is a ferrimagnetic material composed of multiple magnetic domains. Magnetite particles become a single domain as the particle size decreases below 100 nm, where coercivity is maximised. When the particle size is smaller than 20 nm, the magnetisation of magnetite nanoparticles is randomised so that they become superparamagnetic. Reprinted with permission from Ref. [38]. Copyright (2015) American Chemical Society.

A major advantage of SPIONs is that they can be guided under the influence of an external magnetic field gradient to direct towards a given target zone. For the effective magnetic guiding of SPIONS, the magnetic force produced by the external magnetic field must overcome the drag force associated with the carrier fluid. The difference between the velocity of the magnetic nanoparticle and the velocity of the fluid ($\Delta\vec{v}$) can be expressed by Eq. 5.1 [41, 42].

$$\Delta\vec{v} = \frac{R^2 \Delta\chi}{9\mu_0\eta}\nabla(\vec{B}\,.\,\vec{B}) \tag{5.1}$$

where R is the radius of the particle, $\Delta\chi$ is the difference between the magnetic susceptibility of the particle and of the diamagnetic fluid and η is the viscosity of the fluid. The constant μ_0 is the magnetic permeability of free space and B is the magnetic flux density. From the above equation it follows that larger MNPs with higher magnetic susceptibility yield larger velocities. In other words, larger particles can be easily guided. However, the size of the MNPs should remain small enough to ensure the superparamagnetism regime.

The application of an external alternating magnetic field (AMF) to magnetic iron oxide nanoparticles leads to the production of energy, in the form of heat, which leads to a local increase in the temperature. Such an effect can be exploited to use these materials as mediators in magnetic hyperthermia, used as a complementary approach to chemotherapy and radiotherapy [43]. The permeability of the BBB is known to increase in response to a physiologically relevant temperature increase (38°C–39°C) [44]. SPIONs under the influence of a low-radiofrequency field produce moderate heat which increases the permeability of the BBB in a local and reversible process which was observed in rats [13].

The physics behind magnetic heating is beyond the scope of this chapter and can be found in specialised literature [6, 42, 45, 46]. In summary, in larger particles which are composed of several magnetic domains, the production of heat is due to hysteresis losses. In SPIONs, which are single-domain particles, the mechanism is different. In this case, the magnetic moment of the nanoparticle aligns with the alternating direction of the external magnetic field and releases energy when the particle moment relaxes back to the original direction (Fig. 5.3). This mechanism is called Néel relaxation [45]. For both types of particles, larger and smaller, heating can take place under rotation of the particle within the surrounding fluid (Brownian relaxation). In SPIONs, Néel relaxation predominates over Brownian relaxation, while for larger particles and low-viscosity media, the Brown mechanism dominates.

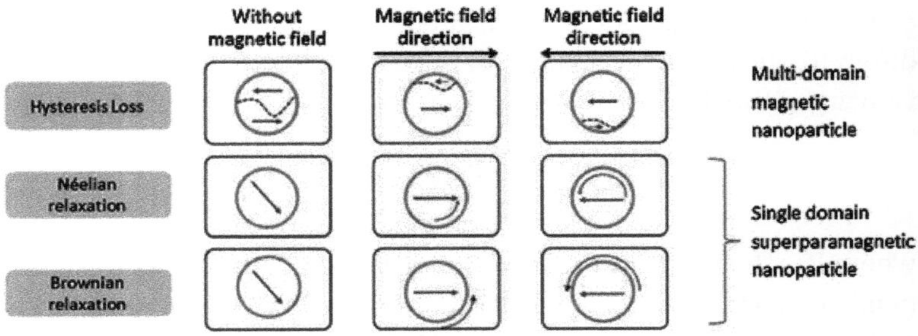

Figure 5.3 Different heat generation models in a magnetic nanoparticle in response to an alternative magnetic field. The short, straight arrows represent the magnetic moment direction, the curved arrows represent the movement or change in direction and the dashed lines represent the domain boundaries in multidomain particles [46] (Creative Commons CC BY).

5.3 Synthesis Procedures

The design of inorganic nanocarriers for in vivo targeting applications is complex because it must take into account all the specifications required by the biological character of the application. This section summarises the most common chemical methods for the synthesis of gold and magnetic iron oxides for biomedical applications. The benefits and drawbacks of each synthetic method are also identified.

5.3.1 Gold Nanoparticles

A number of synthetic strategies have been developed for the synthesis of colloidal Au NPs with uniform morphology, narrow size distribution and tailored properties, as extensively reviewed elsewhere [27, 47–50]. Generally, the synthesis of Au NPs can be performed using chemical, physical or biological methods [15]. Examples of wet-chemical methods are the chemical reduction of Au salts, electrochemical pathways and the decomposition of organometallic compounds. From these methods, chemical reduction is the easiest to prepare stable colloidal Au NPs with desirable sizes and shapes. The process can be divided into two major steps, nucleation and successive growth of nanoparticles. The formation of nuclei occurs by reduction of Au(III) species with a reducing agent, and the collision between ions, atoms and clusters promotes particle growth [51]. The size- and shape-controlled growth of Au NPs depends on the reaction conditions, such as the concentration of reactants, surface capping, temperature and duration of the growth stage. The most common shape of these nanoparticles is spherical because of isotropic growth on the surface of Au nuclei or particles. Even so, Au NPs can be synthesised into triangle, rod, cube, star, wire and flower shapes if anisotropic growth is promoted [21, 52]. The earliest-reported methods for the synthesis of spheroidal nanoparticles were developed by Faraday, Turkevich and Brust [53, 54]. Turkevich developed in 1951 a single-phase aqueous method based on the reduction of a gold salt by citrate [55].

The Turkevich method is still one of the most common synthetic approaches used for preparing Au NPs for bioapplications, including for brain drug delivery [20, 56]. In this method, trisodium citrate is used both as a reducing and as a stabilising agent and is added to boiling chloroauric acid ($HAuCl_4$) solution under vigorous stirring. A red-wine solution is obtained at the end of the reaction because of the formation of Au NPs with an average diameter of around 20 nm, with a negatively charged surface and electrostatically stabilised by citrate ions [55]. The size of the nanoparticles can be adjusted by varying the citrate/Au(III) molar ratio. At high ratio values, the nucleation is faster and dominant and leads to the formation of smaller NPs [57], which is desirable to enhance the permeability of Au NPs through the BBB [19]. Small (<10 nm) and monodisperse Au NPs can be prepared by simply reversing the order of addition of the reactants. Thus, the addition of the $HAuCl_4$ solution to the citrate solution favours the nucleation and stabilisation of Au NPs [58]. Despite the electrostatic stabilisation, citrate-stabilised particles obtained using the Turkevich method can aggregate during storage or subsequent functionalisation steps. Large molecules such as surfactants and mercaptoalkanoic acids can be used to functionalise the surface and prevent the aggregation of Au NPs [27].

Smaller spherical Au NPs, with an average size of 2 nm and narrow size distribution, can be obtained using sodium borohydride ($NaBH_4$), which is a stronger reducing agent, following the Brust–Schiffrin method, a two-phase method which yields thiolatestabilised Au NPs in an organic phase [53]. However, the resulting Au NPs are hydrophobic. To confer water compatibility, the surface of the Au NPs must be further modified with hydrophilic capping agents such as PEG [59].

More recently, multibranched Au NPs are attracting attention as brain-penetrating nanocarriers [10]. Such nanoparticles can be synthesised using seed-mediated methods [60]. Briefly, spherical gold seed particles are firstly prepared using the Turkevich method. Subsequently the Au seeds are added to the aqueous growth solution, which is a solution which contains $HAuCl_4$ and the surfactant cetyltrimethylammonium bromide (CTAB), among other components. The dimension and number of branches could be varied under various combinations of the [seed]/[Au^{3+}] ratio [60]. Alternative methods to synthesise branched Au NPs involving less toxic stabilisers have been developed [61, 62].

5.3.2 Magnetic Nanoparticles

The synthesis of MNPs for biomedical applications encompasses several requirements regarding the particle size, surface composition and colloidal stability under physiological conditions which are intrinsic to each specific application [12, 63–65]. These requirements pose some challenges in terms of synthetic methods. A number of synthetic strategies were developed for the synthesis of magnetic iron oxide nanoparticles with uniform morphology, narrow size distribution and tailored properties, as extensively reviewed elsewhere [38, 66, 67]. In brief, the most common methods for the synthesis of colloidal magnetite nanoparticles include the co-precipitation method [68–70], oxidative hydrolysis [71, 72], hydrothermal treatment [73–75] and the thermal decomposition of iron-containing molecular precursors [76, 77]. The most usual and straightforward method for synthesising superparamagnetic Fe_3O_4 nanoparticles is the co-precipitation of Fe^{2+} and Fe^{3+} aqueous solutions (molar ratio 2:1) by the addition of a base (pH 8–14) in a non-oxidising atmosphere. The global chemical reaction is depicted in Eq. 5.2.

$$Fe^{2+} + 2Fe^{3+} + 8OH^{-} \rightarrow Fe_3O_4 + 4H_2O \tag{5.2}$$

Control of the size, shape and composition of the magnetic iron oxides prepared via co-precipitation depends on the type of salts used (e.g. chlorides, sulfates, nitrates), the Fe^{3+}/Fe^{2+} ratio, the reaction temperature, the pH value and ionic strength of the medium [67]. The main advantage of the co-precipitation process is that a large amount of nanoparticles can be synthesised. By varying the reaction conditions, particles with a size ranging from 2 to 17 nm can be obtained [67]. However, this method does not provide a tight control of the particle size and usually a polydisperse size distribution is obtained. This route, if performed in constrained domains such as microemulsions, is more efficient to control particle size and shape [78]. Nevertheless, nonhydrolytic high-temperature methods usually provide highly crystalline particles, size monodispersity and enhanced magnetic properties. For example, magnetite nanoparticles prepared via thermal decomposition have saturation magnetisation values at room temperature within 65–75 emu/g [79, 80], which are higher than those reported for particles synthesised via co-precipitation (30–60 emu/g) [78, 81]. The method consists of the thermal decomposition of iron organic precursors in the presence of organic solvents and surfactants. Examples of precursors used include iron complexes such as iron cupferronate, iron pentacarbonyl and iron(III) acetylacetonate. Surfactants such as oleic acid and hexadecylamine provide colloidal stability to the particles. Once the nucleation has occurred through the decomposition of the percursor, particles grow at high temperature without additional nucleation events, leading to the formation of monodispersed nanoparticles [38, 67, 82]. The size and morphology of the nanoparticles can be finely controlled by adjusting not only the reaction times and the temperature but also the concentration and ratios of the reactants, namely the relative amounts of precursor and surfactants. The method presents some disadvantages such as a long reaction time, high reaction temperatures and toxicity of many of the reactants. More important, the synthesis using thermal decomposition methods yields hydrophobic iron oxide nanoparticles which are compatible only with organic solvents. Therefore, for their use in biomedical applications, further steps are needed to make them hydrophilic. The surface modification using postsynthetic methods such as ligand exchange reactions and encapsulation with amphiphilic polymers [38] is the most common strategy.

5.4 Surface Modification Strategies towards Brain Delivery

Surface modification and bioconjugation of bare inorganic nanoparticles are necessary to make them suitable for various bioapplications [83–86]. Appropriate surface functionalisation increases the colloidal stability of nanoparticles in biological or physiological media and improves their biocompatibility and biospecificity for targeting bioapplications [87]. Several biodistribution studies have shown that undecorated inorganic nanoparticles have low success in crossing the BBB. For example, only 0.075% of citrate-stabilised 15 nm Au NPs cross the BBB after intravenous administration in mice [88]. The percentage decreased to 0.036% and 0.023% for 50 and 100 nm particle size. After parenteral administration of sterically stabilised 10 and 25 nm core size SPIONs in mice, increased iron levels were detected in all tissues except for the brain [89]. These results suggest that the transport efficacy of SPIONs is not better. Adequate surface modification of the inorganic nanoparticles with endogenous ligands has been shown to improve the transport of nanoparticles across the BBB via the receptor-mediated transcytosis (RMT) mechanism [6, 90]. The entire process consists first of receptor–ligand recognition at the luminal side and then endosome formation, which transports the ligand across the endothelial cell, and exocytosis at the other side of the membrane (Fig. 5.4) [91]. Commonly used endogenous ligands are transferrin [18, 59], lactoferrin [92] and insulin [93]. The proper optimisation of the nanoparticle avidity to the targeted receptor is essential to achieve efficient BBB transcytosis using the receptor-mediated mechanism [94]. This was demonstrated in a study using Au NPs decorated with transferrin [18]. It was found that the brain accumulation of the nanoparticles was dependent on the transferrin level. Nanoparticles decorated with a high level of transferrin remained attached to the brain endothelial cells without strong transcytosis, whereas those with less transferrin were able to interact with the transferrin receptors on the luminal side of the BBB and detach at the brain side.

Cell-penetrating peptides as TAT peptides are also employed in the decoration of inorganic nanoparticles to enhance brain delivery and targeting brain tumours [9, 95, 96]. A few reports have demonstrated that drug-loaded polymeric nanoparticles coated with the non-ionic surfactant polysorbate 80 (PS80) can cross the BBB and be taken up by brain endothelial cells [97, 98]. Subsequently, a similar surface modification strategy has been adopted for MNPs [99, 100].

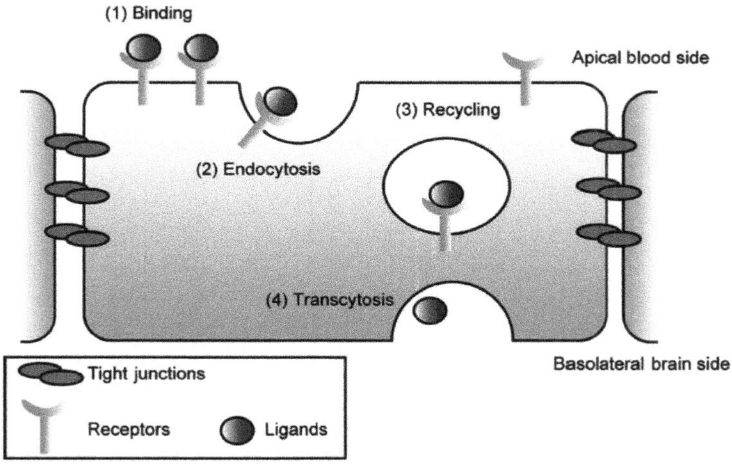

Figure 5.4 Schematic diagram of the process of receptor-mediated transcytosis. Reprinted from Ref. [91], Copyright (2019), with permission from Elsevier.

5.5 Nanoparticles for Brain Delivery

In this section selected examples of recent systems for brain delivery based on magnetic iron oxides and Au NPs are reviewed.

5.5.1 Gold Nanoparticles

Citrate-stabilised Au NPs conjugated with the amphipathic peptide CLPFFD could increase the in vivo penetration of these particles into the rat brain without causing apparent changes in BBB integrity, possibly by receptor-mediated transcytosis mechanisms [56]. The peptide CLPFFD is derived from the β-amyloid peptide, which recognises toxic β-amyloid aggregates (Aβ) involved in Alzheimer's disease and crosses the BBB. Further enhancement of the permeability was achieved after conjugation of Au NPs with a peptide which recognises the transferrin receptor [20]. The conjugated Au NPs could recognise Aβ aggregates (Fig. 5.5), which demonstrates the potential of these nanoplatforms for the development of treatments for neurodegenerative diseases.

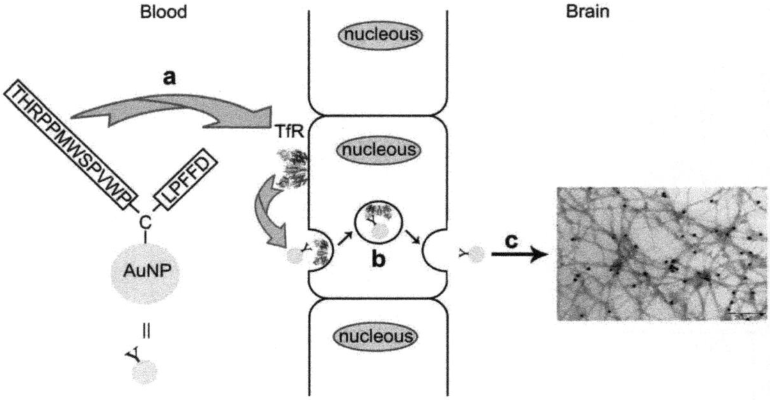

Figure 5.5 Scheme to rationalise the design of the Au NP–THR–LPFFD conjugate. (a) The peptide THR–CLPFFD anchored to the Au NP. This peptide contains the THR sequence which recognises the transferrin receptor and LPFFD which recognise Aβ aggregates. (b) Transport of the endocytic vesicle through the endothelial cells of the blood–brain barrier. (c) Recognition and binding of the conjugate to Aβ aggregates inside the central nervous system. The transferrin receptor is abbreviated as TfR. Reprinted from Ref. [20], Copyright (2012), with permission from Elsevier.

Other surface decoration approaches have been employed. For example, wheat germ agglutinin (WGA) horse radish peroxidase chemically conjugated to Au NPs (~5 nm size) could be transported to the brainstem following intramuscular injection into the diaphragm of rats [17]. The WGA functioned as the targeting moiety to guide nanoconjugates bonded to a drug for the treatment of respiratory dysfunctions exclusively to the phrenic motoneurons which control respiratory function. The drug–Au nanosystem was capable of delivering the drug at a much lower dose than the unconjugated drug injected systemically to effectively induce respiratory recovery in rats.

Au NPs (~5 nm size) decorated with cell-penetrating TAT peptide and carrying doxorubicin demonstrated the ability to cross the BBB after systemic injection, improving the survival of mice bearing intracranial xenografts of glioblastoma (GBM), which is one of the most aggressive tumours occurring in the central nervous system [9]. The system was able to efficiently deliver the Gd^{3+} contrast agent across the BBB to reach brain tumours and thus improved the brain tumour imaging with MRI. The same platform led to improved cytotoxicity towards two brain metastatic breast cancer cell lines with a decrease in the IC50 of at least 80% compared to free doxorubicin [95].

The above-described systems involve spherical Au NPs of small dimensions (5–12 nm). Yet, there has been increasing interest for anisotropic gold nanostructures absorbing within the NIR spectral region because of their potential for imaging and hyperthermia. In this context, Yuan et al. [101] have sown that PEGylated gold nanostars with a hydrodynamic size of 80 nm and plasmon maximum at 800 nm could be delivered beyond the brain tumour vasculature after injection in mice. By employing ultrashort-pulsed laser, the authors achieved an enhanced, optically modulated and image-guided delivery of the Au probes and demonstrated the permeabilisation of brain tumour microvasculature. Recent studies have shown that multibranched Au NPs loaded with L-DOTA, which is a drug used to treat Parkinson's disease, are efficiently transported across in vitro BBB models [10]. Lee and co-workers [102] proposed an innovative virus-inspired approach to modify the surface of gold nanorods and enhance their delivery into the brain. The gold nanorods were firstly coated with a mesoporous silica shell closely resembling the spike-like glycoprotein layer of rabies virus and then conjugated to a peptide of rabies virus glycoprotein which interacts specifically with the nicotinic acetylcholine receptor expressed on neuronal cells. Because of the modified peptide surface, the nanorods could target the brain tumour in mice after intravenous administration. Also, the nanorods were able to induce a hyperthermal effect in response to NIR laser irradiation, based on LSPR, to effectively suppress brain tumours in mice. Together, these results support that the rabies virus mimetic gold nanorods are a potential prototype delivery platform for treating brain tumours.

5.5.2 Magnetic Nanoparticles

Huang and co-workers [99] demonstrated the effective passage of tail-vein-injected Tween-SPIONs across the normal BBB in rats under an external magnetic field. SPIONs consisted of Fe_3O_4 nanoparticles, 11.5 nm average size, which were synthesised by thermal decomposition of iron complexes in the presence of PEG and poly(ethylene imine) (PEI) and then further modified with Tween 80 (PS80), which is a hydrophilic non-ionic surfactant. The study confirmed that both the Tween 80 modification and the external magnetic field play crucial roles in the effective passage of SPIONs across the intact BBB. Both Tween-SPIONs in the absence of the field and PEI/PEG-SPIONs in the presence of the field found it difficult to cross the BBB. Furthermore, only the magnetic force could not drag the SPIONs through the BBB, excluding a passive penetration mechanism. It is proposed that Tween-SPIONs enter capillary endothelial cells by an active penetration pathway via receptor-mediated endocytosis facilitated by the external magnetic field. A plausible mechanism is the formation of an apolipoprotein corona around Tween-SPIONs which favours transport through the BBB by low-density lipoprotein receptor-mediated endocytosis (Fig. 5.6).

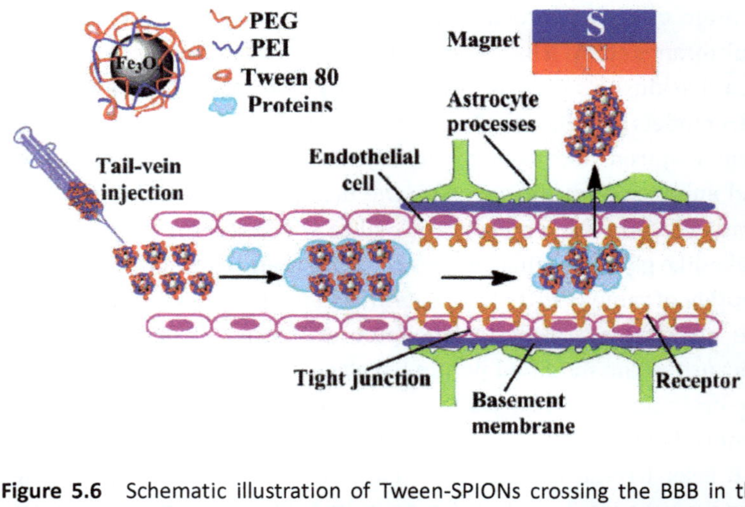

Figure 5.6 Schematic illustration of Tween-SPIONs crossing the BBB in the presence of a magnet. Reprinted with permission from Ref. [99]. Copyright (2016) American Chemical Society.

Engineered MNPs are being developed aiming the treatment of GBM. Having this goal in mind, carriers consisting of Fe_3O_4/PEGylated poly(lactic-co-glycolic acid) composite nanoparticles with superparamagnetic behaviour, loaded with the anticancer paclitaxel (PTX), were prepared [103]. An orthotopic murine GBM model was used to evaluate BBB disruption through MRI. The application of an external magnetic field enhanced the accumulation of PTX-loaded nanoparticles in the brain, as well as the antitumour efficacy, and prolonged the survival rate of mice compared to passive targeting and saline treatments [100]. The results demonstrate the potential of magnetic targeting of PTX/SPIONs as a strategy for GBM chemotherapy. Noteworthy, the coating of these carriers with PS80 did not result in an enhancement of the nanoparticle accumulation in the brain tissues, contrary to what could be expected on the basis of previous studies.

Other types of surface functionalisation have been employed, aiming at the facile penetration of MNPs through the BBB. The functionalisation of silica-coated magnetite nanoparticles with TAT cell-penetrating peptide facilitated the permeability across the in vitro BBB model via a transcellular trafficking mechanism and magnetically mediated dragging. Moreover, the functionalisation with TAT peptide favoured the entry of MNPs into the nucleous of U251 glioma cells co-cultured in the bottom chamber [96]. SPIONs coated with amorphous silica and carbon thin shells were tested in in vitro and in vivo BBB models [104]. The results evidence the ability of these nanoparticles to penetrate the barrier and localise to the brain tissue.

Besides magnetic guiding, MNPs provide the possibility of localised magnetic heating. The effects of AMF-induced hyperthermia of SPIONs (size ~10 nm) with different coatings (citrate-stabilised and coated with cross-linked PEG-polyaspartate) on the BBB permeability was assessed using in vitro BBB models [105]. The temperature increase and the cell medium induced the agglomeration of citrate-SPIONs. These particles were able to enter BBB cells through an endocytosis pathway; however, they did not cross the in vitro BBB model, which indicates a lack of potential therapeutic applications. In contrast, polymer-coated SPIONs displayed enhanced colloidal stability, which was unaffected by temperature increase. Furthermore, polymer-coated SPIONs could cross the BBB model in hyperthermia conditions. Importantly, the AMF-induced hyperthermia enhanced the BBB permeability of polymer-SPIONs more effectively than exogenous temperature increase, without cell death.

Meanwhile, Tabatabaei et al. [13] demonstrated that the thermal energy generated by magnetic heating of superparamagnetic magnetite nanoparticles can increase BBB permeability in rats. The results indicate a substantial but reversible opening of the BBB where magnetic hyperthermia is applied. The magnetic heating was induced remotely by a low-radiofrequency field. The superparamagnetic nanoparticles acted as nanoheaters which deliver the thermal energy uniquely to the endothelium with a higher spatial precision. The authors showed that large molecules of the fluorescent dye Evans blue are able to cross the BBB after application of hyperthermia and that the BBB is able to naturally fully recover afterwards.

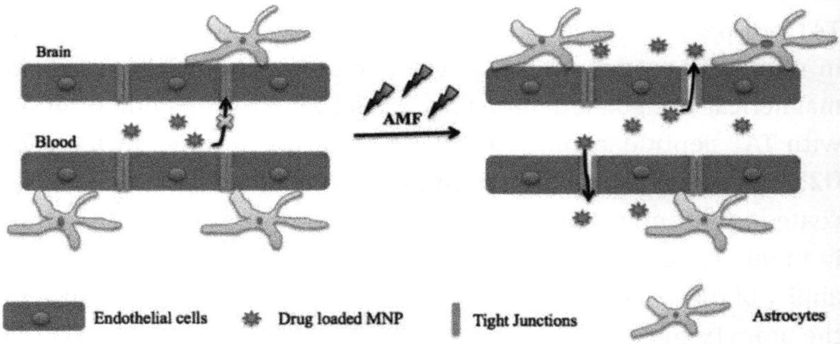

Figure 5.7 Schematic representation of blood–brain barrier disruption by AMF application. The localised heat produced by MNPs on AMF application opens up the tight junction, causing enhanced delivery of the payload. Reprinted with permission from Ref. [106]. Copyright (2019) American Chemical Society.

Lately, several preclinical studies in tumour models presented magnetic hyperthermia as a potential tool, alone or in combination with chemotherapy, for GBM treatment (Fig. 5.7) [106]. Advancements in BBB permeability induced by magnetic nanosystems might contribute towards establishing magnetic hyperthermia as a potential treatment tool for glioma therapy.

5.6 Concluding Remarks

Magnetic iron oxides and Au NPs gained much interest for brain delivery because of their magnetic and plasmonic features which endow them with multiple functionalities which are much useful for clinical applications. By careful design of the surface coating, these inorganic nanoparticles are able to penetrate the BBB and deliver cargoes into the brain. Despite the potential demonstrated by some of the nanoplatforms, issues concerning the neurotoxicity of these nanoparticles must be assessed before clinical translation will be considered. Aspects related to nanoparticle–tissue interaction and impact of hyperthermia on the brain functionality must also be clarified and require further investigation.

Acknowledgements

This work was developed within the scope of the project CICECO-Aveiro Institute of Materials, FCT Ref. UIDB/50011/2020 and UIDP/50011/2020, and the exploratory project IF/00405/2014, financed by national funds through the Fundação para a Ciência e Tecnologia (FCT)/MCTES. A. L. Daniel-da-Silva acknowledges the FCT for the research contract under the Program 'Investigador FCT' 2014.

References

1. Saraiva, C., Praça, C., Ferreira, R., Santos, T., Ferreira, L., Bernardino, L. (2016). Nanoparticle-mediated brain drug delivery: overcoming blood-brain barrier to treat neurodegenerative diseases. *J. Control. Release*, **235**, 34–47.
2. Patel, T., Zhou, J., Piepmeier, J. M., Saltzman, W. M. (2012). Polymeric nanoparticles for drug delivery to the central nervous system. *Adv. Drug Deliv. Rev.*, **64**, 701–705.
3. Vlieghe, P., Khrestchatisky, M. (2013). Medicinal chemistry based approaches and nanotechnology-based systems to improve CNS drug targeting and delivery. *Med. Res. Rev.*, **33**, 457–516.
4. Vieira, D. B., Gamarra, L. F. (2016). Getting into the brain: liposome-based strategies for effective drug delivery across the blood–brain barrier. *Int. J. Nanomed.*, **11**, 5381–5414.

5. D'Agata, F., Ruffinatti, F., Boschi, S., Stura, I., Rainero, I., Abollino, O., Cavalli, R., Guiot, C. (2017). Magnetic nanoparticles in the central nervous system: targeting principles, applications and safety issues. *Molecules*, **23**, 9.

6. Busquets, M., Espargaró, A., Sabaté, R., Estelrich, J. (2015). Magnetic nanoparticles cross the blood-brain barrier: when physics rises to a challenge. *Nanomaterials*, **5**, 2231–2248.

7. Baghirov, H., et al. (2016). Feasibility study of the permeability and uptake of mesoporous silica nanoparticles across the blood-brain barrier. *PLoS One*, **11**, 1–22.

8. Song, Y., Du, D., Li, L., Xu, J., Dutta, P., Lin, Y. (2017). In vitro study of receptor-mediated silica nanoparticles delivery across blood-brain barrier. *ACS Appl. Mater. Interfaces*, **9**, 20410–20416.

9. Cheng, Y., et al. (2014). Blood-brain barrier permeable gold nanoparticles: an efficient delivery platform for enhanced malignant glioma therapy and imaging. *Small*, **10**, 5137–5150.

10. Gonzalez-Carter, D. A., Ong, Z. Y., McGilvery, C. M., Dunlop, I. E., Dexter, D. T., Porter, A. E. (2019). L-DOPA functionalized, multi-branched gold nanoparticles as brain-targeted nano-vehicles. *Nanomedicine*, **15**, 1–11.

11. El-Boubbou, K. (2018). Magnetic iron oxide nanoparticles as drug carriers: clinical relevance. *Nanomedicine*, **13**, 953–971.

12. Blanco-Andujar, C., Walter, A., Cotin, G., Bordeianu, C., Mertz, D., Felder-Flesch, D., Begin-Colin, S. (2016). Design of iron oxide-based nanoparticles for MRI and magnetic hyperthermia. *Nanomedicine*, **11**, 1889–1910.

13. Tabatabaei, S. N., Girouard, H., Carret, A.-S., Martel, S. (2015). Remote control of the permeability of the blood–brain barrier by magnetic heating of nanoparticles: a proof of concept for brain drug delivery. *J. Control. Release*, **206**, 49–57.

14. Giustini, A. J., Petryk, A. A., Cassim, S. M., Tate, J. A., Baker, I., Hoopes, P. J. (2010). Magnetic nanoparticle hyperthermia in cancer treatment. *Nano Life*, **1**, 17–32.

15. Elahi, N., Kamali, M., Baghersad, M. H. (2018). Recent biomedical applications of gold nanoparticles: a review. *Talanta*, **184**, 537–556.

16. Cobley, C. M., Chen, J., Cho, E. C., Wang, L. V., Xia, Y. (2011). Gold nanostructures: a class of multifunctional materials for biomedical applications. *Chem. Soc. Rev.*, **40**, 44–56.

17. Zhang, Y., Walker, J. B., Minic, Z., Liu, F., Goshgarian, H., Mao, G. (2016). Transporter protein and drug-conjugated gold nanoparticles capable of bypassing the blood-brain barrier. *Sci. Rep.*, **6**, 1–8.

18. Wiley, D. T., Webster, P., Gale, A., Davis, M. E. (2013). Transcytosis and brain uptake of transferrin-containing nanoparticles by tuning avidity to transferrin receptor. *Proc. Natl. Acad. Sci.*, **110**, 8662–8667.

19. Etame, A. B., Smith, C. A., Chan, W. C. W., Rutka, J. T. (2011). Design and potential application of PEGylated gold nanoparticles with size-dependent permeation through brain microvasculature. *Nanomedicine*, **7**, 992–1000.

20. Prades, R., et al. (2012). Delivery of gold nanoparticles to the brain by conjugation with a peptide that recognizes the transferrin receptor. *Biomaterials*, **33**, 7194–7205.

21. Li, N., Zhao, P., Astruc, D. (2014). Anisotropic gold nanoparticles: synthesis, properties, applications, and toxicity. *Angew. Chem. Int. Ed.*, **53**, 1756–1789.

22. Ong, Z. Y., Chen, S., Nabavi, E., Regoutz, A., Payne, D. J., Elson, D. S., Dexter, D. T., Dunlop, I. E., Porter, A. E. (2017). Multibranched gold nanoparticles with intrinsic LAT-1 targeting capabilities for selective photothermal therapy of breast cancer. *ACS Appl. Mater. Interfaces*, **9**, 39259–39270.

23. Ruff, J., Hüwel, S., Kogan, M. J., Simon, U., Galla, H. J. (2017). The effects of gold nanoparticles functionalized with ß-amyloid specific peptides on an in vitro model of blood–brain barrier. *Nanomedicine*, **13**, 1645–1652.

24. Meola, A., Rao, J., Chaudhary, N., Sharma, M., Chang, S. D. (2018). Gold nanoparticles for brain tumor imaging: a systematic review. *Front. Neurol.*, **9**, 328.

25. Papavassiliou, G. C. (1979). Optical properties of small inorganic and organic metal particles. *Prog. Solid State Chem.*, **12**, 185–271.

26. Henglein, A. (1993). Physicochemical properties of small metal particles in solution: 'microelectrode' reactions, chemisorption, composite metal particles, and the atom-to-metal transition. *J. Phys. Chem.*, **97**, 5457–5471.

27. Yeh, Y.-C., Creran, B., Rotello, V. M. (2012). Gold nanoparticles: preparation, properties, and applications in bionanotechnology. *Nanoscale*, **4**, 1871–80.

28. Pinheiro, P. C., Daniel-da-Silva, A. L., Nogueira, H. I. S., Trindade, T. (2018). Functionalized inorganic nanoparticles for magnetic

separation and SERS detection of water pollutants. *Eur. J. Inorg. Chem.*, **30**, 3443–3461.

29. Jain, P. K., Huang, X., El-Sayed, I. H., El-Sayed, M. A. (2008). Noble metals on the nanoscale: optical and photothermal properties and some applications in imaging, sensing, biology, and medicine. *Acc. Chem. Res.*, **41**, 1578–1586.
30. Choi, W. Il, Kim, J.-Y., Kang, C., Byeon, C. C., Kim, Y. H., Tae, G. (2011). Tumor regression in vivo by photothermal therapy based on gold-nanorod-loaded, functional nanocarriers. *ACS Nano*, **5**, 1995–2003.
31. Shen, S., Tang, H., Zhang, X., Ren, J., Pang, Z., Wang, D., Gao, H., Qian, Y., Jiang, X., Yang, W. (2013). Targeting mesoporous silica-encapsulated gold nanorods for chemo-photothermal therapy with near-infrared radiation. *Biomaterials*, **34**, 3150–3158.
32. Lal, S., Verma, J., Van Noorden, C. J. F. (2014). Nanoparticles for hyperthermic therapy: synthesis strategies and applications in glioblastoma. *Int. J. Nanomed.*, **9**, 2863.
33. El-boubbou, K. (2018). Magnetic iron oxide nanoparticles as drug carriers: preparation, conjugation and delivery. *Nanomedicine*, **13**, 929–952.
34. Canfarotta, F., Piletsky, S. A. (2014). Engineered magnetic nanoparticles for biomedical applications. *Adv. Healthcare Mater.*, **3**, 160–175.
35. Ulbrich, K., Holá, K., Šubr, V., Bakandritsos, A., Tuček, J., Zbořil, R. (2016). Targeted drug delivery with polymers and magnetic nanoparticles: covalent and noncovalent approaches, release control, and clinical studies. *Chem. Rev.*, **116**, 5338–5431.
36. Iv, M., Telischak, N., Feng, D., Holdsworth, S. J., Yeom, K. W., Daldrup-Link, H. E. (2015). Clinical applications of iron oxide nanoparticles for magnetic resonance imaging of brain tumors. *Nanomedicine*, **10**, 993–1008.
37. Roet, M., Hescham, S.-A., Jahanshahi, A., Rutten, B. P. F., Anikeeva, P. O., Temel, Y. (2019). Progress in neuromodulation of the brain; a role for magnetic nanoparticles? *Prog. Neurobiol.*, 1–14.
38. Ling, D., Lee, N., Hyeon, T. (2015). Chemical synthesis and assembly of uniformly sized iron oxide nanoparticles for medical applications. *Acc. Chem. Res.*, **48**, 1276–1285.
39. Mørup, S., Hansen, M. F., Frandsen, C. (2010). Magnetic interactions between nanoparticles. *Beilstein J. Nanotechnol.*, **1**, 182–190.
40. Champagne, P. O., Westwick, H., Bouthillier, A., Sawan, M. (2018). Colloidal stability of superparamagnetic iron oxide nanoparticles in the central nervous system: a review. *Nanomedicine*, **13**, 1385–1400.

41. Pankhurst, Q. A., Connolly, J., Jones, S. K., Dobson, J. (2003). Applications of magnetic nanoparticles in biomedicine. *J. Phys. D: Appl. Phys.*, **36**, 167–181.

42. Daniel-da-Silva, A. L., Silva, N. J. O., Trindade, T., Gil, A. M. (2011). Biocomposites containing magnetic nanoparticles, in *Nanocomposite Particles for Bio-Applications: Materials and Bio-Interfaces*, Trindade, T., Daniel-da-Silva, A. L., eds., Pan Stanford, Singapore, pp. 165–192.

43. Chang, D., Lim, M., Goos, J. A. C. M., Qiao, R., Ng, Y. Y., Mansfeld, F. M., Jackson, M., Davis, T. P., Kavallaris, M. (2018). Biologically targeted magnetic hyperthermia: potential and limitations. *Front. Pharmacol.*, **9**, 831.

44. Kiyatkin, E. A., Sharma, H. S. (2009). Permeability of the blood-brain barrier depends on brain temperature. *Neuroscience*, **161**, 926–939.

45. Rosensweig, R. E. (2002). Heating magnetic fluid with alternating magnetic field. *J. Magn. Magn. Mater.*, **252**, 370–374.

46. Suriyanto, Ng, E. Y. K., Kumar, S. D. (2017). Physical mechanism and modeling of heat generation and transfer in magnetic fluid hyperthermia through Néelian and Brownian relaxation: a review. *Biomed. Eng. Online*, **16**, 36.

47. Zhao, P., Li, N., Astruc, D. (2013). State of the art in gold nanoparticle synthesis. *Coord. Chem. Rev.*, **257**, 638–665.

48. António, M., Nogueira, J., Vitorino, R., Daniel-da-Silva, A. L. (2018). Functionalized gold nanoparticles for the detection of C-reactive protein. *Nanomaterials*, **8**, 200.

49. Liz-Marzán, L. M. (2004). Nanometals: formation and color. *Mater. Today*, **7**, 26–31.

50. Boisselier, E., Astruc, D. (2009). Gold nanoparticles in nanomedicine: preparations, imaging, diagnostics, therapies and toxicity. *Chem. Soc. Rev.*, **38**, 1759–1782.

51. Xia, Y., Xia, X., Peng, H.-C. (2015). Shape-controlled synthesis of colloidal metal nanocrystals: thermodynamic versus kinetic products. *J. Am. Chem. Soc.*, **137**, 7947–7966.

52. Shah, M., Badwaik, V. D., Dakshinamurthy, R. (2014). Biological applications of gold nanoparticles. *J. Nanosci. Nanotechnol.*, **14**, 344–362.

53. Brust, M., Walker, M., Bethell, D., Schiffrin, D. J., Whyman, R. (1994). Synthesis of thiol-derivatised gold nanoparticles in a two-phase liquid–liquid system. *J. Chem. Soc., Chem. Commun.*, 801–802.

54. Kimling, J., Maier, M., Okenve, B., Kotaidis, V., Ballot, H., Plech, A. (2006). Turkevich method for gold nanoparticle synthesis revisited. *J. Phys. Chem. B*, **110**, 15700–15707.

55. Turkevich, J., Stevenson, P. C., Hillier, J. (1951). A study of the nucleation and growth processes in the synthesis of colloidal gold. *Discuss. Faraday Soc.*, **11**, 55.

56. Arias, J. L., Giralt, E., Arias, J. I., Fernández, M. S., Araya, E., Kogan, M. J., Fiedler, J. L., Adura, C., Guerrero, S., Albericio, F. (2010). Improving the brain delivery of gold nanoparticles by conjugation with an amphipathic peptide. *Nanomedicine*, **5**, 897–913.

57. Ho, L. C., Wang, C. W., Roy, P., Chang, H. T. (2014). Sensitive and selective gold nanomaterials based optical probes. *J. Chinese Chem. Soc.*, **61**, 163–174.

58. Sivaraman, S. K., Kumar, S., Santhanam, V. (2011). Monodisperse sub-10 nm gold nanoparticles by reversing the order of addition in Turkevich method: the role of chloroauric acid. *J. Colloid Interface Sci.*, **361**, 543–547.

59. Dixit, S., Novak, T., Miller, K., Zhu, Y., Kenney, M. E., Broome, A.-M. (2015). Transferrin receptor-targeted theranostic gold nanoparticles for photosensitizer delivery in brain tumors. *Nanoscale*, **7**, 1782–1790.

60. Sau, T. K., Murphy, C. J. (2004). Room temperature, high-yield synthesis of multiple shapes of gold nanoparticles in aqueous solution. *J. Am. Chem. Soc.*, **126**, 8648–8649.

61. Barbosa, S., Agrawal, A., Rodríguez-Lorenzo, L., Pastoriza-Santos, I., Alvarez-Puebla, R. A., Kornowski, A., Weller, H., Liz-Marzán, L. M. (2010). Tuning size and sensing properties in colloidal gold nanostars. *Langmuir*, **26**, 14943–14950.

62. Lu, L., Ai, K., Ozaki, Y. (2008). Environmentally friendly synthesis of highly monodisperse biocompatible gold nanoparticles with urchin-like shape. *Langmuir*, **24**, 1058–1063.

63. Wáng, Y. X. J., Idée, J. M., Corot, C. (2015). Scientific and industrial challenges of developing nanoparticle-based theranostics and multiple-modality contrast agents for clinical application. *Nanoscale*, **7**, 16146–16150.

64. Xu, C., Sun, S. (2013). New forms of superparamagnetic nanoparticles for biomedical applications. *Adv. Drug Deliv. Rev.*, **65**, 732–743.

65. Bohara, R. A., Thorat, N. D., Pawar, S. H. (2016). Role of functionalization: strategies to explore potential nano-bio applications of magnetic nanoparticles. *RSC Adv.*, **6**, 43989–44012.

66. Wu, W., Wu, Z., Yu, T., Jiang, C., Kim, W.-S. (2015). Recent progress on magnetic iron oxide nanoparticles: synthesis, surface functional strategies and biomedical applications. *Sci. Technol. Adv. Mater.*, **16**, 23501.

67. Laurent, S., Forge, D., Port, M., Roch, A., Robic, C., Elst, L. V., Muller, R. N. (2008). Magnetic iron oxide nanoparticles: synthesis, stabilization, vectorization, physicochemical characterizations, and biological applications. *Chem. Rev.*, **108**, 2064–2110.

68. Roth, H. C., Schwaminger, S. P., Schindler, M., Wagner, F. E., Berensmeier, S. (2015). Influencing factors in the CO-precipitation process of superparamagnetic iron oxide nano particles: a model based study. *J. Magn. Magn. Mater.*, **377**, 81–89.

69. Pušnik, K., Goršak, T., Drofenik, M., Makovec, D. (2016). Synthesis of aqueous suspensions of magnetic nanoparticles with the co-precipitation of iron ions in the presence of aspartic acid. *J. Magn. Magn. Mater.*, **413**, 65–75.

70. Lin, S., Lin, K., Lu, D., Liu, Z. (2017). Preparation of uniform magnetic iron oxide nanoparticles by co-precipitation in a helical module microchannel reactor. *J. Environ. Chem. Eng.*, **5**, 303–309.

71. Girginova, P. I., Daniel-da-Silva, A. L., Lopes, C. B., Figueira, P., Otero, M., Amaral, V. S., Pereira, E., Trindade, T. (2010). Silica coated magnetite particles for magnetic removal of Hg^{2+} from water. *J. Colloid Interface Sci.*, **345**, 234–240.

72. Oliveira-Silva, R., Da Costa, J. P., Vitorino, R., Daniel-Da-Silva, A. L. (2015). Magnetic chelating nanoprobes for enrichment and selective recovery of metalloproteases from human saliva. *J. Mater. Chem. B*, **3**, 238–249.

73. Cheng, W., Xu, X., Wu, F., Li, J. (2016). Synthesis of cavity-containing iron oxide nanoparticles by hydrothermal treatment of colloidal dispersion. *Mater. Lett.*, **164**, 210–212.

74. Gyergyek, S., Makovec, D., Jagodič, M., Drofenik, M., Schenk, K., Jordan, O., Kovač, J., Dražič, G., Hofmann, H. (2017). Hydrothermal growth of iron oxide NPs with a uniform size distribution for magnetically induced hyperthermia: structural, colloidal and magnetic properties. *J. Alloys Compd.*, **694**, 261–271.

75. Bhavani, P., Rajababu, C. H., Arif, M. D., Reddy, I. V. S., Reddy, N. R. (2017). Synthesis of high saturation magnetic iron oxide nanomaterials via low temperature hydrothermal method. *J. Magn. Magn. Mater.*, **426**, 459–466.

76. Jiang, F., Li, X., Zhu, Y., Tang, Z. (2014). Synthesis and magnetic characterizations of uniform iron oxide nanoparticles. *Phys. B Condens. Matter*, **443**, 1–5.

77. Bartůněk, V., Průcha, D., Švecová, M., Ulbrich, P., Huber, Š., Sedmidubský, D., Jankovský, O. (2016). Ultrafine ferromagnetic iron oxide nanoparticles: facile synthesis by low temperature decomposition of iron glycerolate. *Mater. Chem. Phys.*, **180**, 272–278.

78. Gupta, A. K., Gupta, M. (2005). Synthesis and surface engineering of iron oxide nanoparticles for biomedical applications. *Biomaterials*, **26**, 3995–4021.

79. Roca, A. G., Morales, M. P., O'Grady, K., Serna, C. J. (2006). Structural and magnetic properties of uniform magnetite nanoparticles prepared by high temperature decomposition of organic precursors. *Nanotechnology*, **17**, 2783–2788.

80. Maity, D., Choo, S. G., Yi, J., Ding, J., Xue, J. M. (2009). Synthesis of magnetite nanoparticles via a solvent-free thermal decomposition route. *J. Magn. Magn. Mater.*, **321**, 1256–1259.

81. Goya, G. F., Berquó, T. S., Fonseca, F. C., Morales, M. P. (2003). Static and dynamic magnetic properties of spherical magnetite nanoparticles. *J. Appl. Phys.*, **94**, 3520–3528.

82. Mendoza-Garcia, A., Sun, S. (2016). Recent advances in the high-temperature chemical synthesis of magnetic nanoparticles. *Adv. Funct. Mater.*, **26**, 3809–3817.

83. Couto, C., Vitorino, R., Daniel-da-Silva, A. L. (2017). Gold nanoparticles and bioconjugation: a pathway for proteomic applications. *Crit. Rev. Biotechnol.*, **37**, 238–250.

84. da Costa, J. P., Oliveira-Silva, R., Daniel-da-Silva, A. L., Vitorino, R. (2014). Bionanoconjugation for proteomics applications: an overview. *Biotechnol. Adv.*, **32**, 952–970.

85. Erathodiyil, N., Ying, J. Y. (2011). Functionalization of inorganic nanoparticles for bioimaging applications. *Acc. Chem. Res.*, **44**, 925–935.

86. Hola, K., Markova, Z., Zoppellaro, G., Tucek, J., Zboril, R. (2015). Tailored functionalization of iron oxide nanoparticles for MRI, drug delivery, magnetic separation and immobilization of biosubstances. *Biotechnol. Adv.*, **33**, 1162–1176.

87. Bohara, R. A., Thorat, N. D., Pawar, S. H. (2016). Role of functionalization: strategies to explore potential nano-bio applications of magnetic nanoparticles. *RSC Adv.*, **6**, 43989–44012.

88. Sonavane, G., Tomoda, K., Makino, K. (2008). Biodistribution of colloidal gold nanoparticles after intravenous administration: effect of particle size. *Colloids Surf., B*, **66**, 274–280.

89. Pham, B. T. T., Colvin, E. K., Pham, N. T. H., Kim, B. J., Fuller, E. S., Moon, E. A., Barbey, R., Yuen, S., Rickman, B. H., Bryce, N. S., Bickley, S., Tanudji, M., Jones, S. K., Howell, V. M., Hawkett, B. S. (2018). Biodistribution and clearance of stable superparamagnetic maghemite iron oxide nanoparticles in mice following intraperitoneal administration. *Int. J. Mol. Sci.*, **19**, 205.

90. Velasco-Aguirre, C., Morales, F., Gallardo-Toledo, E., Guerrero, S., Giralt, E., Araya, E., Kogan, M. J. (2015). Peptides and proteins used to enhance gold nanoparticle delivery to the brain: preclinical approaches. *Int. J. Nanomed.*, **10**, 4919–4936.

91. Khan, N. U., Miao, T., Ju, X., Guo, Q., Han, L. (2018). Receptor-mediated transportation through BBB, in *Brain Targeted Drug Delivery Systems: A Focus on Nanotechnology and Nanoparticulates*, Gao, H., Gao, X., eds., Academic Press, London, pp. 129–158.

92. Tomitaka, A., Arami, H., Gandhi, S., Krishnan, K. M. (2015). Lactoferrin conjugated iron oxide nanoparticles for targeting brain glioma cells in magnetic particle imaging. *Nanoscale*, **7**, 16890–16898.

93. Betzer, O., Shilo, M., Motiei, M., Popovtzer, R. (2019). Insulin-coated gold nanoparticles as an effective approach for bypassing the blood-brain barrier, in *Proc. SPIE 10891, Nanoscale Imaging, Sensing, and Actuation for Biomedical Applications XVI*, 108911H, p. 52.

94. Lu, C. T., Zhao, Y. Z., Wong, H. L., Cai, J., Peng, L., Tian, X. Q. (2014). Current approaches to enhance CNS delivery of drugs across the brain barriers. *Int. J. Nanomed.*, **9**, 2241–2257.

95. Morshed, R. A., Muroski, M. E., Dai, Q., Wegscheid, M. L., Auffinger, B., Yu, D., Han, Y., Zhang, L., Wu, M., Cheng, Y., Lesniak, M. S. (2016). Cell-penetrating peptide-modified gold Nanoparticles for the delivery of doxorubicin to brain metastatic breast cancer. *Mol. Pharm.*, **13**, 1843–1854.

96. Zhao, X., Shang, T., Zhang, X., Ye, T., Wang, D., Rei, L. (2016). Passage of magnetic Tat-conjugated $Fe_3O_4@SiO_2$ nanoparticles across in vitro blood-brain barrier. *Nanoscale Res. Lett.*, **11**, 451.

97. Wang, C. X., Huang, L. S., Hou, L. B., Jiang, L., Yan, Z. T., Wang, Y. L., Chen, Z. L. (2009). Antitumor effects of polysorbate-80 coated gemcitabine polybutylcyanoacrylate nanoparticles in vitro and its pharmacodynamics in vivo on C6 glioma cells of a brain tumor model. *Brain Res.*, **1261**, 91–99.

98. Gelperina, S., Maksimenko, O., Khalansky, A., Vanchugova, L., Shipulo, E., Abbasova, K., Berdiev, R., Wohlfart, S., Chepurnova, N., Kreuter, J. (2010). Drug delivery to the brain using surfactant-coated poly(lactide-co-glycolide) nanoparticles: influence of the formulation parameters. *Eur. J. Pharm. Biopharm.*, **74**, 157–163.

99. Huang, Y., Zhang, B., Xie, S., Yang, B., Xu, Q., Tan, J. (2016). Superparamagnetic iron oxide nanoparticles modified with Tween 80 pass through the intact blood-brain barrier in rats under magnetic field. *ACS Appl. Mater. Interfaces*, **8**, 11336–11341.

100. Bianco, J., Joudiou, N., Préat, V., Ganipineni, L. P., Bastiancich, C., Zhao, M., Danhier, P., Gallez, B., Danhier, F., Ucakar, B. (2018). Magnetic targeting of paclitaxel-loaded poly(lactic-*co*-glycolic acid)-based nanoparticles for the treatment of glioblastoma. *Int. J. Nanomed.*, **13**, 4509–4521.

101. Yuan, H., Wilson, C. M., Xia, J., Doyle, S. L., Li, S., Fales, A. M., Liu, Y., Ozaki, E., Mulfaul, K., Hanna, G., Palmer, G. M., Wang, L. V., Grant, G. A., Vo-Dinh, T. (2014). Plasmonics-enhanced and optically modulated delivery of gold nanostars into brain tumor. *Nanoscale*, **6**, 4078–4082.

102. Lee, C., Hwang, H. S., Lee, S., Kim, B., Kim, J. O., Oh, K. T., Lee, E. S., Choi, H.-G., Youn, Y. S. (2017). Rabies virus-inspired silica-coated gold nanorods as a photothermal therapeutic platform for treating brain tumors. *Adv. Mater.*, **29**, 1605563(1–8).

103. Schleich, N., Sibret, P., Danhier, P., Ucakar, B., Laurent, S., Muller, R. N., Jérôme, C., Gallez, B., Préat, V., Danhier, F. (2013). Dual anticancer drug/superparamagnetic iron oxide-loaded PLGA-based nanoparticles for cancer therapy and magnetic resonance imaging. *Int. J. Pharm.*, **447**, 94–101.

104. Wu, V. M., Huynh, E., Tang, S., Uskoković, V. (2019). Brain and bone cancer targeting by a ferrofluid composed of superparamagnetic iron-oxide/silica/carbon nanoparticles (earthicles). *Acta Biomater.*, **88**, 422–447.

105. Dan, M., Bae, Y., Pittman, T. A., Yokel, R. A. (2015). Alternating magnetic field-induced hyperthermia increases iron oxide nanoparticle cell association/uptake and flux in blood-brain barrier models. *Pharm. Res.*, **32**, 1615–1625.

106. Gupta, R., Sharma, D. (2019). Evolution of magnetic hyperthermia for glioblastoma multiforme therapy. *ACS Chem. Neurosci.*, **10**, 1157–1172.

Chapter 6

Hybrid Nanosystems

Pablo Vicente Torres-Ortega,[a,b] Laura Saludas,[a,b]
Jon Eneko Idoyaga,[a] Carlos Rodríguez-Nogales,[a,b]
Elisa Garbayo[a,b] and María José Blanco-Prieto[a,b]
[a]*Department of Pharmaceutical Technology and Chemistry, Faculty of Pharmacy and Nutrition, Universidad de Navarra, C/Irunlarrea 1, 31008 Pamplona, Spain*
[b]*Instituto de Investigación Sanitaria de Navarra, IdiSNA, C/Irunlarrea 3, 31008 Pamplona, Spain*
mjblanco@unav.es, egarbayo@unav.es

Treatments aiming to stop the progression of brain-related disorders are often nonspecific and focused on the resolution of short-term symptoms. The delivery of therapeutics across the blood–brain barrier represents another limiting challenge in the treatment of these diseases. Hybrid nanosystems (HNs), defined as the combination of inorganic and organic compounds in a single nanocarrier, offer a new generation of multifunctional nanoparticles (NPs) with superior biological and structural properties. HNs could contribute not only to the design of more effective therapies for brain disorders but also to the development of new theranostic

Nanoparticles for Brain Drug Delivery
Edited by Carla Vitorino, Andreia Jorge and Alberto Pais

ISBN 978-981-4877-31-2 (Hardcover), 978-1-003-11932-6 (eBook)
www.jennystanford.com

strategies which combine therapeutic and diagnostic functions in a single system.

This chapter aims to give an overview of the enormous possibilities offered by HNs providing better diagnostic imaging agents, biosensors to detect specific biomarkers and enhanced targeted therapies for brain disorders. The focus lies on HNs made of an organic component in which an inorganic compound is loaded, and on formulations constituted by an inorganic core functionalised with an organic element. Their main limitations, future perspectives and the need to evaluate their potential on more relevant in vivo models are also discussed.

Specifically, HNs based on inorganic nanomaterials loaded within organic matrices are playing an important role in brain cancers. Metals as imaging agents and cytotoxic drugs have been predominantly combined for simultaneous imaging and treatment of glioma. Furthermore, an enhanced NP tumour accumulation can be obtained by the application of an external magnetic field directed to the tumour site, due to the inherent magnetic properties of these systems. HNs constituted by an inorganic core coated with functional molecules have also allowed the development of promising diagnostic and theragnostic tools for application in brain tumours. In addition, HNs could contribute to stop the progression of diseases such as Parkinson's or Alzheimer's disease, as well as provide new techniques which would make possible an earlier diagnosis of these neurodegenerative pathologies. Finally, HNs are currently being investigated for the visualisation and treatment of ischaemic areas of the brain to achieve an effective reduction of the brain infarcted regions. The evidence found in a large number of studies confirms that HNs are one of the most promising approaches in the quest for new diagnostic and therapeutic alternatives in brain-related disorders.

6.1 Introduction

Hybrid nanosystems (HNs), defined as the combination of inorganic and organic compounds in a single nanocarrier, offer a new generation of multifunctional nanoparticles (NPs) with superior biological and structural properties [1]. The development of sophisticated HNs represents a great opportunity to bring about significant improvements in the field of diagnosis and treatment of brain-related diseases.

From a broad perspective, HNs can be classified into two different categories according to their structure. Firstly, HNs can be constituted by an organic component (e.g. polymer, lipid) in which an inorganic compound is loaded (superparamagnetic iron oxide [SPIO], gold, silver, etc.) (Fig. 1A). Alternatively, HNs may be formed by an inorganic core (usually metallic) functionalised with an organic material (antibodies, peptides, etc.) (Fig. 1B). The development of this new generation of HNs with enhanced features has attracted considerable attention among researchers and clinicians [2]. HNs are highly versatile and offer the possibility of designing their properties carefully in order to adjust them to specific requirements [3]. The combination of inorganic and organic compounds involves the expansion of the theranostic concept, focused on the simultaneous diagnosis and treatment of diseases, by using a unique multifunctional nanocarrier. Furthermore, this kind of nanostructure may possess exceptional features, as some components have proved to exhibit synergistic effects when combined [2].

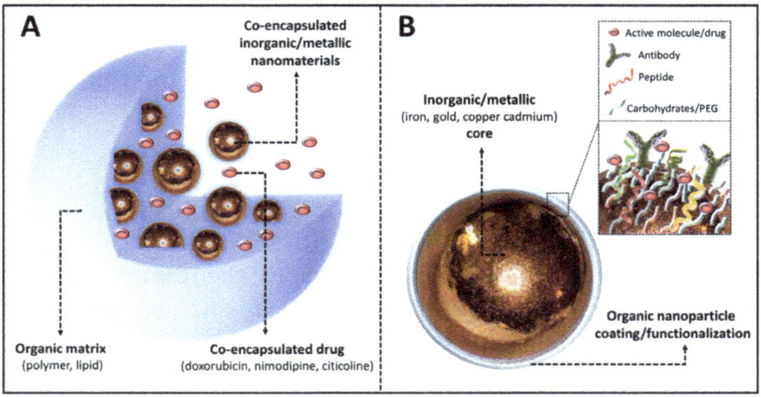

Figure 6.1 Schematic representation of HNs for brain drug delivery and diagnosis. (A) Organic nanomaterials loaded with inorganic materials. (B) Inorganic nanomaterials functionalised with biomolecules.

The field of brain-related disorders has greatly benefited from HNs, paving the way towards precision medicine. For instance, the incorporation of inorganic materials as contrast agents along with chemotherapeutic drugs has revolutionised the in vivo detection of brain tumours and the evaluation of responses to chemotherapeutic treatments. The diagnosis and treatment of brain-related disorders pose a special challenge due to the presence of the blood–brain barrier (BBB) and the extreme sensitivity of the brain tissue to certain molecules and drugs. For this reason, an interesting advantage provided by magnetic HNs is the possibility of directing them to a specific brain area by applying an external magnetic field. Alternation in the application of magnetic fields may increase BBB permeability by magnetic heating, allowing NP passage without damaging this barrier [4], which could be an interesting approach not only in cancer-related strategies but also in neurodegenerative and ischaemic diseases. HNs can be functionalised on their surface with specific antibodies or other ligands in order to attain targeted delivery to a specific tissue. This can improve imaging techniques and avoid peripheral side effects.

In this chapter, we provide an up-to-date framework to explain advances in the field of HNs for brain delivery. In particular, the development and evaluation of HNs for application in brain tumours, neurodegenerative disorders (NDs), and cerebral ischaemia are reviewed and discussed. With this in mind, we focus on HNs made up of an organic component in which an inorganic compound is loaded, and on formulations constituted by an inorganic core functionalised with an organic element.

6.2 Hybrid Nanosystems for Brain Cancer

Brain cancers are neoplasms located in the central nervous system (CNS) characterised by high mortality and poor prognosis. Glioblastoma multiforme (GBM) is the most common and aggressive type among all brain tumours, representing almost 30% of these and 80% of all the malignant ones [5]. Current treatment options are limited in their effectiveness, requiring the development of advanced tumour imaging techniques as well as more effective and less toxic therapeutic strategies [6]. In this regard, HNs may bring new opportunities to improve brain cancer management, overcoming the shortcomings associated with current diagnostic and therapeutic approaches. As shown in Fig. 2A, HNs hold potential for improving the sensitivity and resolution of tumour-imaging agents as well as for increasing chemotherapy efficacy. In fact, there are already Food and Drug Administration (FDA)-approved nanoparticulate systems available for clinical use, such as Feridex (nanosized iron oxide crystals coated with dextran) [7, 8].

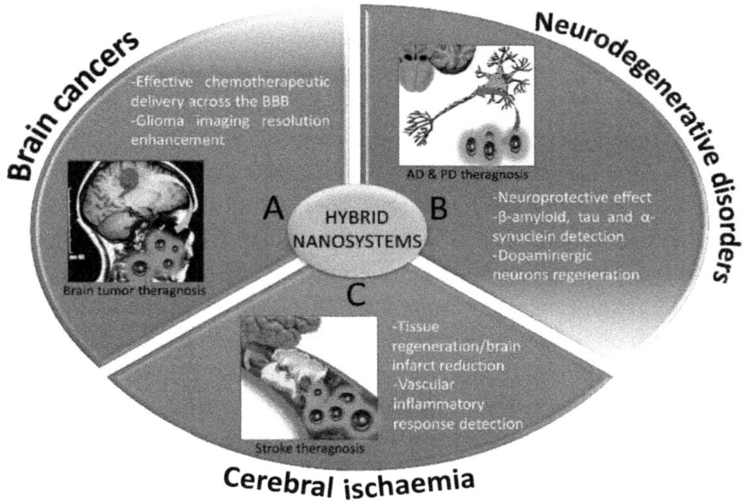

Figure 6.2 Applications of HNs for the management of (A) brain cancers, (B) neurodegenerative disorders and (C) cerebral ischaemia.

HNs based on inorganic nanomaterials incorporated within organic matrices are playing an important role in glioma management. Predominantly, metals as imaging agents and cytotoxic drugs have been co-encapsulated for simultaneous imaging and treatment of glioma. As previously mentioned, enhanced NP tumour accumulation can be obtained by the application of an external magnetic field directed to the tumour site, due to the inherent magnetic properties of these systems. As an example, Zhao et al. took advantage of the magnetic targeting for the site-specific delivery of paclitaxel. For that purpose, Fe_3O_4 ferrofluid and paclitaxel were encapsulated in octadecyl-quaternised carboxymethyl chitosan nanocarriers and the efficacy of the magnetic paclitaxel NPs was evaluated in C6 glioma-bearing rats. Remarkably, an increased median survival rate was observed compared to free paclitaxel after magnetic targeting therapy with the HNs. [9]. Similarly, Ganipineni et al. reported the co-encapsulation of both SPIO and paclitaxel inside poly(lactic-co-glycolic acid) (PLGA)-based NPs for magnetic targeting and treatment. The magnetically focused delivery brought about a significant improvement in the median survival time when these HNs were tested in an orthotopic U87MG glioma-bearing mouse model [10].

Not only iron can be used as an imaging metallic agent for the development of HNs, but so can also other metals such as gold or silver. For example, Zhong et al. utilised Arg-Gly-Asp (RGD)-directed polyethylene glycol (PEG)-b-poly(ε-caprolactone)-lipoic acid ester HNs loaded with gold nanorods (AuNRs) and doxorubicin (DOX) for targeted chemotherapy for glioblastoma. The tumour targetability and therapeutic efficacy of the nanoformulation were evaluated in vivo in U87MG glioma-bearing xenograft mice by labelling the NPs with Cy7, a fluorescent compound which allows the in vivo monitoring of the nanoformulation in the tumour. Fluorescence imaging showed significant tumour accumulation of the cRGD-directed NPs compared to non cRGD-directed formulations. Moreover, NPs in combination with near infrared irradiation exhibited complete tumour growth inhibition with lower side effects than free DOX [11]. Regarding the use of gold as an imaging agent, Song et al. designed hybrid reduced graphene oxide-loaded ultrasmall plasmonic gold nanorod vesicles (rGO-AuNRVe) loaded with DOX. This formulation was tested in U87MG tumour-bearing mice showing effective tumour growth inhibition after low-power-density 808 nm laser irradiation due to the combination of both chemo- and photothermal therapies. Moreover, positron emission tomography (PET) evidenced a large amount of ^{64}Cu-labeled rGO-AuNRVe-DOX in the U87MG tumour with strong photoacoustic signal in the tumour area, which suggests a synergistic effect of photothermal therapy with controlled release of the chemotherapeutic agent [12]. By using a similar approach, Locatelli et al. reported the use of silver as a cytotoxic agent against glioblastoma in combination with the drug alisertib. Both compounds were encapsulated in polymeric NPs and conjugated with the tumour targeting agent chlorotoxin to obtain theranostic nanodevices. An enhanced imaging capacity and tumour reduction were observed when tested in U87MG tumour-bearing mice, which indicates a suitable therapeutic delivery of the cytotoxic compounds in the tumour tissue compared to formulations containing just silver [13].

Many studies have also focused on exploring the potential of HNs formed by an inorganic core coated with functional molecules in brain cancer. Iron oxide NPs (IONPs) and quantum dots (QDs) can be found within this type of nanosystem. In most cases, these formulations led to the development of promising diagnostic tools for application in brain tumours. In this regard, Tomanek et al. determined the accumulation of a targeted contrast agent in tumour vessels using a GBM mouse model. In this case, SPIO coated with dextran and functionalised with anti-insulin-like-growth-factor binding protein 7 single-domain antibody was synthesised. For the in vivo fluorescence follow up study, a near infrared marker (Cy5.5) was also attached to the formulation, and a GBM-targeted contrast agent was obtained. The formulation was administered to U87MGdEGFRvIII tumour-bearing nude mice, leading to HN accumulation in the tumour, as demonstrated by in vivo imaging techniques and magnetic resonance imaging (MRI). These results confirmed that HNs were able to selectively bind to abnormal vessels within a glioblastoma [14]. Nevertheless, this approach needs to be further explored in order to find the optimal pulse sequence for the superparamagnetic-based contrast agent of GBM MRI at the high field. Similarly, Veiseh et al. synthesised a diagnostic nanoprobe consisting of an IONP coated with a biocompatible polymer-based layer of PEG-grafted chitosan, chlorotoxin and near infrared fluorophore (Cy5.5). The MRI capacity of the nanoprobe was tested in transgenic ND2:SmoA1 mice generated on a C57BL/6 background, showing an enhanced contrast on tumour areas of the brain due to the accumulation of the nanoprobe on damaged tissues compared to tumour-free areas of the brain. These results evidenced a high chlorotoxin tumour-targeting capacity and selectivity. Furthermore, the safe BBB-crossing ability of the nanoprobe was also studied, showing an innocuous toxicity profile [15]. Chlorotoxin-labelled magnetic nanovectors were also prepared by Kievit et al. for targeted gene delivery to glioma and for diagnostic purposes [16]. The developed nanovector consisted of an IONP core coated with a copolymer of PEG, chitosan and polyethylenimine. Green fluorescent protein (GFP) encoding DNA and chlorotoxin was attached to this nanovector for optical monitoring of the gene expression and for NP targeting, respectively. In vivo gene delivery was tested on mice bearing C6 xenograft flank tumours. MRI showed the accumulation of nanovectors in the tumour site, whereas the increase in GFP expression on the tumour cells revealed an enhanced nanovector uptake into the cancer cells due to the chlorotoxin [16]. This study offers an interesting point of view on glioma diagnosis. However, further studies should consider the use of an autograft glioma model to evaluate the therapeutic efficacy of the formulation on a clinically relevant glioma model and to prove safety regarding the BBB. The combination of this imaging tool with a chemotherapeutic agent should also be considered for the development of a theragnostic platform.

Other HNs such as bioconjugated QDs have been used for glioma diagnosis. QD are semiconductor particles with a diameter of less than 10 nm, which consist of a cadmium selenide core and a zinc selenide cap with size-dependent electronic and optical properties. As they can emit bright colours, they are used in biological research as fluorescence imaging tools [17]. Interestingly, Veeranarayanan et al. synthesised luminescent single cadmium sulphide (CdS) QD-encapsulated silica NPs which were directed for precision optical bioimaging. CD31 antibody was conjugated to these QDs to obtain a targeted effect. In vitro imaging testing was carried out in both human umbilical vein endothelial cells and in a brain cancer cell line of glioma (G1-1), while the in vivo imaging was performed on medaka fish embryos. In vitro testing showed that both silica-coated and bare QDs exerted no significant cytotoxic effects on endothelial cells, suggesting the safety and biocompatibility of the formulation as a labelling probe. Moreover, in vivo imaging with QDs confirmed the increased biocompatibility of the silica-coated QDs compared to bare QDs as well as their safety and imaging capacity [18]. Similarly, Guo et al. developed intrinsically radioactive [^{64}Cu]CuInS/ZnS QDs for PET and optical imaging of glioma. This formulation was obtained by direct incorporation of ^{64}Cu into CuInS/ZnS nanostructure with $^{64}CuCl_2$ as the synthesis precursor. They were PEGylated in situ obtaining PEGylated radioactive QDs which were then tested in vivo for imaging and biodistribution studies in a xenograft model of human U87 glioblastoma tumour-bearing mice. Importantly, the results provided evidence of high tumour uptake of the formulation and efficient PET/self-illuminating luminescence imaging capacity [19]. The next step should consist of testing the efficacy of the HN in an autograft glioma model which mimics the physiological characteristics of the disease.

Finally, as an example of a theragnostic tool against glioma based on micelles, Groult et al. developed micellar IONPs which were coated through micellation with bioactive glycosides (GC22, IG20 and TFA-GC22). The magnetic and relaxation properties of the HNs were evaluated in vitro showing the suitable values for T2-weighted MRI-based contrast agents. Moreover, the TFA-GC22 coated IONP micelles showed the most promising antitumour activity when tested in the C6 rat glioma cell line [20]. Further in vivo studies will be needed to validate these proof-of principle studies with nanomicellar formulations.

In summary, all the advances described above indicate that HNs hold promise for precise management of glioma and other brain tumours.

6.3 Hybrid Nanosystems for Neurodegenerative Disorders

NDs are a set of diseases characterised by neuronal loss, synaptic dysfunction and the presence of brain deposits of poorly folded proteins [21]. The most common symptoms associated with NDs are the loss of memory and motor and cognitive disability [22]. Alzheimer's disease (AD) and Parkinson's disease (PD) are nowadays the most prevalent NDs. The aging population and the longer lifespan make these pathologies one of the highest challenges of the modern medicine of the 21st century. Moreover, current therapies are only focused on symptomatic aspects of the disease and not on curing or delaying the progression of these pathologies. Besides this problem, there are no techniques able to achieve an early diagnosis [23]. By taking advantage of the characteristics mentioned above, nanomedicine is working on the development of formulations able to cross the BBB, and on new diagnostic techniques [24, 25]. In this regard, HNs may offer novel avenues in the diagnosis and treatment of NDs. As shown in Fig. 6.2B, HNs are currently being investigated for diagnostic imaging of AD and PD, as well as for neuroprotection and tissue repair.

6.3.1 Hybrid Nanosystems for Alzheimer's Disease

Some strategies have recently been developed to explore the potential of HNs based on inorganic nanomaterials combined with organic matrices in neuroprotective treatments for AD. For instance, magnetic particles produced by magnetospirillum bacteria conjugated to carbon nanotubes have demonstrated tremendous potential for AD treatment [26]. These hybrids have a neuroprotective effect due to their intrinsic peroxidase-like catalytic activity, which reduces the reactive oxygen species formation, and also thanks to their capacity to inhibit the formation of β-amyloid when interfering with AB peptides in the Aβ fibril-induced neurotoxic conditions in SH-SY5Y cells [26].

Recent studies have also shown promise using HNs based on an inorganic core functionalised with different organic ligands for AD diagnosis and treatment. In particular, Cheng et al. worked on the development of SPIO NPs functionalised with curcumin, due to the ability of this compound to specifically bind to amyloid plaques. Using this strategy, authors were able to detect the presence of amyloid plaques ex vivo by MRI in the rat brain. Immunohistochemistry analysis confirmed that NPs were localised next to the amyloid plaques, demonstrating the high potential of such tool for AD diagnosis [27]. More interesting is the development of HNs compatible with surface-enhanced Raman spectroscopy (SERS) to detect the presence of AD's own biomarkers. SERS is a vibrational spectroscopy technique used for investigating the complexity of analytic molecules in various fields, such as chemistry and medical sciences. Demeritte et al. devised a magnetic-plasmonic nanoplatform by conjugating iron oxide core–gold plasmonic shell NPs on graphene oxide conjugated with anti-β-amyloid and anti-tau antibodies. These HNs were able to selectively detect both biomarkers in suspensions of citrated whole rabbit blood infected with tau and β amyloid proteins, and to detect β amyloid and tau protein in concentrations as low as 100 fg/ml using SERS technology [28]. Furthermore, the recent demonstration that magnetic-fluorescent Fe_2O_3 NPs loaded with rhodamine or red Congo can detect amyloid-β fibrils and remove them holds great promise for early AD diagnosis. The developed NPs were able to join the $A\beta_{40}$ fibrils synthesised in vitro and could be later detected by MRI and fluorescence microscopy. The removal of $A\beta_{40}$ fibrils was possible due to the application of a magnetic field. These NPs have been successfully investigated in vitro as multimodal imaging agents showing a tremendous potential based on the combination of magnetic properties and fluorescence imaging in one hybrid nanocarrier [29]. Alternatively, QDs offer unique opportunities to develop new strategies for ND theragnosis due to their excellent optical and electronic properties [30]. In this regard, cadmium-selenide/zinc sulphide (CdSe@ZnS) QDs can be used to develop an immunocomplex microarray to detect the AD biomarker apolipoprotein E by excitement of visible light. The efficacy of this assay was proven using ELISA, showing high sensitivity and acceptable precision [31]. This study could serve as an example to support the use of QDs as microarrays for the detection of proteins associated with neurodegenerative pathologies in complex protein mixtures.

HNs based on inorganic nanomaterials functionalised with organic compounds have also demonstrated promising applications in AD treatment. With the purpose of achieving neuroprotection in an AD Aβ1–42 mouse model, Ali et al. designed gold NPs loaded with anthocyanin [32]. These hybrid NPs showed higher efficacy than free anthocyanin against the neurotoxicity induced by Aβ1–42, which was associated with an improvement in the bioavailability and a sustained drug release. Functionally, NPs exerted a neuroprotective effect through the regulation of routes implied in neuroprotection, neuronal survival and neuronal synapse [32]. Another interesting approach is the functionalisation of nanosystems with peptides which provide a high BBB permeability. As an example, Yin et al. showed that sialic acid-modified selenium NPs coated with B6 peptide have tremendous potential in AD [33]. In vitro studies proved that these NPs were able to cross the BBB and were effective against Aß fibrillation. Moreover, they also proved to be effective in decreasing Aß-induced cytotoxicity, in inhibiting Aß aggregation and in disaggregating Aß fibrils [33]. Relatedly, Nday et al. focused on the oxidative stress produced by metallic species such as Cu (II) in AD. To obtain hybrid NPs with antioxidant potential, hybrid silica NPs modified with PEG or cetyltrimethylammonium bromide (CTAB) and loaded with the natural flavonoid quercetin (QC) were developed. The QC-PEG NPs produced a slightly better neuronal cell survival than QC-CTAB NPs. Moreover, the potential of those systems was evaluated in vitro showing antioxidant protective effects of QC against the oxidative stress mediated by Cu (II) [34]. Of particular interest was the investigation of the effectiveness of ceria-containing uncoated and coated hydroxyapatite-based galantamine in ovariectomised AD albino rats, which showed histological improvements with recovery of cerebral neurons and disappearance of amyloid plaques [35].

6.3.2 Hybrid Nanosystems for Parkinson's Disease

The use of HNs based on magnetic NPs incorporated within an organic matrix is attractive for PD treatment. For example, Ji et al. developed an interesting strategy based on Fe_3O_4 magnetic nanoliposomes loaded with nimodipine [36]. In this study, magnetic NPs demonstrated unique properties to guide these nanoliposomes to the targeted tissue by the application of an external magnetic field [36]. In addition, authors incorporated into the study a diagnostic value known as fractional anisotropy (FA), which is a useful measure of brain connectivity [37]. It was previously shown that the FA values measured by MRI may be related to microstuctural changes which happen in the *substantia nigra* [38]. Ji et al. observed a higher FA value and number of positive TH cells after intraperitoneal administration of the magnetic nanoliposomes in the 6-hydroxydopamine (6-OHDA) PD rat model compared to the free nimodipine and control groups [36]. Along similar lines, other studies have found a decrease in the FA associated with dopaminergic neuron loss [39, 40]. These results support the point that these HNs have a significant potential to cross the BBB and to provide a neuroprotective effect, constituting a promising targeting therapy for PD.

Efforts have also focused on the development of PD diagnostic tools using inorganic nanomaterials functionalised with biomolecules. In this regard, the development of functionalised hybrid NPs used as reactive for immunomagnetic reduction (IMR) assays has been investigated. For instance, Fe_3O_4 NPs functionalised with antibodies against α-synuclein were useful to quantify α-synuclein at ultralow concentrations in human plasma using an ultrasensitive IMR assay by correlating the signal obtained with a concentration of α-synuclein. This assay found clear differences in α-synuclein plasma concentration between healthy patients, patients suffering from PD and patients suffering from parkinsonian dementia. [41]. However, more research is needed to establish an IMR assay combined with functionalised hybrid NPs as an effective and accurate method to quantify plasmatic biomarkers such as α-synuclein. More recently, a further step toward PD diagnosis was reported based on α-synuclein immunoquantification by surface-based fluorescence intensity distribution analysis assay (sFIDA). To this end, α-synuclein NPs of silica were developed with a size within the established ranges of oligomers of α-synuclein and with a high number of epitopes. This approach validated the developed NPs as a calibration standard in the detection and quantification of α-synuclein in cerebrospinal fluid [42]. These advances can help us to determine whether the quantification of this biomarker is useful or not for PD diagnosis. In another interesting example, an NP-based biobarcode strategy for PD diagnosis was reported [43]. This technology is based on the use of sensors encoded with multifunctional oligonucleotides modified with a detection antibody, magnetic particles functionalised with a capture antibody and a DNA detection method. In this study, gold NPs were conjugated with a dopamine antibody and with double-stranded DNA [44]. These HNs were used in an immunoassay to detect dopamine by SERS able to detect dopamine in the *midbrain* and *striatum* of 1-methyl-4-phenyl-1,2,3,6-tetrahydropyridine (MPTP)-treated mice, finding that dopamine Raman intensity decreased by 56.77% and 61.12% on days 7 and 21, respectively [43]. Although this seems to be an effective method to detect the dopamine loss produced by MPTP in mice, the success of this bio-barcode strategy will depend on its ability to detect pathological changes in dopamine levels in early stages of PD in humans with high accuracy.

Finally, within this group of HNs based on inorganic nanomaterials functionalised with biomolecules, there is a study devoted to PD treatment which seeks to modify the expression of key PD proteins using superparamagnetic NPs functionalised with nerve growth factor and combined with interfering RNA [45]. The intraperitoneal injection of the HN provided an effective repair in a PD mouse model, being able to slow dopaminergic neuron degeneration, to increase TH expression and to downregulate α-synuclein expression [45].

Together, these examples highlight the potential of HNs to lead exciting breakthroughs in the diagnosis and treatment of ND.

6.4 Hybrid Nanosystems for Cerebral Ischaemia

Stroke is the second leading cause of death worldwide. Early confirmation of the diagnosis allows the prompt delivery of appropriate treatment, which is generally based on the administration of thrombolytic agents such as tissue plasminogen activator or antiplatelet drugs combined with neuroprotective molecules such as memantine or citicoline. In this perspective, neuroimaging techniques based on nanotechnology may allow marked progress in stroke treatment and prevention, HN carrier systems being particularly relevant [46, 47]. As shown in Fig. 2C, HNs are currently being investigated for the visualisation of the stroke-affected areas and the effective reduction of the brain infarcted regions.

Many of the studies performed to date have investigated the use of HNs constituted by an organic nanovehicle in which an inorganic compound is loaded. A good example is the development of CdSe@ZnS/ZnS QDs loaded in polymeric micelles for stroke imaging. In this study, a fluorescence imaging probe for targeted diagnosis acidic pathological areas was prepared through self-assembly of QDs and pH-responsive methoxy polyethylene glycol-poly-(B-amino ester/amidoamine)-dodecylamine multiblock copolymers. Interestingly, the micelle state was retained at physiological pH, whereas QDs were released in response to low pH and targeted imaging. The in vivo fluorescence imaging analysis performed in a rat model of cerebral ischaemia confirmed that this system can be employed as a pH-triggerable targeting imaging probe for stroke detection [48]. Within this group of studies based on an organic vehicle comprising an inorganic structure, other studies have focused on developing theranostic hybrid nanoplatforms for simultaneous visualisation of the penumbra area and for the administration of neuroprotective drugs. For instance, the development of anti-HSP72 vectorised stealth cholesterol/DSPC immunoliposomes containing rhodamine or gadolinium as imaging probes and citicoline as neuroprotective agent were reported by Agulla et al. [49]. HSP72 protein is specifically expressed in at-risk tissue up to 7-days following ischaemia and is therefore, a suitable biomarker of the peri-infarct region in the ischaemic brain. Interestingly, 80% of vectorised liposomes were located on the peripheral of the ischaemic lesion. Moreover, animals treated with citicoline loaded-liposomes presented lesion volumes up to 30% smaller than animals treated with the non-encapsulated drug, which demonstrated the potential which nanotechnology offers in cases of stroke. In another study, Feczkó et al. developed theranostic albumin nanocarriers loaded with nerve growth factor and ultrasmall particles of iron oxide (USPIO). The NP surface was functionalised with apolipoprotein E to facilitate active transport into the brain. When tested in an in vivo rat model of stroke, the nanocarrier was able to decrease infarct size compared to control vehicle [50]. Therefore, multifunctional hybrid NPs could be considered as potential theranostic agents for stroke.

Modification of inorganic nanomaterials with biomolecules has also been used to enhance the imaging properties of contrast agents. For example, dextran iron-oxide NPs targeted with P-selectin binding peptide were investigated to visualise endothelial activation in post-stroke neuroinflammation [51]. The contrast agent developed successfully detected endothelial activation in a mouse model of cerebral ischaemia. Another example of a hybrid nanoplatform for in vivo inflammation detection was used by S.I. van Kasteren et al. who explored the possibility of using carbohydrate-functionalised NPs for direct detection of the endothelial markers E-/P-selectin in a clinically-relevant model of stroke. Conjugating carbohydrates to NPs helped specifically to target transmembrane proteins overexpressed in early brain inflammation, which may prove very useful for the pre-symptomatic diagnosis and treatment of brain diseases [52]. In another study, a nanohybrid tool based on the conjugation of a peptide which targets vascular cell adhesion molecule-1 to USPIO NPs was developed to detect the vascular inflammatory response by MRI [53]. Finally, although most of the studies to date have been focused on neuroprotection, we should note the use of HNs for clot visualisation and dissolution. In this regard, the use of a computed tomography imaging agent based on glycol-chitosan coated gold NPs conjugated with fibrin-targeting peptides for cerebral thromboembolism visualisation and imaging guided-thrombolytic therapy has been reported. The HNs allowed the effective detection and quantification of the cerebral thrombi and the monitoring of the tissue plasminogen activator-mediated thrombolytic effect in a mouse model of embolic stroke [54]. In summary, it is therefore evident that HNs may offer improved options for stroke management.

6.5 Conclusions

Over the past few years, the area of brain-related disorders has experienced great advances. However, the lack of early diagnostic tools and effective treatments remains an important problem. This chapter highlights the tremendous possibilities offered by HNs to bring new opportunities in the form of better diagnostic imaging agents, biosensors to detect specific biomarkers and enhanced targeted therapies. In this regard, the most popular inorganic component used to develop HNs is iron. Nevertheless, other inorganic materials have also been used, such as gold, silver, cadmium, copper and silica. The wide variety of materials and hybrid NPs systems which could be used for the treatment of brain diseases allows us to see how versatile this approach is to achieve effective treatment for these diseases.

In the case of HNs for brain cancer theragnosis, some studies demonstrate that their use as magnetic targeting agents is of particular importance. Magnetic targeting of NPs to the tumour site has resulted in a raised NP tumour accumulation, with a significant increase of median survival in some animal models. In the area of NDs, the development of HNs provides several advantages for the treatment of this set of diseases. These systems are an effective strategy to ensure the passage of the drugs through the BBB and to allow their controlled release. In addition, the functionalisation of nanomaterials with specific biomolecules able to interact with endogenous receptors in the BBB could be a useful strategy for this purpose. Furthermore, HNs used for the detection of specific PD and AD biomarkers hold great promise for the development of new diagnostic techniques in the future. Promisingly, HNs could also represent suitable systems for stroke detection, as well as for the design of new effective therapeutics.

Despite the promising future of HNs, this technology is still at a premature stage and further studies should demonstrate its efficacy on more accurate in vivo models before its translation to clinical trials. Furthermore, the relative toxicity of inorganic compounds is still one of the main concerns for the use of these systems in brain-related disorders and rigorous evaluation of the possible toxicity and negative effects associated with these systems is necessary [55]. Approaches to develop reproducible methodologies and feasible scale-up synthesis of hybrid nanomaterials are also needed. A regulatory framework should also be defined in order to progress in this technology. Therefore, further efforts should be focused on the development of suitable specific guidelines able to harmonise related issues with safety, efficacy evaluation and manufacturing processes.

Finally, the growing interest and the abundant evidence found in a large number of studies confirm that HNs are one of the most promising approaches in the quest for new diagnostic and therapeutic alternatives in brain-related disorders.

Acknowledgements

P. Torres thanks the Spanish Ministry of Education (programa FPU (FPU17/01212)) and L. Saludas 'Asociación de Amigos de la Universidad de Navarra' and 'Obra Social la Caixa' for the fellowship grants.

References

1. Yao, H.-B., Gao, M.-R., Yu, S.-H. (2010). Small organic molecule templating synthesis of organic–inorganic hybrid materials: their nanostructures and properties. *Nanoscale*, **2**, 323–334.
2. Nguyen, K. T., Zhao, Y. (2015). Engineered hybrid nanoparticles for on-demand diagnostics and therapeutics. *Acc. Chem. Res.*, **48**(12), 3016–3025.
3. Li, M., Luo, Z., Zhao, Y. (2016). Hybrid nanoparticles as drug carriers for controlled chemotherapy of cancer. *Chem. Rec.*, **16**, 1833–1851.
4. D'Agata, F., Ruffinatti, F. A., Boschi, S., Stura, I., Rainero, I., Abollino, O., Cavalli, R., Guiot, C. (2017). Magnetic nanoparticles in the central nervous system: targeting principles, applications and safety issues. *Molecules*, **23**, 9.
5. Weller, M., Wick, W., Aldape, K., Brada, M., Berger, M., Pfister, S. M., Nishikawa, R., Rosenthal, M., Wen, P. Y., Stupp, R., Reifenberger, G. (2015). Glioma. *Nat. Rev. Dis. Prim.*, **1**, 1–18.
6. Nie, S., Xing, Y., Kim, G. J., Simons, J. W. (2007). Nanotechnology applications in cancer. *Annu. Rev. Biomed. Eng.*, **9**, 257–288.
7. Pillai, G. (2014). Nanomedicines for cancer therapy: an update of FDA approved and those under various stages of development. *SOJ Pharm. Pharm. Sci.*, **1**(2), 13.

8. Ventola, C. L. (2017). Progress in nanomedicine: approved and investigational nanodrugs. *P T*, **42**, 742–755.
9. Zhao, M., Liang, C., Li, A., Chang, J. I. N., Wang, H., Yan, R., Zhang, J., Tai, J. (2010). Magnetic paclitaxel nanoparticles inhibit glioma growth and improve the survival of rats bearing glioma xenografts. *Anticancer Res.*, **30**, 2217–2224.
10. Ganipineni, L. P., Ucakar, B., Joudiou, N., Bianco, J., Danhier, P., Danhier, F. (2018). Magnetic targeting of paclitaxel-loaded poly(lactic-co-glycolic acid)-based nanoparticles for the treatment of glioblastoma. *Int. J. Nanomed.*, **13**, 4509–4521.
11. Zhong, Y., Wang, C., Cheng, R., Cheng, L., Meng, F., Liu, Z., Zhong, Z. (2014). cRGD-directed, NIR-responsive and robust AuNR/PEG–PCL hybrid nanoparticles for targeted chemotherapy of glioblastoma in vivo. *J. Control. Release*, **195**, 63–71.
12. Song, J., Yang, X., Jacobson, O., Lin, L., Huang, P., Niu, G., Ma, Q., Chen, X. (2017). Sequential drug release and enhanced photothermal and photoacoustic effect of hybrid reduced graphene oxide-loaded ultrasmall gold nanorod vesicles for cancer therapy. *ACS Nano*, **9**, 9199–9209.
13. Locatelli, E., Naddaka, M., Uboldi, C., Loudos, G., Fragogeorgi, E., Molinario, V., Pucci, A., Tsotakos, T., Psimadas, D., Ponti, J., Franchini, M. C. (2014). Targeted delivery of silver nanoparticles and alisertib: in vitro and in vivo synergistic effect against glioblastoma. *Nanomedicine*, **9**, 839–849.
14. Tomanek, B., Iqbal, U., Blasiak, B., Abulrob, A., Albaghdadi, H., Matyas, J. R., Ponjevic, D., Sutherland, G. R. (2012). Evaluation of brain tumor vessels specific contrast agents for glioblastoma imaging. *Neuro. Oncol.*, **14**, 53–63.
15. Veiseh, O., Sun, C., Fang, C., Bhattarai, N., Gunn, J., Kievit, F., Du, K., Pullar, B., Lee, D., Ellenbogen, R. G., Olson, J., Zhang, M. (2009). Specific targeting of brain tumors with an optical/MR imaging nanoprobe across the blood brain barrier. *Cancer Res.*, **69**, 6200–6207.
16. Kievit, F. M., Veiseh, O., Fang, C., Bhattarai, N., Lee, D., Ellenbogen, R. G., Zhang, M. (2010). Chlorotoxin labeled magnetic nanovectors for targeted gene delivery to glioma. *ACS Nano*, **4**, 4587–4594.
17. Wang, E. C., Wang, A. Z. (2014). Nanoparticles and their applications in cell and molecular biology. *Integr Biol.*, **6**, 9–26.
18. Veeranarayanan, S., Poulose, A. C., Mohamed, M. S., Nagaoka, Y., Iwai, S., Nagakame, Y., Kashiwada, S., Yoshida, Y., Maekawa, T., Kumar, D. S.

(2012). Synthesis and application of luminescent single CdS quantum dot encapsulated silica nanoparticles directed for precision optical bioimaging. *Int. J. Nanomed.*, **7**, 3769–3786.

19. Guo, W., Sun, X., Jacobson, O., Yan, X., Min, K., Srivatsan, A., Niu, G., Kiesewetter, D. O., Chang, J., Chen, X. (2015). Intrinsically radioactive [^{64}Cu]CuInS/ZnS quantum dots for PET and optical imaging: improved radiochemical stability and controllable cerenkov luminesecence. *ACS Nano*, **9**, 488–495.
20. Groult, H., García-Álvarez, I., Romero-Ramírez, L., Nieto-Sampedro, M., Herranz, F., Fernández-Mayoralas, A., Ruiz-Cabello, J. (2018). Micellar iron oxide nanoparticles coated with anti-tumor glycosides. *Nanomaterials*, **8**, 1–14.
21. Ramanathan, S., Archunan, G., Sivakumar, M., Tamil Selvan, S., Fred, A. L., Kumar, S., Gulyás, B., Padmanabhan, P. (2018). Theranostic applications of nanoparticles in neurodegenerative disorders. *Int. J. Nanomed.*, **13**, 5561–5576.
22. Gitler, A. D., Dhillon, P., Shorter, J. (2017). Neurodegenerative disease: models, mechanisms, and a new hope. *Dis. Model. Mech.*, **10**, 499–502.
23. Del Rey, N. L.-G., Quiroga-Varela, A., Garbayo, E., Carballo-Carbajal, I., Fernández-Santiago, R., Monje, M. H. G., Trigo-Damas, I., Blanco-Prieto, M. J., Blesa, J. (2018). Advances in Parkinson's disease: 200 years later. *Front. Neuroanat.*, **12**, 113.
24. Torres-Ortega, P. V., Saludas, L., Hanafy, A. S., Garbayo, E., Blanco-Prieto, M. J., (2019). Micro- and nanotechnology approaches to improve Parkinson's disease therapy. *J. Control. Release*, **295**, 201–213.
25. Garbayo, E., Mendoza, A., Blanco-Prieto, M. (2014). Diagnostic and therapeutic uses of nanomaterials in the brain. *Curr. Med. Chem.*, **21**, 4100–4131.
26. Shin, J., Lee, S., Cha, M. (2017). Neuroprotective effect of single-wall carbon nanotubes with built-in peroxidase-like activity against β-amyloid-induced neurotoxicity. *Medchemcomm*, **8**, 625–632.
27. Cheng, K. K., Chan, P. S., Fan, S., Kwan, S. M., Yeung, K. L., Wáng, Y. X. J., Chow, A. H. L., Wu, E. X., Baum, L. (2015). Curcumin-conjugated magnetic nanoparticles for detecting amyloid plaques in Alzheimer's disease mice using magnetic resonance imaging (MRI). *Biomaterials*, **44**, 155–172.
28. Demeritte, T., Priya Viraka Nellore, B., Kanchanapally, R., Sekhar Sinha, S., Pramanik, A., Reddy Chavva, S., Chandra Ray, P. (2015). Hybrid graphene oxide based plasmonic-magnetic multifunctional

nanoplatform for selective separation and label-free identification of Alzheimer's disease biomarkers HHS public access. *ACS Appl. Mater. Interfaces*, **7**, 13693–13700.

29. Skaat, H., Margel, S. (2009). Synthesis of fluorescent-maghemite nanoparticles as multimodal imaging agents for amyloid-β fibrils detection and removal by a magnetic field. *Biochem. Biophys. Res. Commun.*, **386**, 645–649.
30. Matea, C. T., Mocan, T., Tabaran, F., Pop, T., Mosteanu, O., Puia, C., Iancu, C., Mocan, L. (2017). Quantum dots in imaging, drug delivery and sensor applications. *Int. J. Nanomed.*, **12**, 5421–5431.
31. Morales-Narvaéz, E., Montón, H. M., Fomicheva, A., Merkoç, A. (2012). Signal enhancement in antibody microarrays using quantum dots nanocrystals: application to potential Alzheimer's disease biomarker screening. *Anal. Chem.*, **84**, 6821–6827.
32. Ali, T., Kim, M. J., Rehman, S. U., Ahmad, A., Kim, M. O. (2017). Anthocyanin-loaded PEG-gold nanoparticles enhanced the neuroprotection of anthocyanins in an Aβ1-42 mouse model of Alzheimer's disease. *Mol. Neurobiol.*, **54**, 6490–6506.
33. Yin, T., Yang, L., Liu, Y., Zhou, X. Sun, J., Liu, J. (2015). Sialic acid (SA)-modified selenium nanoparticles coated with a high blood-brain barrier permeability peptide-B6 peptide for potential use in Alzheimer's disease. *Acta Biomater.*, **25**, 172–183.
34. Nday, C. M., Halevas, E., Jackson, G. E., Salifoglou, A. (2015). Quercetin encapsulation in modified silica nanoparticles: potential use against Cu(II)-induced oxidative stress in neurodegeneration. *J. Inorg. Biochem.*, **145**, 51–64.
35. Wahba, S. M. R., Darwish, A. S., Kamal, S. M. (2016). Ceria-containing uncoated and coated hydroxyapatite-based galantamine nanocomposites for formidable treatment of Alzheimer's disease in ovariectomized albino-rat model. *Mater. Sci. Eng. C*, **65**, 151–163.
36. Ji, B., Wang, M., Gao, D., Xing, S., Li, L., Liu, L., Zhao, M., Qi, X., Dai, K. (2017). Combining nanoscale magnetic nimodipine liposomes with magnetic resonance image for Parkinson's disease targeting therapy. *Nanomedicine*, **12**, 237–253.
37. Grieve, S. M., Williams, L. M., Paul, R. H., Clark, C. R. Gordon, E. (2007). Cognitive aging, executive function, and fractional anisotropy: a diffusion tensor MR imaging study. *Am. J. Neuroradiol.*, **28**, 226–235.
38. Spalletta, G., Pontieri, F. E., Piras, F., Péran, P., Stefani, A., Peppe, A., Démonet, J.-F., Celsis, P., Rascol, O., Assogna, F., Quattrocchi, C.,

Cherubini, A., Sabatini, U., Pierantozzi, M., Caltagirone, C. (2010). Magnetic resonance imaging markers of Parkinson's disease nigrostriatal signature. *Brain*, **133**, 3423–3433.

39. Soria, G., Aguilar, E., Tudela, R., Mullol, J., Planas, A. M., Marin, C. (2011). In vivo magnetic resonance imaging characterization of bilateral structural changes in experimental Parkinson's disease: a T2 relaxometry study combined with longitudinal diffusion tensor imaging and manganese-enhanced magnetic resonance imaging in the 6-hydroxydopamine rat model. *Eur. J. Neurosci.*, **33**, 1551–1560.
40. Boska, M. D., Hasan, K. M., Kibuule, D., Banerjee, R., McIntyre, E., Nelson, J. A., Hahn, T., Gendelman, H. E., Mosley, R. L. (2007). Quantitative diffusion tensor imaging detects dopaminergic neuronal degeneration in a murine model of Parkinson's disease. *Neurobiol. Dis.*, **26**, 590–596.
41. Yang, S.-Y., Chiu, M.-J., Lin, C.-H., Horng, H.-E., Yang, C.-C., Chieh, J.-J., Chen, H.-H., Liu, B.-H. (2016). Development of an ultra-high sensitive immunoassay with plasma biomarker for differentiating Parkinson disease dementia from Parkinson disease using antibody functionalized magnetic nanoparticles. *J. Nanobiotechnol.*, **14**, 41.
42. Herrmann, Y., Bujnicki, T., Zafiu, C., Kulawik, A., Kühbach, K., Peters, L., Fabig, J., Willbold, J., Bannach, O., Willbold, D. (2017). Nanoparticle standards for immuno-based quantitation of α-synuclein oligomers in diagnostics of Parkinson's disease and other synucleinopathies. *Clin. Chim. Acta*, **466**, 152–159.
43. An, J. H., Choi, D.-K., Lee, K.-J., Choi, J.-W. (2015). Surface-enhanced Raman spectroscopy detection of dopamine by DNA targeting amplification assay in Parkisons's model. *Biosens. Bioelectron.*, **67**, 739–746.
44. Broto, M., Galve, R., Marco, M.-P. (2017). Sandwich NP-based biobarcode assay for quantification C-reactive protein in plasma samples. *Anal. Chim. Acta*, **992**, 112–118.
45. Niu, S., Zhang, L. K., Zhang, L., Zhuang, S., Zhan, X., Chen, W. Y., Du, S., Yin, L., You, R., Li, C. H., Guan, Y. Q. (2017). Inhibition by multifunctional magnetic nanoparticles loaded with alpha-synuclein RNAi plasmid in a Parkinson's disease model. *Theranostics*, **7**, 344–356.
46. Kyle, S., Saha, S. (2014). Nanotechnology for the detection and therapy of stroke. *Adv. Healthcare Mater.*, **3**, 1703–1720.
47. Kaviarasi, S., Yuba, E., Harada, A., Krishnan, U. M. (2019). Emerging paradigms in nanotechnology for imaging and treatment of cerebral ischemia. *J. Control. Release*, **300**, 22–45.

48. Yang, H. Y., Fu, Y., Jang, M.-S., Li, Y., Yin, W. P., Ahn, T. K., Lee, J. H., Chae, H., Lee, D. S. (2017). CdSe@ZnS/ZnS quantum dots loaded in polymeric micelles as a pH-triggerable targeting fluorescence imaging probe for detecting cerebral ischemic area. *Colloids Surf., B*, **155**, 497–506.

49. Agulla, J., Brea, D., Campos, F., Sobrino, T., Argibay, B., Al-Soufi, W., Blanco, M., Castillo, J., Ramos-Cabrer, P. (2014). In vivo theranostics at the peri-infarct region in cerebral ischemia. *Theranostics*, **4**, 90–105.

50. Feczkó, T., Piiper, A., Ansar, S., Blixt, F. W., Ashtikar, M., Schiffmann, S., Ulshöfer, T., Parnham, M. J., Harel, Y., Israel, L. L., Lellouche, J.-P., Wacker, M. G. (2019). Stimulating brain recovery after stroke using theranostic albumin nanocarriers loaded with nerve growth factor in combination therapy. *J. Control. Release*, **293**, 63–72.

51. Jin, A. Y., Tuor, U. I., Rushforth, D., Filfil, R., Kaur, J., Ni, F., Tomanek, B., Barber, P. A. (2009). Magnetic resonance molecular imaging of post-stroke neuroinflammation with a P-selectin targeted iron oxide nanoparticle. *Contrast Media Mol. Imaging*, **4**, 305–311.

52. van Kasteren, S. I., Campbell, S. J., Serres, S., Anthony, D. C., Sibson, N. R., Davis, B. G. (2009). Glyconanoparticles allow pre-symptomatic in vivo imaging of brain disease. *Proc. Natl. Acad. Sci.*, **106**, 18–23.

53. Fréchou, M., Beray-Berthat, V., Raynaud, J.-S., Mériaux, S., Gombert, F., Lancelot, E., Plotkine, M., Marchand-Leroux, C., Ballet, S., Robert, P., Louin, G., Margaill, I. (2013). Detection of vascular cell adhesion molecule-1 expression with USPIO-enhanced molecular MRI in a mouse model of cerebral ischemia. *Contrast Media Mol. Imaging*, **8**, 157–164.

54. Kim, J. Y., Ryu, J. H., Schellingerhout, D., Sun, I. C., Lee, S. K., Jeon, S., Kim, J., Kwon, I. C., Nahrendorf, M., Ahn, C. H., Kim, K., Kim, D. E. (2015). Direct imaging of cerebral thromboemboli using computed tomography and fibrin-targeted gold nanoparticles. *Theranostics*, **5**, 1098–1114.

55. Li, J., Chang, X., Chen, X., Gu, Z., Zhao, F., Chai, Z., Zhao, Y. (2014). Toxicity of inorganic nanomaterials in biomedical imaging. *Biotechnol. Adv.*, **32**, 727–743.

Chapter 7

Drug Nanocrystals

M. Ermelinda S. Eusébio,[a] Ricardo A. E. Castro[a,b] and João Canotilho[a,b]
[a]*Coimbra Chemistry Center, Department of Chemistry, University of Coimbra, Coimbra, Portugal*
[b]*Faculty of Pharmacy, University of Coimbra, Coimbra, Portugal*
quierme@ci.uc.pt

Drug nanocrystals are solid drug nanosized particles, covered with a thin layer of a stabiliser, which are, a priori, classified in the low-nano-toxicological-risk group. In this chapter, the most relevant physicochemical properties of drug nanocrystals are discussed (saturation solubility, dissolution rate) and methods for their preparation presented (top-down, bottom-up and combination techniques). The key issue of nanocrystals stability is discussed and examples of drug brain delivery using nanocrystals exemplified for different administration routes.

7.1 Introduction

Drug nanocrystals, according to the most common concept within the scientific community, are particles of nanometric size (ranging

Nanoparticles for Brain Drug Delivery
Edited by Carla Vitorino, Andreia Jorge and Alberto Pais

ISBN 978-981-4877-31-2 (Hardcover), 978-1-003-11932-6 (eBook)
www.jennystanford.com

from a few nm to 1000 nm) composed of the active pharmaceutical ingredient (API) arranged in a crystalline structure [1–6]. They are most commonly produced as nanosuspensions in a liquid medium, usually stabilised by a thin adsorbed layer (typically 2–5 nm thick) formed of either a surfactant or a sterically stabilising polymer [3, 4]. The United States Food and Drug Administration (USFDA) [7], European Commission (EC) and European Medicines Agency (EMA) [8, 9] all propose a smaller size limit of <100 nm in their nanoparticle definitions, which encompasses only those particles which can be internalised through endocytosis by all cells in the body – therefore also including the blood–brain barrier (BBB) – and not only by the mononuclear phagocytic system (MPS). The term nanocrystal has been extended by some authors to also describe suspensions of nanosized, partially crystalline and – in some cases – even amorphous drugs [1, 4, 10–13], although, strictly speaking, this wider definition is not correct.

Compared with other nanomedicines, the main distinguishing characteristic of drug nanocrystals results from the fact that their composition is almost 100% drug without additional matrix materials. Consequently, nanocrystals have the potential to circumvent two of the problems often associated with other kinds of nanoparticles, namely to achieve high loading capacity for the drug and to significantly reduce the amount of excipients. Nanocrystal stabilisers can consist of polymers or surfactants which have gained regulatory acceptance for the intended administration route; moreover, these are used in small amounts, thereby eliminating one potential contributory factor to the toxicological effects of nanomedicines. Additionally, most nanocrystals are classified as class I or class III under the Nanotoxicological Classification System (NCS) proposed by Keck and Müller [14], based on particle size and biopersistence. Nanocrystals are considered biodegradable, as dissolution will occur in the amount of available aqueous media. Toxicity will ultimately be that of the API. However, it should not be overlooked that, despite being biodegradable, nanocrystals can eventually have undesired effects prior to complete dissolution; consequently, careful evaluation is advisable even for these a priori low-toxicity nanoparticles [1, 6, 24]. The two classes, NCS I and III, distinguish those nanocrystals which can be internalised by all cells via endocytosis (those <100 nm) from those which cannot [14].

Table 7.1 Pharmaceutical nanocrystals: approved and investigational nanodrugs [2, 15–23]

Brand name	INN name	Therapeutic indication	Dosage form/ administration route	Company	Approval date/clinical trials
		Central nervous system (CNS)			
Xeplion®	Paliperidone palmitate	Antipsychotic	Extended-release injectable suspension /i.m.	Janssen-Cilag International N.V.	EMA, 2011
Invega Sustenna®	Paliperidone palmitate	Antipsychotic	Extended-release injectable suspension /i.m.	Elan/Johnson & Johnson	FDA, 2009
Zypadhera®	Olanzapine pamoate	Schizophrenia	Extended-release injectable suspension/i.m.	Eli Lilly Nederland B.V	EMA, 2008
Focalin XR®	Dexmethylphenidate HCl	Antipsychotic	Extended release capsules/ oral	Novartis	FDA, 2001
Ritalin LA®	Methylphenidate HCl	Antipsychotic	Extended release capsules/ oral	Novartis	FDA, 2002
		Cancer			
Theralux®	Thymectacin	Colon cancer	Extended-release injectable suspension/i.v.	Celmed Biociences	Phase II
Panzem® NCD	2-methoxyestradiol	Ovarian cancer	Tablet/oral	EntreMed	Phase II
Nanotax® NT	Paclitaxel	Refractory peritoneal cancer	Injectable/i.peritoneal	Crititech	Phase I

(Continued)

Table 7.1 (*Continued*)

Brand name	INN name	Therapeutic indication	Dosage form/ administration route	Company	Approval date/clinical trials
		Nausea and vomiting			
Emend®	Aprepitant	Antiemetic	Capsule/oral	Elan/Merck	FDA, 2003
Cesamet®	Nabilone	Antiemetic	Capsule/oral	Lilly	FDA, 2005
		Dyslipidemias			
Cholib®	Fenofribate/Simvastatin	Antihyperlipidemic	Tablet/oral	Abbott Healthcare	EMA, 2013
Triglide®	Fenofribate	Antihyperlipidemic	Tablet/oral	SkyePharma/ First Horizon Pharmaceuticals	FDA, 2005
Tricor®	Fenofribate	Antihyperlipidemic	Tablet/oral	Elan/Abbott	FDA, 2004
Lipidil®	Fenofribate	Antihyperlipidemic	Capsule/oral	Laboratoires Fournier SAS	FDA, 1993
Lipanthyl®	Fenofribate	Antihyperlipidemic	Capsule/oral	Abbott Products SAS	EMA, 1991
		Microorganisms			
Silcryst™	NPI 32101	Antibacterial	Cream/topical	Nucryst Pharmaceuticals	FDA, 2007

Brand name	INN name	Therapeutic indication	Dosage form/ administration route	Company	Approval date/clinical trials
Acticoat Absorvent (with Silcryst™ Nanocrystals)	NPI 32101	Antimicrobial barrier	Dressing/topical	Smith & Nephew´s U.S.	FDA, 2005
Gris-Peg®	Griseofulvin	Antifungal	Tablet/oral	Novartis	FDA, 1982
			Asthma		
Budesonide	Budesonide	Antiasthmatic	Powder/pulmonary	Apotex	FDA, 2014
Theodur®	Theophylline	Asthma, COPD	Tablet, capsule/oral	Mitsubishi Tanabe Pharma	FDA, 2008
			Heart and blood vessels		
Verelan PM®	Verapamil HCl	Hypertension	Capsule/oral	Schwarz Pharma	FDA, 1998
Herbesser®	Diltiazem HCl	Hypertension	Tablet/oral	Mitsubishi	FDA, 2002
			Pain		
Ryanodex®	Dantrolene sodium	Malignant hyperthermia	Injectable suspension/i.v.	Eagle Pharmaceuticals	FDA, 2014
Zenaflex®	Tizanidine HCL	Muscle relaxant	Capsule/oral	Acorda	FDA, 2002
Avinza®	Morphine sulfate	Moderate to severe pain	Capsule/oral	King Pharma	FDA, 2002

(*Continued*)

Table 7.1 *(Continued)*

Brand name	INN name	Therapeutic indication	Dosage form/ administration route	Company	Approval date/clinical trials
			Appetite		
Megace ES®	Megestrol acetate	Appetite stimulant	Suspension/oral	Elan/Par Pharmaceutical	FDA, 2005
			Eye		
Azopt®	Brizolamide	Ocular hypertension	Suspension/ocular	Alcon	FDA, 1998
			Inflammation		
Naprelan®	Naproxen sodium	NSAID	Tablet/oral	Wyeth	FDA, 2006
			Immune system		
Rapamune®	Sirolimus (rapamycin)	Immunosuppressant	Suspension, tablet/oral	Elan/Wyeth	FDA, 2000

The most special physicochemical properties of nanocrystals are their increased surface area and the resulting increased saturation solubility, both of which affect dissolution rates. Of course, appropriate strategies must be developed to effectively reach the target, in this case the blood–brain barrier.

Drug nanocrystals were first reported in patents published by the beginning of the 1990s [25–27]. The first nanocrystal drug product – the immunosuppressant Rapamune® by Elan/Wyeth – was launched relatively soon thereafter, in 2000 [6, 28]. This was a consequence of the relatively easy and cost-effective large-scale production of nanocrystals, in conjunction with their other advantages [29, 30]. Other examples of nanocrystals which have reached the market are summarised in Table 7.1 [4, 19–22], with relevance to the antihypercholesterolemia Tricor®, containing the API fenofibrate, which was the first nanoblockbuster product [6, 23]. The first products to be launched which act on the brain were the antipsychotic drug Ritalin LA® and Invega Sustenna® used in schizophrenia management.

7.2 Relevant Nanocrystal Physicochemical Properties

The biopharmaceutics classification system (BCS) proposed by Amidon et al. [31, 32] categorises APIs according to some in vitro properties which have consequences for in vivo performance, namely aqueous solubility and membrane permeability. BCS class II drugs have limited oral bioavailability due to their low aqueous solubility, despite having high permeability. Low molecular weight, MW, lipophilic drugs, with MW up to 400–600 Da [33–35], should be able to cross the lipophilic BBB by passive diffusion. However, the necessary lipophilic characteristics result in low aqueous solubility, making many of these drugs BCS class II. The developability classification system (DCS) proposed by Butler and Dressman in 2010 [36, 37] further divides these APIs into those with dissolution-rate-limited oral bioavailability (i.e., DCS class IIa drugs) and those which are solubility-limited (i.e., DCS class IIb). For BCS class IV drugs, both low permeability and low solubility limit oral bioavailability.

It is estimated that more than 40% of marketed APIs are BCS class II or IV [35, 38–40]. Moreover, advances in high-throughput screening methods have led to many new drug candidates, but these show increasing prevalence of solubility/dissolution rate problems [40–42]. Formulations must be developed to overcome issues of very low bioavailability after oral administration, or to avoid excessively large injection volumes if parenteral administration is considered, which may also lead to undesirable side effects, when traditional formulations consisting of solutions of the solubilised drug are used.

Nanocrystals are an attractive formulation strategy for poorly water-soluble drugs and those for which dissolution is the rate-limiting step for drug absorption [29, 41, 43, 44], as size reduction to the nanometric scale has both thermodynamic and kinetic implications.

For nanocrystals, due to the large surface-area-to-volume ratio, interfacial effects have to be taken into account and the chemical potential of the pure substance, μ, is given by Eq. 7.1, considering a spherical particle:

$$\mu = \mu_\infty + \frac{2\gamma V_\mathrm{m}}{r} \tag{7.1}$$

where μ_∞ is the chemical potential as the radius $r \to \infty$, γ is interfacial tension and V_m is the molar volume.

These interfacial effects give rise to increased solubility of nanoparticles compared to microsized ones, as expressed by the Ostwald–Freundlich equation (Eq. 7.2) for spherical particles:

$$\ln\frac{S}{S_\infty} = \frac{2\gamma V_\mathrm{m}}{rRT} \tag{7.2}$$

where S is the solubility of a nanocrystal of radius r at temperature T, S_∞ is the solubility of a solid consisting of large particles and R is the gas constant. Solubility increases with decreasing size, but the effect will be of relevance for particle sizes <200 nm [45, 46]. The increased saturation solubility of nanocrystals results in more pronounced concentration gradients at biological barriers, contributing to increased drug uptake in molecular form by passive diffusion. Melting temperature and enthalpy are examples of other thermodynamic properties which change (decrease) for nanocrystals when compared to larger counterparts [47–50].

Besides thermodynamic solubility, dissolution rate is also influenced by particle size reduction to the nanoscale (see Fig. 7.1). The dissolution of a solid in a liquid medium may be understood as a process in which several barriers must be overcome. Firstly, a solid–liquid interface needs to be produced (wetting); next, the intermolecular interactions in the solid must be broken; the solid molecules are solvated at the interface; finally, they diffuse from the solid–liquid interface into the bulk solution. The second and fourth steps are obviously affected by nanoscaling, due to both the lower energy required for lattice breakdown and also a more favourable diffusion process. The rate of dissolution may be expressed by the Noyes–Whitney equation [51], modified by Nernst and Brunner, as in Eq. 7.3:

$$\frac{dC}{dt} = \frac{AD}{h_{\mathrm{D}}}(C_{\mathrm{s}} - C) \tag{7.3}$$

where dC/dt is the dissolution rate, A is the area of the particles exposed to the solvent, D is the diffusion coefficient, h_{D} is the thickness of the diffusion layer, C_{s} the equilibrium solubility and C the concentration of the drug in solution at time t. The dissolution rate increases due to larger surface area and – for particles small enough – also due to greater saturation solubility. Moreover, the hydrodynamic boundary layer thickness, h_{H}, is also dependent on particle size, as shown by the Prandtl equation (Eq. 7.4) being smaller for nanosized crystals (Fig. 7.1):

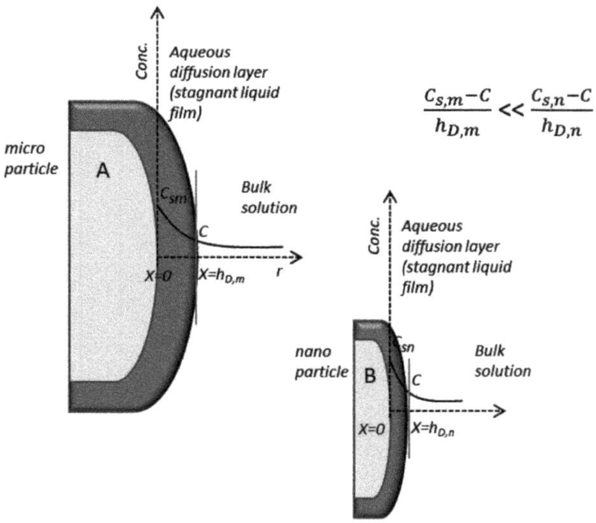

Figure 7.1 Micro- and nanoparticle solid drug dissolution in a solvent liquid phase ($C_{\mathrm{s,m}}$ and $C_{\mathrm{s,n}}$: equilibrium solubilities of micro- and nanoparticles, respectively; $h_{\mathrm{D,m}}$ and $h_{\mathrm{D,n}}$: thickness of the diffusion layers for micro- and of nanoparticles, respectively).

$$h_{\mathrm{H}} = k\left(\frac{L^{\frac{1}{2}}}{v^{\frac{1}{3}}}\right) \tag{7.4}$$

In Eq. 7.4, k is a constant, L the length of the particle surface in the direction of flow and v the relative velocity of the flowing liquid surrounding the particle.

Moreover, increased surface wettability is expected because of the presence of the stabilisers, also contributing to a higher dissolution rate. Increased adhesion to surfaces/cell membranes is another special feature of nanocrystals, resulting obviously from their larger surface area.

7.3 Preparation of Nanocrystals

Currently, two main approaches are employed in producing nanocrystals (see Fig. 7.2): top-down methods, in which large crystals are broken down until reaching a mean particle size, usually not <200 nm [6]; and bottom-up, a controlled solution crystallisation process often giving rise to mean particle sizes <100 nm. In 2003, the first combined use of these two techniques was reported, which also gave rise to mean particle sizes <100 nm [6].

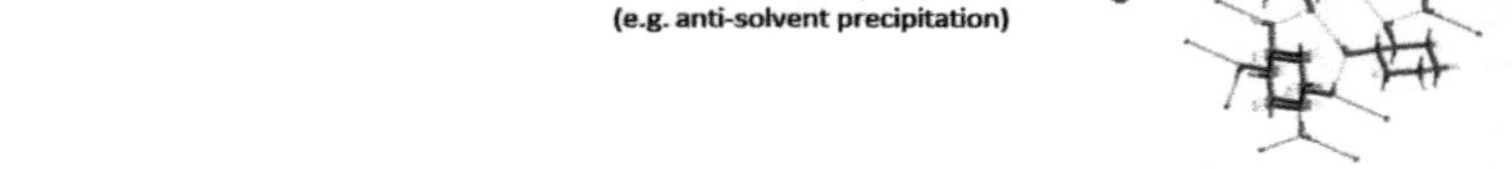

Figure 7.2 Schematic representation of methods of nanocrystal preparation: by size reduction of large crystals (top-down) and by growing crystals from the component molecules (bottom-up). Bottom-up processes are more adequate to give rise to small-sized crystals than top-down processes, if conditions for multiple crystallisation nucleus formation are provided, with reduced crystal growth, and Ostwald ripening prevented.

Table 7.2 presents examples of drug nanocrystals with a mean particle size around or smaller than 100 nm. It is worth mentioning that these examples are dominated by bottom-up techniques.

Table 7.2 Examples of nanocrystals with dimensions around 100 nm which were synthesised to be used in the brain (*) or which can potentially be used in the brain (#). Other examples are presented to show the potentiality of other approaches

API	Therapeutic indication	Method	Mean diameter (nm)	Refs.
		Bottom-up evaporation		
Danazol	Endometriosis	Spray-freezing into liquid (SFL)	100	[63]
		Bottom-up precipitation		
Lysozime#	Antimicrobial enzyme	Supercritical antisolvent (SAS)	70–100	[64], #[65]
Rifampicin	Antibiotic	SAS	70–170	[66], #[67]
Puerarin*	Anti-Parkinson	SAS	83	*[68]
Paeoniflorin*	Anti-Parkinson	SAS	140	*[69]
Dextran#	Antithrombotic	SAS	50	[70], #[71]
Cefuroxime axetil#	Antibiotic	Sonoprecipitation	80	[72], #[73]
Cefixime#	Antibiotic	High-gravity antisolvent precipitation (HGAP)	57	[74], #[75, 76]
Salbutamol sulfate	Asthma	HGAP	100	[77]
Cefixime#	Antibiotic	High-gravity reactive precipitation (HGRP)	45	[78], #[76]
Raloxifene#	Treat osteoporosis	Rapid expansion of supercritical solution (RESS)	19	[79], #[80]
Theophylline	Bronchodilator	RESS	85	[81]

(*Continued*)

Table 7.2 (*Continued*)

API	Therapeutic indication	Method	Mean diameter (nm)	Refs.
Retinyl palmitate in poly (L-lactide)	Ester of vitamin A	Rapid expansion of supercritical solution into a liquid solvent (RESOLV)	40–110	[82]
Ibuprofen#	NSAID	RESOLV	40–50	[83], #[84]
Phenytoin#	Antiepileptic	Rapid expansion of supercritical solution with solid co-solvent (RESS-SC)	75–120	[85], #[86]
Paclitaxel#	Anticancer	Flash nanoprecipitation (FNP)	86	[87], #[88]
Doxorubicin#	Anticancer	FNP	50	[89], #[90]
Top-down				
Griseofulvin	Antifungal	Nanocrystals® technology	<100	[91]
Probucol#	Antihyperlipidemic	Nanocrystals® technology	77	[92], #[93]
PX-18#	Phospholipase A2 inhibitor	High-pressure homogenisation (HPH)	50	[94], #[95]
Top-down and bottom-up combination				
Hydrocortisone#	Corticosteroid	Nanoedge-like	80	[96], #[97]
Prednisolone#	Corticosteroid	H69	22	[98], #[97]
Amphotericin B#	Antifungal	H96	62	[98], #[99]

BU, bottom-up; TP, top-down; CTPBU, combination of top-down and bottom-up; H69, cavi-precipitation/HPH; H96, freeze-drying/HPH; RESS, rapid expansion of supercritical solutions; RESOLVE; rapid expansion of supercritical solutions into liquid solvents; RESS-SC, rapid expansion of supercritical solution with solid cosolvent; SAS, supercritical antisolvent.

7.3.1 Top-Down Techniques

Several commercial products rely on top-down methods [43, 52]. This is a successful industrial technique due to its good reproducibility and scalability [53], but it has some drawbacks which require alternative approaches [54]. The scale-up of these high-energy processes is difficult and often limited by the formation of amorphous phases, degradation and, in many cases, residual metal contents [55]. The main top-down processes for nanocrystal preparation are described in the following sections.

7.3.1.1 Wet media milling

Wet milling is used to produce nanosized crystals as dry milling is not efficient enough. Wet milling means that the drug particles are dispersed in a surfactant/stabiliser solution and then the obtained macrosuspension is submitted to milling energy, with cleavage, abrasion and fracturing being the main mechanisms of size reduction [45, 56, 57]. Parameters which influence the median obtained particle size include milling duration (which follows a first-order decay function), milling speed, bead (type, dimension and number) and drug loading [23]. Low- and high-energy milling approaches can be used. The first method takes longer, yielding nanosuspensions containing particles with a narrow size distribution [19]. High-energy milling approaches result from industrial demands. Nanocrystals® technology [25], is one of the most successful nanosizing techniques. Several market nanosuspensions which are formulated as capsules, suspensions, or tablets are prepared using this technology [2, 19, 23, 58].

7.3.1.2 High-pressure homogenisation

Homogenisation can be performed by dispersing a drug in an aqueous medium at room temperature (Dissocubes®) or in non-aqueous media such as liquid polyethylene glycol (PEG) or oils at low temperatures (Nanopure®). These methods were originally developed by Müller and co-workers [2, 6, 59]. The size reduction is achieved by employing a high-pressure piston (up to 1500 bar) to force the dispersion through a very narrow gap (of diameter 5–25 μm). Up to 20 high-pressure homogenisation, HPH cycles can be performed [6]. Cavitation, collisions between particles and shear forces contribute to size reduction [58, 60].

7.3.2 Bottom-Up Techniques

In bottom-up processes, nanocrystals are grown from solutions. To obtain nanosized crystals, the two steps of the crystallisation process, nucleation and crystal growth, must be controlled [61, 62]. Crystallisation must be conducted under experimental conditions which favour high nucleation rates, in order to obtain a large number of crystalline nuclei. The rate of homogeneous nucleation, *J*, according to the classical theory of nucleation, is described by an Arrhenius-type velocity equation, and is controlled by temperature, *T*, interfacial tension, γ, and supersaturation, *SS*, as shown in Eq. 7.5 (for spherical particles) [61],

$$J = A_r \exp\left[-\frac{16\pi\gamma^3 v^2}{3k^3T^3(\ln SS^2)}\right] \tag{7.5}$$

Here, *v* is molecular volume. Therefore, in bottom-up processes for nanocrystal preparation, high supersaturation ratios are used, which facilitates a large number of nuclei, thus decreasing supersaturation and limiting crystal growth rates. Small crystals with a narrow size distribution can be expected if several parameters are optimised: drug concentration, choices of solvent, antisolvent (if used), stabiliser and temperature. However, highly-supersaturated solutions are quite prone to forming nanoamorphous suspensions; additionally, the reproducibility of the process may be compromised by the presence of heterogeneous nucleation sites which are difficult to control.

Bottom-up techniques are low-cost processes with lower energy consumption and more basic equipment requirements than top-down methods. Smaller particle sizes are achievable and bottom-up methods can be applied to thermolabile active pharmaceutical ingredients. However, reproducibility and scalability may be limiting factors, and at present only a few nanocrystal drug products in the market are prepared using bottom-up processes (GrisPEG® griseofulvin in PEG8000 and Cesamet® nabilone in PVP); see Table 7.1 [100].

Bottom-up approaches obtain nanocrystals either by solvent evaporation or by precipitation as detailed in the next sections.

7.3.2.1 Bottom-up: evaporation methods

7.3.2.1.1 *Spray-freezing into liquid*

A solution containing API and surfactant is sprayed into a cryogenic liquid. The resulting frozen solid particles are collected and lyophilised [63, 101, 102]. Freeze-drying is used to obtain dry powders which can be used in formulations with enhanced shelf lives [103]. Amorphous nanostructures tend to result, as observed in experiments conducted for danazol, in which 100 nm diameter particles were obtained, using a small amount of surfactant [63].

7.3.2.1.2 *Spray-drying: Nano Spray Dryer B-90*

A Nano Spray Dryer B-90 (Büchi, Flawil, Switzerland) may be used to obtain particles within the 200 nm to 5 μm range [104]. Several examples of this method are reported in the literature, although none with mean particle sizes less than 100 nm [105–108]. The API solution is nebulised by a thin, stainless steel membrane with micron-sized holes (4.0–7.0 μm), which is excited by a piezoelectric actuator at ultrasonic frequencies (80–140 kHz). Microdroplets are ejected at high speed, which are then dried by a drying gas (flow 80–160 l min^{-1}) at the inlet temperature (maximum 120°C). The resulting particles accumulate at the wall of the collecting electrode [109, 110].

7.3.2.2 Bottom-up: precipitation methods

7.3.2.2.1 *Solvent–antisolvent*

Using this technique, a drug is dissolved in an organic solvent and the crystallisation process is then controlled by precipitation with an antisolvent, which is miscible with the organic solvent, in the presence of a stabiliser. A basic disadvantage of many precipitation processes is the use of organic solvents, which subsequently need to be removed, thereby increasing costs [46].

7.3.2.2.2 *Supercritical fluid*

Rapid expansion of supercritical solutions (RESS) [58, 100] uses CO_2 as the supercritical fluid, as it is easy to obtain in its supercritical state (T_c = 31.1°C; p_c = 72.9 atm), inexpensive, nontoxic and easy to

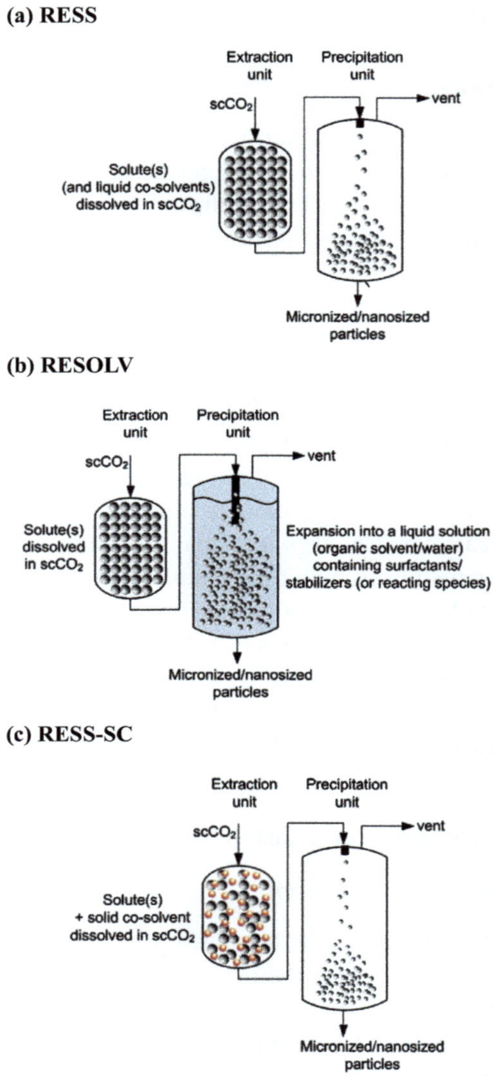

Figure 7.3 Schematic representation of (a) RESS, (b) RESOL and (c) RESS-SC processes. Adapted from Ref. [113], Copyright (2018), with permission from Elsevier.

remove by reducing the pressure. The resulting solution is rapidly expanded into a low-pressure area through a narrow nozzle; see

Fig. 7.3a [111]. Alternatively, the supercritical solution may be rapidly expanded into a liquid solvent (RESOLV) containing a surfactant, as in Fig. 7.3b [112]. These techniques are only appropriate for hydrophobic drugs which are soluble in supercritical CO_2 [112]. Consequently, variants such as supercritical solution with solid co-solvent (RESS-SC), have been used to overcome this limitation, (Fig. 7.3c). The solid, normally menthol and more recently vanillin, is firstly dissolved in supercritical CO_2 and then this fluid will dissolve the drug. The solid co-solvent nanoparticles (drug/menthol) produced by rapid expansion are then submitted to freeze-drying or lyophilisation to remove the menthol [113].

Supercritical antisolvent (SAS) uses supercritical fluid CO_2 as the antisolvent. The drug is dissolved in an organic solvent which is miscible with supercritical CO_2; the drug is then precipitated by adding supercritical CO_2 into the solution or vice versa [54, 111].

These methods (mainly continuous methods) have not yet been applied on an industrial scale. However, they have great potential in terms of crystal quality (degree of crystallinity and purity) and cost savings, which are issues of major interest to the pharmaceutical sector [113].

7.3.2.2.3 *Sonoprecipitation*

Ultrasonic waves cause faster and uniform nucleation and are applied when the antisolvent is mixed with the solution. The resulting drug mean particle sizes will depend on the duration, intensity and frequency of the ultrasonic waves; on the volume of solution; and ultrasonic probe size and its immersion depth [58, 111]. One major limitation is the current lack of equipment suitable for scaling-up such processes [111].

7.3.2.2.4 *High-gravity precipitation*

High-gravity precipitation can be operated in two modes, depending on the liquid streams distributing into the rotating packed bed (see Fig. 7.4): high-gravity antisolvent precipitation (HGAP) or high-gravity reactive precipitation (HGRP). In HGAP, two liquid streams (drug solution and antisolvent) are mixed at the centre of a rotating packed bed, where the mixture is subjected to high gravity due to centrifugal forces. The mixture is forced to pass the packed bed before leaving the reactor [77, 111, 114–117]. This method normally uses organic solvents. In the alternative HGRP process, which is applied to acidic drugs for instance, a basic aqueous drug solution and an acid aqueous solution are mixed, generating, in situ, the acidic form of the drug. Very recently, Zhang et al and Kuang et al. achieved sizes smaller than 100 nm with both approaches [74, 78].

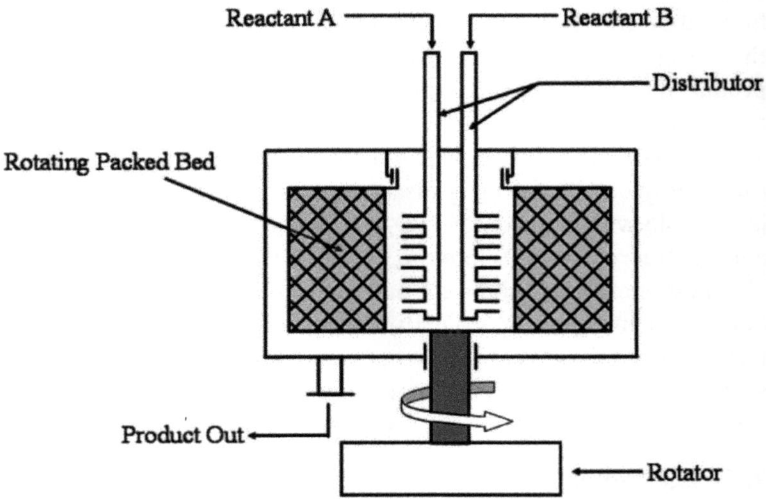

Figure 7.4 Schematic representation of the HGRP process. Reprinted from Ref. [111], Copyright (2011), with permission from Elsevier.

7.3.2.2.5 *Flash nanoprecipitation*

In the flash nanoprecipitation technique, a hydrophobic drug is typically dissolved with a block copolymer in a water-miscible organic solvent. This solution and water (antisolvent) are injected separately into a small chamber at high velocity. The high velocity generates turbulent mixing, causing the drug and the polymer to co-precipitate very rapidly, forming nanoparticles. The block copolymer should be amphiphilic: the hydrophobic block encapsulates drug molecules, preventing particle growth, and the hydrophilic layer around the nanoparticles inhibits aggregation [87, 118, 119].

7.3.3 Combination of Top-Down and Bottom-Up Techniques

Since 2003, combined approaches emerged as a new trend in the field of nanocrystal preparation [98]. These comprise two steps: pretreatment of the sample using a bottom-up process and then a high-energy step involving high-pressure homogenisation. In the NANOEDGE® approach, the first step is microprecipitation, in H69 technique a cavitation-precipitation step, in H42 a spray-drying step, in H96 a freeze-drying one. Combinative Technology (CT) is a combination of two top-down techniques, a media milling step followed by high-pressure homogenisation [58, 98, 120].

7.4 Stability of Nanocrystals

Nanocrystal stability is a key issue for pharmaceutical development. The small-sized particles, with high surface energy, are in a thermodynamically unstable state, such that aggregation and Ostwald ripening may occur. Additionally, the solid form obtained after the nanosizing process – the drug molecular arrangement in the solid phase – may also be a source of instability.

7.4.1 Aggregation and Ostwald Ripening

To prevent aggregation, nanocrystallisation must be carried out in the presence of stabilisers [121]. These are adsorbed at the particle surface and stabilisation may be achieved by electrostatic repulsion among particles, by steric effects, or by a combination of both. Electrostatic stabilisers typically include ionic surfactants and polymers (e.g., sodium dodecyl sulphate [122, 123], sodium alginate [54]) [124–126]. For electrostatic stabilisation of nanocrystals, the zeta potential should be in excess of 30 mV [1]. Concerning brain delivery, some authors report that negatively charged particles should be used, as highly positively charged nanoparticles displayed toxicity to the BBB [127]. Electrostatic stabilisation is effective in aqueous media, but problems may arise when converting into dry solid forms. Moreover, stability may also be affected by changes in both pH and ionic strength. Steric stabilisation is not dependent on these effects, although it shows a greater temperature dependency [1], and may be used to prepare nanocrystals both in aqueous and non-aqueous media. For steric stabilisation, non-ionic amphiphilic surfactants or polymers are used (e.g., Tween 80, poloxamers, polyvinyl alcohol, polyvinylpyrrolidone [123–125]). Nanosuspensions may also be made more stable by combining electrostatic and steric effects in the same stabiliser molecule [118] or combining non-ionic and ionic stabilisers [128].

At present, stabiliser selection is essentially a process of trial and error, although research is ongoing to correlate API physicochemical properties with the best stabiliser [129–131].

Ostwald ripening is another potential source of physical instability for nanosuspensions [132]. Due to the tendency of a solid phase to achieve the minimum surface Gibbs energy, particle growth will occur in nanosuspensions, resulting from saturation solubility differences between smaller and larger particles: saturation solubility increases as particle size decreases (Eq. 7.2, for spherical particles), such that smaller particles tend to dissolve whereas larger ones grow due to diffusional mass exchange. The relevance of the Ostwald ripening increases with higher polydispersity index (PDI).

It is worth mentioning that, after intravenous administration, the eventual gradual loss of the stabilising agents may result in agglomeration and Ostwald ripening, which will have consequences for the dissolution rate and may, in extreme cases, give rise to embolism.

7.4.2 Solid Forms: Polymorphs, Amorphous Phases and Solvates

Different molecular arrangements of an API in the solid phase, polymorphs, amorphous phases, solvates, co-crystals and salts may give rise to differences in API physicochemical properties [133–142], including aqueous solubility and dissolution rate. The observations by Aguiar et al. [143] regarding the polymorphism of chloramphenicol palmitate and the strong influence of ritonavir polymorphism during postmarket stage [144] represent seminal findings for the pharmaceutical industry concerning API solid-form/property relationships. Strictly speaking, polymorphs refer to different crystalline structures of the same molecular species, with different molecular arrangements or conformations in the solid state [145, 146]. Obviously, this does not include amorphous phases with their random molecular arrangement. Pharmaceutical solvates are multicomponent solid forms made up of the API and solvent molecules. These three solid forms are all included in what the FDA operationally defines as API polymorphs [147]. Different solid forms will have different thermodynamic stabilities (except at the temperature and pressure values where a reversible transition between specific forms may occur).

Amorphous phases, which are quite often obtained both by top-down and bottom-up nanosizing processes, are always higher-energy solid forms. Therefore, despite having higher saturation solubility, its inherent thermodynamic instability makes the use of an amorphous nanosuspension dependent on the kinetic barrier for conversion to a stable crystalline phase, which in turn will be dependent on environmental conditions.

Concerning thermodynamic stability, crystalline polymorphs may be monotropically or enantiotropically related [133, 146]. In the first case, one solid form is always metastable relative to the other; in the second case, both polymorphs, at a given pressure, will have stability domains within different temperatures ranges. Instability of nanocrystals may also result if metastable crystalline forms are obtained in the nanosizing process; these may convert to the stable form with different physicochemical properties. Naturally, if solvates are obtained, then stability conditions of the multicomponent solid must be assured.

Suspensions subjected to top-down methods may also result in crystalline polymorphs or solvates, different from the starting solid form. For instance, high-pressure homogenisation of the anticancer compound SN30191 resulted in phase transition of the initial polymorph II into polymorph I at intermediate pressure values, while with further pressure increase a hydrate was obtained [148]; after HPH of two suspensions, each made up of a different diclofenac polymorph, DCF1 (metastable form at ambient conditions) and DCF2, no change in solid form was observed when diclofenac DCF1 was used, whereas HPH of DCF2 suspension gives rise to polymorph DCF1 [149].

The solid form crystallised from solutions is always quite dependent on the experimental conditions [133, 134, 146]. This is also the case for nanocrystals obtained by bottom-up processes. For instance, indomethacin crystallisation by solvent evaporation in a nano-spray dryer gave rise to a mixture of two polymorphs [150].

Identification of the solid form obtained after nanocrystal synthesis is therefore of utmost importance. X-ray powder diffraction, differential scanning calorimetry, thermogravimetry and infrared spectroscopy are methods of choice for characterising API solid forms [133, 134, 141, 151].

7.5 Nanocrystals for Brain Drug Delivery

7.5.1 Oral Administration

The oral route of drug administration has by far the highest patient compliance, an issue of particular relevance if long-term treatment has to be considered, such as for neuropsychiatric disorders. After oral administration, nanocrystals will most probably dissolve in the gastrointestinal tract before intracellular uptake can occur [152–154]. The rapid dissolution rate (also affected by the higher saturation solubility if crystals are sufficiently small) will result in a higher concentration gradient at the gut endothelial barrier, contributing to higher API oral bioavailability. Compared with larger particles, nanocrystals show greater adhesion to the mucus layer, which is considered a key factor in their more reproducible oral bioavailability, with lower intra- and intersubject pharmacokinetic variability [155, 156]. Additionally, nanocrystals have been reported to reduce differences between fasted and fed dissolution rates for poorly water-soluble drugs, due to enhanced fasted dissolution rate [22, 30, 157].

Several nanocrystalline-based products for oral administration have reached the market, as shown in Table 7.1. Concerning nanocrystals for oral brain drug delivery two marketed products were identified (see Table 7.1), but promising research has been reported in the literature. Some examples are gathered below.

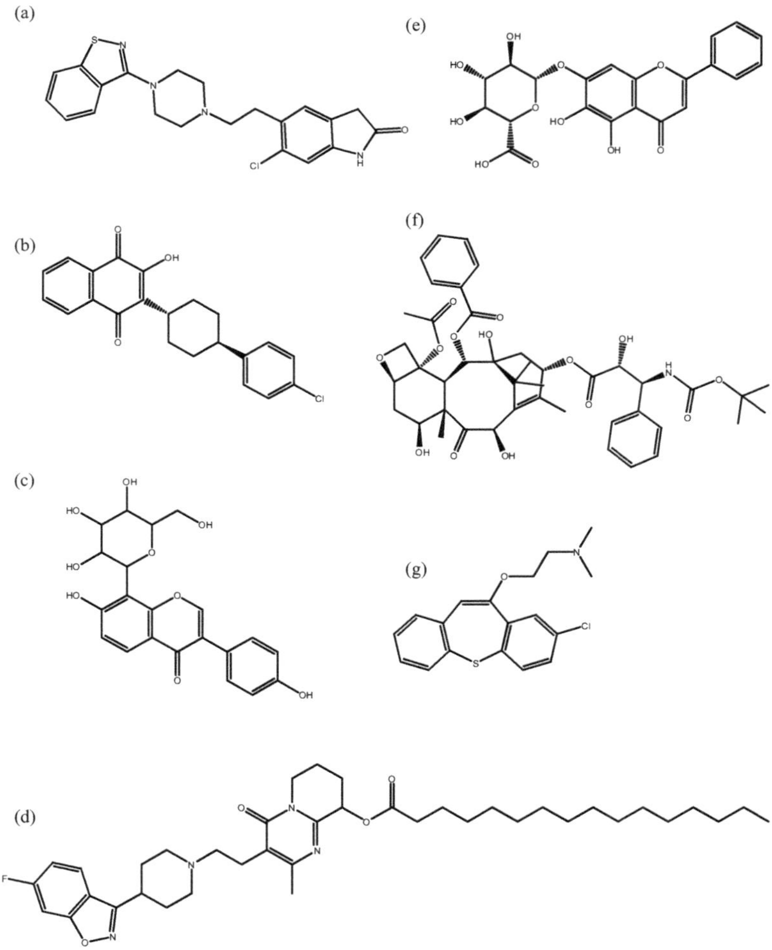

Figure 7.5 Molecular structures of APIs referred in the text as examples: (a) ziprasidone, (b) atovaquone, (c) puerarin, (d) paliperidone palmitate, (e) baicalin, (f) docetaxel and (g) zotepine.

Thombre et al. [157–159] investigated nanosuspensions of both ziprasidone free base and its hydrochloride (Fig 7.5a) an antipsychotic drug used in the treatment of schizophrenia and bipolar disorder. A significant food effect is reported on the dissolution rate of this drug [35]. A free base nanosuspension with mean particle diameters of about 270 nm was prepared by milling, using poloxamer 338, polysorbate 80 and lecithin as stabilisers. The nanosuspension afforded a considerable drug load of 210 mg/ml and, in in vivo pharmacokinetic studies carried out in beagle dogs, showed increased oral bioavailability when compared to the commercial product and enhanced fasted bioavailability [159]. For the hydrochloride, nanocrystals (size range 20–100 nm) could be obtained after annealing the amorphous nanosuspension obtained by spray-drying with hydroxypropyl methylcellulose acetate succinate (HPMCAS) from methanol solution.

These also showed improved oral absorption in the fasted state and no significant difference between fasted and fed absorption (which were reported for the free base nanosuspension) [157]. This is of particular relevance for enhancing treatment efficiency and avoiding drug-induced toxicity, which is particularly risky for non-compliant patients.

The effect of the stabiliser on the performance of orally administered nanosuspensions for brain drug delivery was evident from the results reported by Shubar et al. [160]. The authors investigated atovaquone (Fig. 7.5b), an API with very low aqueous solubility which is used for toxoplasmic encephalitis therapy [122]. Atovaquone nanosuspensions were prepared by high-pressure homogenisation using poloxamer 188, P188 and sodium docecyl sulfate (SDS) as stabilisers. Particles with mean sizes of 440 and 469 nm and a polydispersity index of 0.25 and 0.39, respectively, were obtained, with a considerable negative surface charge of −76 mV for the SDS-coated particles. In vivo experiments in mice, comparing the performance of the two nanosuspensions and of the commercial micronised suspension, indicated that SDS-coated nanocrystals, at a lower dose, were able to significantly increase atovaquone concentration, both in the serum and in the brain, thereby reducing parasite loads and the number of inflammatory foci in the brain. The P188-coated nanocrystals showed similar behaviour to the commercial formulation.

Xiong et al. [68] prepared puerarin nanocrystals (PU-NCs) (Fig. 7.5c), a BCS class IV potential anti-Parkinson compound [161] by antisolvent precipitation, using factor design to reach the lowest particle size and polydispersity index as well as convenient stability. Variables taken into account included the type and concentration of the stabilisers, drug concentration and antisolvent-to-solvent ratio.

Table 7.3 Pharmacokinetic parameters of PU-NCs in plasma and brain ($n = 6$ and $n = 4$, respectively)[a]

Pharmacokinetic parameters	Control group	PU-NCs group
	Plasma	
$T_{1/2}$/h	2.34 ± 0.38	2.80 ± 0.19[b]
T_{max}/h	4.33 ± 0.82	1.83 ± 0.41[b]
C_{max}/ng ml^{-1}	306.32 ± 43.04	2186.75 ± 161.92[c]
$AUC_{0\to t}$/ng h ml^{-1}	2635.27 ± 247.11	12648.20 ± 813.26[c]
$MRT_{0\to t}$/h	6.70 ± 0.88	5.24 ± 0.57[c]
F/%	100	480
	Brain	
$T_{1/2}$/h	1.59 ± 0.13	1.17 ± 0.11
T_{max}/h	5.83 ± 0.45	4.27 ± 0.24[b]
C_{max}/ng g^{-1}	84.98 ± 7.85	322.13 ± 28.35[c]
$AUC_{0\to t}$/ng h g^{-1}	565.90 ± 53.21	2408.51 ± 392.76[c]
$MRT_{0\to t}$/h	7.02 ± 0.59	6.31 ± 0.56[b]
	Brain/Plasma Ratio	
DTE	0.21	0.19

Source: Reprinted with permission from Ref. [68]. Copyright (2019) American Chemical Society.

[a]Data are presented as means ± standard deviation.

[b]$p < 0.05$.

[c]$p < 0.01$ vss the control group (PU alone administered rats).

$T_{1/2}$, elimination half-time; T_{max}, time to achieve the peak concentration; C_{max}, peak concentration in plasma or brain; $AUC_{0\to t}$, area under the concentration–time curve from time zero to t; $MRT_{0\to t}$, mean residence time; F, relative bioavailability of PU-NCs relative to the control group; DTE, AUC_{brain}/AUC_{plasma}.

The chosen stabiliser was Pluronic F68 (mean nanocrystal size equal to about 85 nm, PDI = 0.048), and X-ray powder diffraction and differential scanning calorimetry confirmed that antisolvent precipitation gave rise to a crystalline material, the same polymorph used in the solution preparation. A drug loading of about 73% was achieved. The interactions between the API and the stabiliser were investigated by molecular dynamics simulation, with van der Waals interactions playing a major role as expected. Additionally, the plasma and brain pharmacokinetic parameters were obtained in a study with Sprague–Dawley rats which were orally administered these PU-NCs or with the same dose of the active dispersed in 0.5% carboxymethylcellulose sodium solution (control group). The relevant values are shown in Table 7.3. Both the peak concentrations, C_{max}, and the areas under the concentration–time curve, AUC, are considerably higher for PU-NCs in both plasma and the brain when compared to the control group, with the maximum concentrations being achieved in a shorter period of time.

To obtain information on the eventual intestinal and brain uptake of intact nanocrystals following oral administration, Xiong et al. [68] performed in vivo fluorescence resonance energy transfer (FRET) imaging on zebrafish, loading DiO (3,3'-dioctadecyloxacarbocyanine perchlorate) and DiI (1,1'-dioctadecyl-3,3,3',3'-tetramethylindocarbocyanine perchlorate), a fluorophore donor/acceptor pair in the nanocrystals (DiO excitation λ = 420 nm; DiI emission λ = 565 nm). The results (see Fig. 7.6) were interpreted as indicating the permeability of the intact nanocrystals across both the intestinal and blood–brain barriers.

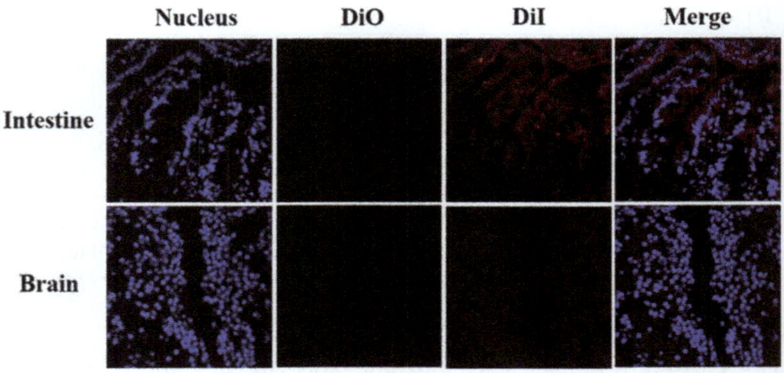

Figure 7.6 Histological changes on zebrafish intestine and brain, as observed by FRET imaging using confocal laser scanning microscopy, after administering DiO/DiI/PU-NCs. DiO and DiI signals are represented by green and red fluorescence, respectively. Cell nuclei are stained using Hoechst 33258. Reprinted with permission from Ref. [68]. Copyright (2019) American Chemical Society.

7.5.2 Parenteral Administration

Some nanocrystal-based products for poorly water-soluble drugs have been formulated for parenteral administration [162] (Table 7.1). Invega Sustenna® was the first injectable nanocrystal product, approved by FDA, brought to market, an aqueous nanosuspension of the antipsychotic paliperidone palmitate (Fig. 7.5d) which allows delivery of the drug in small volume via intramuscular injection. The parent drug, paliperidone, does not have solubility issues: the use of a nanosuspension of the drug palmitate enables limiting its solubility such that sustained release of the drug is achieved, allowing once-monthly administration, with improved patient compliance [163, 164]. The optimum particle size of nanosuspension products may depend on the intended propose, and for extended release of paliperidone Leng et al. [165] showed that nanosuspensions of paliperidone palmitate with sizes about 1000 nm have improved pharmacokinetic parameters when compared to a 500 nm batch.

Following parenteral administration, nanocrystal BBB delivery by cellular internalisation may be envisaged. By this mechanism, nanocrystals of sizes less than 100 nm will be able to enter the blood-brain barrier, dissolve and deliver the drug to the brain. However, before reaching the BBB, the phagocytotic uptake of nanocrystals by the monocluear phagocytic system, which was shown to be promoted by adsorption of opsonins such as immunoglobulin G, fibrinogen, must be circumvented [6, 33]. If sufficiently small, nanocrystals may eventually dissolve before being uptaken by the MPS [166]. Another restriction results from the efflux transporters at the BBB, such as the *P*-glycoprotein pump [6, 167]. A target strategy, directing the nanocrystals to the BBB, and able to promote internalisation, must be considered. This may be achieved by targeting the receptors overexpressed at the BBB, such as insulin receptor, transferrin receptors, or low-density lipoprotein receptor [168–170].

To circumvent interaction of the nanocrystals with macrophages, the adsorption of opsonins must be avoided. This can be achieved by modifying the nanocrystal surface, by choosing an appropriate stabiliser. An approach has been proposed [171] based on nanoparticle surface modification to promote selective protein adsorption, favouring those which can play the role of carrier to the

BBB. The literature reports several examples of nanoparticles in which, after appropriate surface modification, opsonin absorption was superseded by that of apolipoprotein E which targets the low-density lipoprotein BBB receptor [172–174].

As an example, Liu et al. [175] prepared nanocrystals of baicalin (Fig. 7.5e), a substance with potential for stroke and Alzheimer treatment [176], by high-pressure homogenisation using several stabilisers (polysorbate 80, TW80, poloxamer P188, poloxamer P407, RH40 and D-α-tocopherol polyethylene glycol succinate, TPGS). Particles were obtained with 50% drug load and sizes approximately 250 nm. Among the different nanosuspensions, in vitro absorption of proteins from human plasma was dependent on the nature of the stabiliser: for baicalin nanocrystals coated with TW80, TPGS, or a mixture of both stabilisers, relatively low amounts of opsonins were adsorbed, whereas high amounts of apolipoproteins were found. Pharmacokinetic studies comparing the performance of baicalin solution with TW80 and TW80+TPGS nanosuspensions were conducted in rats. Better results were obtained for TW80+TPGS-coated particles, with a four-fold increase in brain-targeting efficiency relative to the baicalin solution.

Another interesting approach was recently proposed by Chai et al. [177]. The authors used biomimetic nanocarriers made up of a nanocrystal core coated by red blood cell membranes modified according to the target. Their results concern nanocrystals of docetaxel (Fig. 7.5f), a low-aqueous-solubility chemotherapeutic drug, coated with red blood cell membranes in which the peptide c(RGDyK) was incorporated (modified red blood cell membrane-coated nanocrystals, MRBC-CNCs). This peptide targets integrins on tumour cells and neovasculature. Coated particles of about 70 nm were obtained. In vivo safety in nude mice was investigated for the bare nanocrystals (NCs), the MRBC-CNCs and the docetaxel intravenous infusion. The nanocrystals were not sufficiently stable to prevent in vivo agglomeration [178], and embolism occurred. This was circumvented with MRBC-CNCs, which showed also fewer side effects than the intravenous infusion. Additionally, an in vivo orthotropic glioma model was used in mice. The results showed higher drug accumulation in the tumour and higher median survival time using MRBC-CNCs, when compared with both intravenous infusion and nonmodified red blood cell membrane-coated

nanocrystals. The use of nanocrystals allows high drug loading and therefore higher concentration of the drug at the tumour, and the membrane coating was crucial for increased nanocrystal stability, biocompatibility, higher tumour accumulation and therapeutic efficacy.

7.5.3 Nasal Administration

Intranasal administration (IN) is an attractive, non-invasive route which can be used to directly target the brain via the olfactory and trigeminal neural systems, therefore bypassing the blood–brain barrier. Other interesting features of this administration route include rapid absorption and circumvention of the first-pass metabolism [179–182]; however, important drawbacks include active mucociliary clearance and the limited volumes which can be used in intranasal delivery [181, 182]. Furthermore, it has also been noted that this administration route lacks validated translational animal models [183, 184].

The work by Pailla et al. [185] is an example, from the few found in the literature, of the potential for using nanocrystals in intranasal brain drug delivery. These authors investigated brain distribution in Wistar rats of the BCS class II antipsychotic zotepine (Fig. 7.5g) following intranasal administration of nanosuspensions of the drug. Two kinds of nanosuspensions were prepared, one by sonoprecipitation and the other by a combination technique (antisolvent precipitation followed by high-pressure homogenisation), with particle sizes of 519 ± 10 nm and 330 ± 13 nm and a PDI of 0.272 ± 0.023 and 0.208 ± 0.029, respectively. A mixture of three stabilisers (Pluronic F-127, hydroxypropyl methyl cellulose E15 and soya lecithin) proved to be the best choice for particle size stability. Pharmacokinetic parameters were evaluated for both nanosuspensions after intranasal administration, and for zotepine solution administered by both intranasal (IN) and intravenous (IV) routes. The AUC ratio of brain (AUC_{brain}) versus plasma (AUC_{plasma}) was similar for both nanosuspensions (AUC_{brain}/AUC_{plasma} = 55) and much higher than those obtained for IN zotepine (AUC_{brain}/AUC_{plasma} = 0.87) and IV zotepine ($dAUC_{brain}/AUC_{plasma}$ = 0.17) solutions. For the nanosuspensions, $C_{max,brain}$ was 14 ± 2 μg ml^{-1}, compared with 2.1 ± 0.4 μg ml^{-1} for the IN solution and 2.3 ± 0.7 μg ml^{-1} for the IV solution. The results highlight the effective brain targeting achieved with these zotepine nanosuspensions administered by the intranasal route.

7.6 Concluding Remarks

Drug nanocrystals are an appealing approach to enhance dissolution rate and bioavailability of poorly soluble drugs which have also been applied for sustained release and drug targeting. High drug loading, with reduced amount of additional matrix materials, the possibility of variable administration routes and easy scale-up fabrication are additional interesting features of drug nanocrystals for brain delivery. Effective brain targeting will certainly be the object of additional future investigation as well as the understanding of the mechanisms of nanocrystals stabilisation. Stabilisation of nanocrystals is a crucial issue in the development of drug nanocrystal products and, to date, the choice of the stabilisers is a time-consuming trial-and-error process.

References

1. Peltonen, L. (2013). Drug nanocrystals, in *Fundamentals of Pharmaceutical Nanoscience*, Uchegbu, I. F., ed., Springer, New York, p. 277.
2. Malamatari, M., Taylor, K. M. G., Malamataris, S., Douroumis, D., Kachrimanis, K. (2018). Pharmaceutical nanocrystals: production by wet milling and applications. *Drug Discov. Today*, **23**, 534–547.
3. Müller, R. H., Shegokar, R., Gohla, S., Keck, C. M. (2011). Nanocrystals: production, cellular drug delivery, current and future products, in *Intracellular Delivery: Fundamentals and Applications*, Prokop, A., ed., Springer Netherlands, Dordrecht, pp. 411–432.
4. Junghanns, J., Muller, R. H. (2008). Nanocrystal technology, drug delivery and clinical applications. *Int. J. Nanomed.*, **3**, 295–309.
5. Peltonen, L., Hirvonen, J. (2018). Drug nanocrystals - versatile option for formulation of poorly soluble materials. *Int. J. Pharm.*, **537**, 73–83.
6. Müller, R. H., Gohla, S., Keck, C. M. (2011). State of the art of nanocrystals: special features, production, nanotoxicology aspects and intracellular delivery. *Eur. J. Pharm. Biopharm.*, **78**, 1–9.

7. FDA (2014). Guidance for Industry - Considering whether an FDA-regulated product involves the application of nanotechnology. Food and Drug Administration. Available at: http://www.fda.gov/media/88423/download, Accessed on: 2019/10/29.
8. Commission-Recommendation (2011). Commission recommendation of 18 October 2011 on the definition of nanomaterial 2011/696/EU. *Off. J. Eur. Union L.*, **275**, 38–40.
9. Ossa, D. (2014). Quality aspects of nano-based medicines SME workshop: focus on quality for medicines containing chemical entities London. Available at: http://www.ema.europa.eu/docs/en_GB/document_library/Presentation/2014/2004/WC500165444.pdf, Accessed on: 2019/12/20.
10. Hasegawa, Y., Higashi, K., Yamamoto, K., Moribe, K. (2015). Direct evaluation of molecular states of piroxicam/poloxamer nanosuspension by suspended-state NMR and Raman spectroscopies. *Mol. Pharm.*, **12**, 1564–1572.
11. Lindfors, L., Skantze, P., Skantze, U., Westergren, J., Olsson, U. (2007). Amorphous drug nanosuspensions. 3. Particle dissolution and crystal growth. *Langmuir*, **23**, 9866–9874.
12. Jog, R., Burgess, D. J. (2017). Pharmaceutical amorphous nanoparticles. *J. Pharm. Sci.*, **106**, 39–65.
13. Wang, M., Rutledge, G. C., Myerson, A. S., Trout, B. L. (2012). Production and characterization of carbamazepine nanocrystals by electrospraying for continuous pharmaceutical manufacturing. *J. Pharm. Sci.*, **101**, 1178–1188.
14. Keck, C. M., Muller, R. H. (2013). Nanotoxicological classification system (NCS): a guide for the risk-benefit assessment of nanoparticulate drug delivery systems. *Eur. J. Pharm. Biopharm.*, **84**, 445–448.
15. Ventola, C. L. (2017). Progress in nanomedicine: approved and investigational nanodrugs. *Pharm. Ther.*, **42**, 742–755.
16. Bansal, S., Bansal, M. B., Kumria, R. (2012). Nanocrystals: current strategies and trends. *J. Pharm. Biomed. Sci.*, **3**, 406–419.
17. Silva, A. C., Gonzalez-Mira, E., Lobo, J. M., Amaral, M. H. (2013). Current progresses on nanodelivery systems for the treatment of neuropsychiatric diseases: Alzheimer's and schizophrenia. *Curr. Pharm. Des.*, **19**, 7185–7195.
18. Gülsün, T., Gürsoy, R. N., Öner, L. (2009). Nanocrystal technology for oral delivery of poorly water-soluble drugs. *FABAD J. Pharm. Sci.*, **34**, 55–65.

19. Moschwitzer, J. P. (2013). Drug nanocrystals in the commercial pharmaceutical development process. *Int. J. Pharm.*, **453**, 142–156.

20. Hafner, A., Lovric, J., Lakos, G. P., Pepic, I. (2014). Nanotherapeutics in the EU: an overview on current state and future directions. *Int. J. Nanomed.*, **9**, 1005–1023.

21. Choi, Y. H., Han, H. K. (2018). Nanomedicines: current status and future perspectives in aspect of drug delivery and pharmacokinetics. *J. Pharm. Investig.*, **48**, 43–60.

22. Gao, L., Liu, G. Y., Ma, J. L., Wang, X. Q., Zhou, L., et al. (2013). Application of drug nanocrystal technologies on oral drug delivery of poorly soluble drugs. *Pharm. Res.*, **30**, 307–324.

23. Shegokar, R., Muller, R. H. (2010). Nanocrystals: industrially feasible multifunctional formulation technology for poorly soluble actives. *Int. J. Pharm.*, **399**, 129–139.

24. Rycroft, T., Trump, B., Poinsatte-Jones, K., Linkov, I. (2018). Nanotoxicology and nanomedicine: making development decisions in an evolving governance environment. *J. Nanopart. Res.*, **20**, 52.

25. Liversidge, G. G., Cundy, K. C., Bishop, J. F., Czekai, D. A. (1992). Surface modified drug nanoparticles. US Patent 5145684.

26. Müller, R. H., Becker, R., Kruss, B., Peters, K. (1999). Pharmaceutical nanosuspensions for medicament administration as systems with increased saturation solubility and rate of solution. US Patent 5858410A.

27. Khan, S., Pace, G. W. (2002). Composition and method of preparing microparticles of water-insoluble substances. US Patent 6337092B1.

28. Jarvis, M., Krishnan, V., Mitragotri, S. (2019). Nanocrystals: a perspective on translational research and clinical studies. *Bioeng. Transl. Med.*, **4**, 5–16.

29. Gao, L., Liu, G. Y., Ma, J. L., Wang, X. Q., Zhou, L., et al. (2012). Drug nanocrystals: in vivo performances. *J. Control. Release*, **160**, 418–430.

30. Kawakami, K. (2012). Modification of physicochemical characteristics of active pharmaceutical ingredients and application of supersaturatable dosage forms for improving bioavailability of poorly absorbed drugs. *Adv. Drug Deliv. Rev.*, **64**, 480–495.

31. Amidon, G. L., Lennernas, H., Shah, V. P., Crison, J. R. (1995). A theoretical basis for a biopharmaceutic drug classification: the correlation of in-vitro drug product dissolution and in-vivo biovailability. *Pharm. Res.*, **12**, 413–420.

32. Yu, L. X., Amidon, G. L., Polli, J. E., Zhao, H., Mehta, M. U., et al. (2002). Biopharmaceutics classification system: the scientific basis for biowaiver extensions. *Pharm. Res.*, **19**, 921–925.

33. Masserini, M. (2013). Nanoparticles for brain drug delivery. *ISRN Biochem.*, **2013**, 1–18.

34. Wong, H. L., Wu, X. Y., Bendayan, R. (2012). Nanotechnological advances for the delivery of CNS therapeutics. *Adv. Drug Deliv. Rev.*, **64**, 686–700.

35. Dening, T. J., Rao, S., Thomas, N., Prestidge, C. A. (2016). Oral nanomedicine approaches for the treatment of psychiatric illnesses. *J. Control. Release*, **223**, 137–156.

36. Butler, J. M., Dressman, J. B. (2010). The developability classification system: application of biopharmaceutics concepts to formulation development. *J. Pharm. Sci.*, **99**, 4940–4954.

37. Rosenberger, J., Butler, J., Dressman, J. (2018). A refined developability classification system. *J. Pharm. Sci.*, **107**, 2020–2032.

38. Lipinski, C. A., Lombardo, F., Dominy, B. W., Feeney, P. J. (2012). Experimental and computational approaches to estimate solubility and permeability in drug discovery and development settings. *Adv. Drug Deliv. Rev.*, **64**, 4–17.

39. Di, L., Kerns, E. H., Carter, G. T. (2009). Drug-like property concepts in pharmaceutical design. *Curr. Pharm. Des.*, **15**, 2184–2194.

40. Kawabata, Y., Wada, K., Nakatani, M., Yamada, S., Onoue, S. (2011). Formulation design for poorly water-soluble drugs based on biopharmaceutics classification system: basic approaches and practical applications. *Int. J. Pharm.*, **420**, 1–10.

41. Merisko-Liversidge, E., Liversidge, G. G., Cooper, E. R. (2003). Nanosizing: a formulation approach for poorly-water-soluble compounds. *Eur. J. Pharm. Sci.*, **18**, 113–120.

42. Gardner, C. R., Walsh, C. T., Almarsson, O. (2004). Drugs as materials: valuing physical form in drug discovery. *Nat. Rev. Drug Discovery*, **3**, 926–934.

43. Sun, L. M., Hu, Y. Z., Zhang, L. B. (2018). Recent trends in nanocrystals for pharmaceutical applications. *Curr. Pharm. Des.*, **24**, 2394–2402.

44. Singh, M. K., Pooja, D., Ravuri, H. G., Gunukula, A., Kulhari, H., et al. (2018). Fabrication of surfactant-stabilized nanosuspension of naringenin to surpass its poor physiochemical properties and low oral bioavailability. *Phytomedicine*, **40**, 48–54.

45. Junyaprasert, V. B., Morakul, B. (2015). Nanocrystals for enhancement of oral bioavailability of poorly water-soluble drugs. *Asian J. Pharm. Sci.*, **10**, 13–23.

46. Kipp, J. E. (2004). The role of solid nanoparticle technology in the parenteral delivery of poorly water-soluble drugs. *Int. J. Pharm.*, **284**, 109–122.

47. Fu, Q. S., Cui, Z. X., Xue, Y. Q., Duan, H. J. (2018). Research of size- and shape-dependent thermodynamic properties of the actual melting process of nanoparticles. *J. Phys. Chem. C*, **122**, 15713–15722.

48. Wang, Y., Xue, Y. Q., Fu, Q. S. (2020). Size dependence of the integral melting enthalpy and entropy of nanoparticles. *J. Nanosci. Nanotechnol.*, **20**, 934–940.

49. Jiang, Q., Shi, H. X., Zhao, M. (1999). Melting thermodynamics of organic nanocrystals. *J. Chem. Phys.*, **111**, 2176–2180.

50. Chiarappa, G., Piccolo, A., Colombo, I., Hasa, D., Voinovich, D., et al. (2017). Exploring the shape influence on melting temperature, enthalpy, and solubility of organic drug nanocrystals by a thermodynamic model. *Cryst. Growth Des.*, **17**, 4072–4083.

51. Noyes, A. A., Whitney, W. R. (1897). The rate of solution of solid substances in their own solutions. *J. Am. Chem. Soc.*, **19**, 930–934.

52. Dolores, R. S., Kieran, H. G., Anne Marie, H. (2015). Emerging nanonisation technologies: tailoring crystalline versus amorphous nanomaterials. *Curr. Top. Med. Chem.*, **15**, 2327–2340.

53. Liu, T., Müller, R. H., Möschwitzer, J. P. (2015). Effect of drug physico-chemical properties on the efficiency of top-down process and characterization of nanosuspension. *Expert Opin. Drug Deliv.*, **12**, 1741–1754.

54. Sinha, B., Müller, R. H., Möschwitzer, J. P. (2013). Bottom-up approaches for preparing drug nanocrystals: formulations and factors affecting particle size. *Int. J. Pharm.*, **453**, 126–141.

55. Keck, C. M., Müller, R. H. (2006). Drug nanocrystals of poorly soluble drugs produced by high pressure homogenisation. *Eur. J. Pharm. Biopharm.*, **62**, 3–16.

56. Fontana, F., Figueiredo, P., Zhang, P., Hirvonen, J. T., Liu, D., et al. (2018). Production of pure drug nanocrystals and nano co-crystals by confinement methods. *Adv. Drug Deliv. Rev.*, **131**, 3–21.

57. Loh, Z. H., Samanta, A. K., Sia Heng, P. W. (2015). Overview of milling techniques for improving the solubility of poorly water-soluble drugs. *Asian J. Pharm. Sci.*, **10**, 255–274.

58. Al-Kassas, R., Bansal, M., Shaw, J. (2017). Nanosizing techniques for improving bioavailability of drugs. *J. Control. Release*, **260**, 202–212.

59. Müller, R. H., Mäder, K., Krause, K. (2000). Verfahren zur schonenden Herstellung von hochfeinen micro-/nanopartikeln. PCT/EP00/06535.

60. Sachin Kumar, S., Yogyata, V., Monica, G., Sibasis, B., Varun, G., et al. (2016). Nanosuspension: principles, perspectives and practices. *Curr. Drug Deliv.*, **13**, 1222–1246.

61. Mullin, J. W. (2001). *Crystallization*, Butterworth-Heinemann, Oxford.

62. Lu, Y., Chen, Y., Gemeinhart, R. A., Wu, W., Li, T. L. (2015). Developing nanocrystals for cancer treatment. *Nanomedicine*, **10**, 2537–2552.

63. Hu, J., Johnston, K. P., Williams, R. O., 3rd (2004). Rapid dissolving high potency danazol powders produced by spray freezing into liquid process. *Int. J. Pharm.*, **271**, 145–154.

64. Chang, S.-C., Lee, M.-J., Lin, H.-M. (2008). Role of phase behavior in micronization of lysozyme via a supercritical anti-solvent process. *Chem. Eng. J.*, **139**, 416–425.

65. Nordling-David, M. M., Rachamin, E., Grad, E., Golomb, G. (2018). Lysozyme transport to the brain by liposomes. *Prec. Nanomed.*, **1**, 146–161.

66. Reverchon, E., De Marco, I., Della Porta, G. (2002). Rifampicin microparticles production by supercritical antisolvent precipitation. *Int. J. Pharm.*, **243**, 83–91.

67. Hedberg, A., Hårdemark, H. G., Olsson-Liljequist, B., Sjölin, J. (2004). Penetration of fusidic acid and rifampicin into cerebrospinal fluid in low-grade inflammatory meningitis caused by Staphylococcus epidermidis. *Clin. Microbiol. Infec.*, **10**, 765–768.

68. Xiong, S., Liu, W., Li, D. L., Chen, X. J., Liu, F., et al. (2019). Oral delivery of puerarin nanocrystals to improve brain accumulation and anti-Parkinsonian efficacy. *Mol. Pharm.*, **16**, 1444–1455.

69. Wu, C., Li, B., Zhang, Y., Chen, T., Chen, C., et al. (2019). Intranasal delivery of paeoniflorin nanocrystals for brain targeting, *Asian J. Pharm. Sci.*, doi:10.1016/j.ajps.2019.11.002.

70. Reverchon, E., Della Porta, G., De Rosa, I., Subra, P., Letourneur, D. (2000). Supercritical antisolvent micronization of some biopolymers. *J. Supercrit. Fluids*, **18**, 239–245.

71. Dufour, J. P., Russell-Lodrigue, K. E., Doyle-Meyers, L., Falkenstein, K. P., Blair, R. V., et al. (2018). Hydrocephalus after intrathecal administration of dextran to rhesus macaques (Macaca mulatta). *Comp. Med.*, **68**, 227–232.

72. Dhumal, R. S., Biradar, S. V., Yamamura, S., Paradkar, A. R., York, P. (2008). Preparation of amorphous cefuroxime axetil nanoparticles by

sonoprecipitation for enhancement of bioavailability. *Eur. J. Pharm. Biopharm.*, **70**, 109–115.

73. Hosmann, A., Ritscher, L. C., Burgmann, H., Oesterreicher, Z., Jäger, W., et al. (2018). Concentrations of cefuroxime in brain tissue of neurointensive care patients. *Antimicrob. Agents Chemother.*, **62**, e02164–02117.

74. Kuang, Y.-Y., Zhang, Z.-B., Xie, M.-L., Wang, J.-X., Le, Y., et al. (2015). Large-scale preparation of amorphous cefixime nanoparticles by antisolvent precipitation in a high-gravity rotating packed bed. *Ind. Eng. Chem. Res.*, **54**, 8157–8165.

75. Sullins, A. K., Abdel-Rahman, S. M. (2013). Pharmacokinetics of antibacterial agents in the CSF of children and adolescents. *Paediatr. Drugs*, **15**, 93–117.

76. Craig, W. A., Andes, D. R. (2015). Cephalosporins, in *Mandell, Douglas, and Bennett's Principles and Practice of Infectious Diseases*, 8th ed., Bennett, J. E., Dolin, R., Blaser, M. J., eds., Elsevier Health Sciences, Philadelphia, pp. 278–292.

77. Chiou, H., Li, L., Hu, T., Chan, H. K., Chen, J. F., et al. (2007). Production of salbutamol sulfate for inhalation by high-gravity controlled antisolvent precipitation. *Int. J. Pharm.*, **331**, 93–98.

78. Zhang, Z.-B., Xie, M.-L., Kuang, Y.-Y., Wang, J.-X., Le, Y., et al. (2016). Preparation of amorphous drug nanoparticles by high-gravity reactive precipitation technique. *Chem. Eng. Process.*, **104**, 253–261.

79. Keshavarz, A., Karimi-Sabet, J., Fattahi, A., Golzary, A., Rafiee-Tehrani, M., et al. (2012). Preparation and characterization of raloxifene nanoparticles using Rapid Expansion of Supercritical Solution (RESS). *J. Supercrit. Fluids*, **63**, 169–179.

80. Kindler, J., Weickert, C. S., Schofield, P. R., Lenroot, R., Weickert, T. W. (2016). Raloxifene increases prefrontal activity during emotional inhibition in schizophrenia based on estrogen receptor genotype. *Eur. Neuropsychopharmacol.*, **26**, 1930–1940.

81. Uchida, H., Nishijima, M., Sano, K., Demoto, K., Sakabe, J., et al. (2015). Production of theophylline nanoparticles using rapid expansion of supercritical solutions with a solid cosolvent (RESS-SC) technique. *J. Supercrit. Fluids*, **105**, 128–135.

82. Sane, A., Limtrakul, J. (2009). Formation of retinyl palmitate-loaded poly(l-lactide) nanoparticles using rapid expansion of supercritical solutions into liquid solvents (RESOLV). *J. Supercrit. Fluids*, **51**, 230–237.

83. Pathak, P., Meziani, M. J., Desai, T., Sun, Y.-P. (2006). Formation and stabilization of ibuprofen nanoparticles in supercritical fluid processing. *J. Supercrit. Fluids*, **37**, 279–286.
84. Parepally, J. M., Mandula, H., Smith, Q. R. (2006). Brain uptake of nonsteroidal anti-inflammatory drugs: ibuprofen, flurbiprofen, and indomethacin. *Pharm. Res.*, **23**, 873–881.
85. Thakur, R., Gupta, R. B. (2006). Formation of phenytoin nanoparticles using rapid expansion of supercritical solution with solid cosolvent (RESS-SC) process. *Int. J. Pharm.*, **308**, 190–199.
86. Nevitt, S. J., Tudur Smith, C., Marson, A. G. (2019). Phenobarbitone versus phenytoin monotherapy for epilepsy: an individual participant data review. *Cochrane Database Syst. Rev.*, **7**(7), CD002217.
87. Zhu, Z. (2014). Flash nanoprecipitation: prediction and enhancement of particle stability via drug structure. *Mol. Pharm.*, **11**, 776–786.
88. Fellner, S., Bauer, B., Miller, D. S., Schaffrik, M., Fankhanel, M., et al. (2002). Transport of paclitaxel (Taxol) across the blood-brain barrier in vitro and in vivo. *J. Clin. Invest.*, **110**, 1309–1318.
89. Tam, Y. T., To, K. K., Chow, A. H. (2016). Fabrication of doxorubicin nanoparticles by controlled antisolvent precipitation for enhanced intracellular delivery. *Colloids Surf., B*, **139**, 249–258.
90. Keeney, J. T. R., Ren, X., Warrier, G., Noel, T., Powell, D. K., et al. (2018). Doxorubicin-induced elevated oxidative stress and neurochemical alterations in brain and cognitive decline: protection by MESNA and insights into mechanisms of chemotherapy-induced cognitive impairment ("chemobrain"). *Oncotarget*, **9**, 30324–30339.
91. Li, M., Yaragudi, N., Afolabi, A., Dave, R., Bilgili, E. (2015). Sub-100nm drug particle suspensions prepared via wet milling with low bead contamination through novel process intensification. *Chem. Eng. Sci.*, **130**, 207–220.
92. Tanaka, Y., Inkyo, M., Yumoto, R., Nagai, J., Takano, M., et al. (2012). Nanoparticulation of probucol, a poorly water-soluble drug, using a novel wet-milling process to improve in vitro dissolution and in vivo oral absorption. *Drug. Dev. Ind. Pharm.*, **38**, 1015–1023.
93. Jung, Y. S., Park, J. H., Kim, H., Kim, S. Y., Hwang, J. Y., et al. (2016). Probucol inhibits LPS-induced microglia activation and ameliorates brain ischemic injury in normal and hyperlipidemic mice. *Acta Pharm. Sin.*, **37**, 1031–1044.
94. Pardeike, J., Müller, R. H. (2010). Nanosuspensions: a promising formulation for the new phospholipase A2 inhibitor PX-18. *Int. J. Pharm.*, **391**, 322–329.

95. Wang, Q., Sun, A. Y., Pardeike, J., Müller, R. H., Simonyi, A., et al. (2009). Neuroprotective effects of a nanocrystal formulation of sPLA2 inhibitor PX-18 in cerebral ischemia/reperfusion in gerbils. *Brain Res.*, **1285**, 188–195.

96. Ali, H. S. M., York, P., Blagden, N. (2009). Preparation of hydrocortisone nanosuspension through a bottom-up nanoprecipitation technique using microfluidic reactors. *Int. J. Pharm.*, **375**, 107–113.

97. Dietrich, J., Rao, K., Pastorino, S., Kesari, S. (2011). Corticosteroids in brain cancer patients: benefits and pitfalls. *Expert Rev. Clin. Pharmacol.*, **4**, 233–242.

98. Salazar, J., Muller, R. H., Schwitzer, J. P. (2014). Combinative particle size reduction technologies for the production of drug nanocrystals. *J. Pharm.*, **2014**, 1–14.

99. Elgamal, E. A., Murshid, W. R. (2000). Intracavitary administration of amphotericin B in the treatment of cerebral aspergillosis in a non immune-compromised patient: case report and review of the literature. *Br. J. Neurosurg.*, **14**, 137–141.

100. de Waard, H., Frijlink, H. W., Hinrichs, W. L. (2011). Bottom-up preparation techniques for nanocrystals of lipophilic drugs. *Pharm. Res.*, **28**, 1220–1223.

101. Ige, P. P., Baria, R. K., Gattani, S. G. (2013). Fabrication of fenofibrate nanocrystals by probe sonication method for enhancement of dissolution rate and oral bioavailability. *Colloids Surf., B*, **108**, 366–373.

102. Barron, M. K., Young, T. J., Johnston, K. P., Williams, R. O., 3rd (2003). Investigation of processing parameters of spray freezing into liquid to prepare polyethylene glycol polymeric particles for drug delivery. *AAPS PharmSciTech*, **4**, 1–13.

103. Wais, U., Jackson, A. W., He, T., Zhang, H. (2016). Nanoformulation and encapsulation approaches for poorly water-soluble drug nanoparticles. *Nanoscale*, **8**, 1746–1769.

104. BÜCHI Labortechnik AG (2019). Nano spray dryer B-90 HP. Available at: https://www.buchi.com/en/products/spray-drying-and-encapsulation/nano-spray-dryer-b-90-hp, Accessed on: 2019/11/03.

105. Martena, V., Censi, R., Hoti, E., Malaj, L., Di Martino, P. (2012). A new nanospray drying method for the preparation of nicergoline pure nanoparticles. *J. Nanopart. Res.*, **14**, 1–10.

106. Li, X., Anton, N., Arpagaus, C., Belleteix, F., Vandamme, T. F. (2010). Nanoparticles by spray drying using innovative new technology: the Buchi nano spray dryer B-90. *J. Control. Release*, **147**, 304–310.

107. Gigliobianco, M. R., Casadidio, C., Censi, R., Di Martino, P. (2018). Nanocrystals of poorly soluble drugs: drug bioavailability and physicochemical stability. *Pharmaceutics*, **10**, 1–29.

108. Baba, K., Nishida, K. (2013). Steroid nanocrystals prepared using the nano spray dryer B-90. *Pharmaceutics*, **5**, 107–114.

109. Heng, D., Lee, S. H., Ng, W. K., Tan, R. B. (2011). The nano spray dryer B-90. *Expert Opin. Drug Deliv.*, **8**, 965–972.

110. Schmid, K., Arpagaus, C., Friess, W. (2011). Evaluation of the nano spray dryer B-90 for pharmaceutical applications. *Pharm. Dev. Technol.*, **16**, 287–294.

111. Chan, H. K., Kwok, P. C. (2011). Production methods for nanodrug particles using the bottom-up approach. *Adv. Drug Deliv. Rev.*, **63**, 406–416.

112. Campardelli, R., Baldino, L., Reverchon, E. (2015). Supercritical fluids applications in nanomedicine. *J. Supercrit. Fluids*, **101**, 193–214.

113. Padrela, L., Rodrigues, M. A., Duarte, A., Dias, A. M. A., Braga, M. E. M., et al. (2018). Supercritical carbon dioxide-based technologies for the production of drug nanoparticles/nanocrystals: a comprehensive review. *Adv. Drug Deliv. Rev.*, **131**, 22–78.

114. Chen, J.-F., Zhang, J.-Y., Shen, Z.-G., Zhong, J., Yun, J. (2006). Preparation and characterization of amorphous cefuroxime axetil drug nanoparticles with novel technology: high-gravity antisolvent precipitation. *Ind. Eng. Chem. Res.*, **45**, 8723–8727.

115. Zhong, J., Shen, Z., Yang, Y., Chen, J. (2005). Preparation and characterization of uniform nanosized cephradine by combination of reactive precipitation and liquid anti-solvent precipitation under high gravity environment. *Int. J. Pharm.*, **301**, 286–293.

116. Zhao, H., Wang, J.-X., Wang, Q.-A., Chen, J.-F., Yun, J. (2007). Controlled liquid antisolvent precipitation of hydrophobic pharmaceutical nanoparticles in a microchannel reactor. *Ind. Eng. Chem. Res.*, **46**, 8229–8235.

117. Zhao, H., Wang, J., Zhang, H., Shen, Z., Yun, J., et al. (2009). Facile preparation of danazol nanoparticles by high-gravity anti-solvent precipitation (HGAP) method. *Chin. J. Chem. Eng.*, **17**, 318–323.

118. Zhu, Z., Margulis-Goshen, K., Magdassi, S., Talmon, Y., Macosko, C. W. (2010). Polyelectrolyte stabilized drug nanoparticles via flash nanoprecipitation: a model study with beta-carotene. *J. Pharm. Sci.*, **99**, 4295–4306.

119. Tao, J., Chow, S. F., Zheng, Y. (2019). Application of flash nanoprecipitation to fabricate poorly water-soluble drug nanoparticles. *Acta Pharm. Sin. B*, **9**, 4–18.

120. Zhongyao, C., Yumei, L., Zul, K., Xin, M., Jianjun, C., et al. (2018). Nanocrystals technology for pharmaceutical science. *Curr. Pharm. Des.*, **24**, 2497–2507.

121. Van Eerdenbrugh, B., Van den Mooter, G., Augustijns, P. (2008). Top-down production of drug nanocrystals: nanosuspension stabilization, miniaturization and transformation into solid products. *Int. J. Pharm.*, **364**, 64–75.

122. Rolan, P. E., Mercer, A. J., Weatherley, B. C., Holdich, T., Meire, H., et al. (1994). Examination of some factors responsible for a food-induced increase in absorption of atovaquone. *Br. J. Clin. Pharmacol.*, **37**, 13–20.

123. Hyerim, Y., Hyeongmin, K., Sumin, J., Hyeyeon, S., Shofa Khoirun, N., et al. (2018). Pharmaceutical strategies for stabilizing drug nanocrystals. *Curr. Pharm. Des.*, **24**, 2362–2374.

124. Peltonen, L., Tuomela, A., Hirvonen, J. (2016). Polymeric stabilizers for drug nanocrystals, in *Handbook of Polymers for Pharmaceutical Technologies, Vol 4: Bioactive and Compatible Synthetic/Hybrid Polymers*, Thakur, V. K., Thakur, M. K., eds., Scrivener Publishing Llc, Beverly, pp. 67–87.

125. Tuomela, A., Hirvonen, J., Peltonen, L. (2016). Stabilizing agents for drug nanocrystals: effect on bioavailability. *Pharmaceutics*, **8**, 1–18.

126. Yang, H., Kim, H., Jung, S., Seo, H., Nida, S. K., et al. (2018). Pharmaceutical strategies for stabilizing drug nanocrystals. *Curr. Pharm. Des.*, **24**, 2362–2374.

127. Lockman, P. R., Koziara, J. M., Mumper, R. J., Allen, D. D. (2004). Nanoparticle surface charges alter blood-brain barrier integrity and permeability. *J. Drug Targeting*, **12**, 635–641.

128. Bilgili, E., Li, M., Afolabi, A. (2016). Is the combination of cellulosic polymers and anionic surfactants a good strategy for ensuring physical stability of BCS Class II drug nanosuspensions? *Pharm. Dev. Technol.*, **21**, 499–510.

129. George, M., Ghosh, I. (2013). Identifying the correlation between drug/stabilizer properties and critical quality attributes (CQAs) of nanosuspension formulation prepared by wet media milling technology. *Eur. J. Pharm. Sci.*, **48**, 142–152.

130. Van Eerdenbrugh, B., Vermant, J., Martens, J. A., Froyen, L., Van Humbeeck, J., et al. (2009). A screening study of surface stabilization

during the production of drug nanocrystals. *J. Pharm. Sci.*, **98**, 2091–2103.

131. Lestari, M. L., Muller, R. H., Moschwitzer, J. P. (2015). Systematic screening of different surface modifiers for the production of physically stable nanosuspensions. *J. Pharm. Sci.*, **104**, 1128–1140.

132. Nutan, M. T. H., Reddy, I. K. (2010). General principles of suspensions, in *Pharmaceutical Suspensions*, Kulshreshtha, A., Singh, O., Wall, G., eds., Springer, New York, pp. 39–65.

133. Hilfiker, R., von Raumer, M. (2019). *Polymorphism in the Pharmaceutical Industry*, Wiley-VCH, Weinheim.

134. Castro, R. A. E., Maria, T. M. R., Évora, A. O. L., Feiteira, J. C., Silva, M. R., et al. (2010). A new insight into pyrazinamide polymorphic forms and their thermodynamic relationships. *Cryst. Growth Des.*, **10**, 274–282.

135. Maria, T. M. R., Castro, R. A. E., Silva, M. R., Ramos, M. L., Justino, L. L. G., et al. (2013). Polymorphism and melt crystallisation of racemic betaxolol, a β-adrenergic antagonist drug. *J. Therm. Anal. Calorim.*, **111**, 2171–2178.

136. Maria, T. M. R., Castro, R. A. E., Bebiano, S. S., Ramos Silva, M., Matos Beja, A., et al. (2010). Polymorphism of trans-1,4-cyclohexanediol: conformational isomorphism. *Cryst. Growth Des.*, **10**, 1194–1200.

137. Évora, A. O. L., Castro, R. A. E., Maria, T. M. R., Rosado, M. T. S., Ramos Silva, M., et al. (2011). Pyrazinamide-diflunisal: a new dual-drug co-crystal. *Cryst. Growth Des.*, **11**, 4780–4788.

138. Castro, R. A. E., Ribeiro, J. D. B., Maria, T. M. R., Ramos Silva, M., Yuste-Vivas, C., et al. (2011). Naproxen cocrystals with pyridinecarboxamide isomers. *Cryst. Growth Des.*, **11**, 5396–5404.

139. Évora, A. O. L., Castro, R. A. E., Maria, T. M. R., Silva, M. R., ter Horst, J. H., et al. (2014). A thermodynamic based approach on the investigation of a diflunisal pharmaceutical co-crystal with improved intrinsic dissolution rate. *Int. J. Pharm.*, **466**, 68–75.

140. Aakeröy, C. B., Sinha, A. S. (2018). *Co-crystals: Preparation, Characterization and Applications*, The Royal Society of Chemistry, London.

141. Évora, A. O. L., Castro, R. A. E., Maria, T. M. R., Ramos Silva, M., Canotilho, J., et al. (2019). Lamotrigine: design and synthesis of new multicomponent solid forms. *Eur. J. Pharm. Sci.*, **129**, 148–162.

142. Stahl, P. H., Wermuth, C. G. (2008). *Handbook of Pharmaceutical Salts Properties, Selection, and Use*, Wiley-VCH, Zurich.

143. Aguiar, A. J., Krc Jr., J., Kinkel, A. W., Samyn, J. C. (1967). Effect of polymorphism on the absorption of chloramphenicol from chloramphenicol palmitate. *J. Pharm. Sci.*, **56**, 847–853.

144. Bauer, J., Spanton, S., Henry, R., Quick, J., Dziki, W., et al. (2001). Ritonavir: an extraordinary example of conformational polymorphism. *Pharm. Res.*, **18**, 859–866.

145. McCrone, W. C. (1965). Polymorphism, in *Physics and Chemistry of the Organic Solid State*, Fox, D., Labes, M. M., Weissberger, A., eds., Wiley Interscience, New York, pp. 725–767.

146. Bernstein, J. (2002). *Polymorphism in Molecular Crystal*, Oxford University Press.

147. FDA (2007). Guidance for Industry - ANDAs:Pharmaceutical solid polymorphism: chemistry, manufacturing, and controls information. Food and Drug Administration. Available at: http://www.fda.gov/media/71375/download, Accessed on: 2019/10/29.

148. Sharma, P., Zujovic, Z. D., Bowmaker, G. A., Marshall, A. J., Denny, W. A., et al. (2011). Evaluation of a crystalline nanosuspension: polymorphism, process induced transformation and in vivo studies. *Int. J. Pharm.*, **408**, 138–151.

149. Lai, F., Sinico, C., Ennas, G., Marongiu, F., Marongiu, G., et al. (2009). Diclofenac nanosuspensions: influence of preparation procedure and crystal form on drug dissolution behaviour. *Int. J. Pharm.*, **373**, 124–132.

150. Martena, V., Censi, R., Hoti, E., Malaj, L., Di Martino, P. (2012). Indomethacin nanocrystals prepared by different laboratory scale methods: effect on crystalline form and dissolution behavior. *J. Nanopart. Res.*, **14**, 1–14.

151. Peltonen, L. (2018). Practical guidelines for the characterization and quality control of pure drug nanoparticles and nano-cocrystals in the pharmaceutical industry. *Adv. Drug Deliv. Rev.*, **131**, 101–115.

152. Florence, A. T., Hillery, A. M., Hussain, N., Jani, P. U. (1995). Factors affecting the oral uptake and translocation of polystyrene nanoparticles - histological and analytical evidence. *J. Drug Targeting*, **3**, 65–70.

153. Jani, P., Halbert, G. W., Langridge, J., Florence, A. T. (1990). Nanoparticle uptake by the rat gastrointestinal mucosa - quantification and particle-size dependency. *J. Pharm. Pharmacol.*, **42**, 821–826.

154. Florence, A. T. (1997). The oral absorption of micro- and nanoparticulates: neither exceptional nor unusual. *Pharm. Res.*, **14**, 259–266.

155. Liversidge, G. G., Conzentino, P. (1995). Drug particle-size reduction for decreasing gastric irritancy and enhancing absorption of naproxen in rats. *Int. J. Pharm.*, **125**, 309–313.

156. Liversidge, G. G., Cundy, K. C. (1995). Particle-sise reduction for improvement of oral bioavailability of hydrophobic drugs. 1. Absolute oral bioavailability of nanocrystalline danazol in beagle dogs. *Int. J. Pharm.*, **125**, 91–97.

157. Thombre, A. G., Caldwell, W. B., Friesen, D. T., McCray, S. B., Sutton, S. C. (2012). Solid nanocrystalline dispersions of ziprasidone with enhanced bioavailability in the fasted state. *Mol. Pharm.*, **9**, 3526–3534.

158. Thombre, A. G., Herbig, S. M., Alderman, J. A. (2011). Improved ziprasidone formulations with enhanced bioavailability in the fasted state and a reduced food effect. *Pharm. Res.*, **28**, 3159–3170.

159. Thombre, A. G., Shah, J. C., Sagawa, K., Caldwell, W. B. (2012). In vitro and in vivo characterization of amorphous, nanocrystalline, and crystalline ziprasidone formulations. *Int. J. Pharm.*, **428**, 8–17.

160. Shubar, H. M., Lachenmaier, S., Heimesaat, M. M., Lohman, U., Mauludin, R., et al. (2011). SDS-coated atovaquone nanosuspensions show improved therapeutic efficacy against experimental acquired and reactivated toxoplasmosis by improving passage of gastrointestinal and blood-brain barriers. *J. Drug Targeting*, **19**, 114–124.

161. Liu, S. Y., Qu, X. H., Jin, G. H., Nie, F., Liu, F., et al. (2018). Puerarin promoted proliferation and differentiation of dopamine-producing cells in Parkinson's animal models. *Biomed. Pharmacother.*, **106**, 1236–1242.

162. Sun, B., Yeo, Y. (2012). Nanocrystals for the parenteral delivery of poorly water-soluble drugs. *Curr. Opin. Solid State Mater. Sci.*, **16**, 295–301.

163. Bishara, D. (2010). Once-monthly paliperidone injection for the treatment of schizophrenia. *Neuropsychiatr. Dis. Treat.*, **6**, 561–572.

164. Gopal, S., Gassmann-Mayer, C., Palumbo, J., Samtani, M. N., Shiwach, R., et al. (2010). Practical guidance for dosing and switching paliperidone palmitate treatment in patients with schizophrenia. *Curr. Med. Res. Opin.*, **26**, 377–387.

165. Leng, D. L., Chen, H. M., Li, G. J., Guo, M. R., Zhu, Z. L., et al. (2014). Development and comparison of intramuscularly long-acting paliperidone palmitate nanosuspensions with different particle size. *Int. J. Pharm.*, **472**, 380–385.

166. Gao, L., Zhang, D. R., Chen, M. H., Duan, C. X., Dai, W. T., et al. (2008). Studies on pharmacokinetics and tissue distribution of oridonin nanosuspensions. *Int. J. Pharm.*, **355**, 321–327.

167. Teleanu, D. M., Chircov, C., Grumezescu, A. M., Volceanov, A., Teleanu, R. I. (2018). Blood-brain delivery methods using nanotechnology. *Pharmaceutics*, **10**, 16.

168. Gao, H. L. (2016). Progress and perspectives on targeting nanoparticles for brain drug delivery. *Acta Pharm. Sin. B*, **6**, 268–286.

169. Wiley, D. T., Webster, P., Gale, A., Davis, M. E. (2013). Transcytosis and brain uptake of transferrin-containing nanoparticles by tuning avidity to transferrin receptor. *Proc. Natl. Acad. Sci. U. S. A.*, **110**, 8662–8667.

170. Jiang, W. L., Xie, H., Ghoorah, D., Shang, Y. L., Shi, H. J., et al. (2012). Conjugation of functionalized SPIONs with transferrin for targeting and imaging brain glial tumors in rat model. *PLoS One*, **7**, 1–6.

171. R. H. Müller, S. H. (1989). Surface modelling of microparticles as parenteral systems with high tissue affinity, in *Bioadhesion-Possibilities and Future Trends*, Gurny, R., Junginger, H. E., eds., Wissenschaftliche Verlagsgesellschaft, Stuttgart, pp. 202–214.

172. Kreuter, J., Shamenkov, D., Petrov, V., Ramge, P., Cychutek, K., et al. (2002). Apolipoprotein-mediated transport of nanoparticle-bound drugs across the blood-brain barrier. *J. Drug Targeting*, **10**, 317–325.

173. Scholer, N., Krause, K., Kayser, O., Muller, R. H., Borner, K., et al. (2001). Atovaquone nanosuspensions show excellent therapeutic effect in a new murine model of reactivated toxoplasmosis. *Antimicrob. Agents Chemother.*, **45**, 1771–1779.

174. Shubar, H. M., Dunay, I. R., Lachenmaier, S., Dathe, M., Bushrab, F. N., et al. (2009). The role of apolipoprotein E in uptake of atovaquone into the brain in murine acute and reactivated toxoplasmosis. *J. Drug Targeting*, **17**, 257–267.

175. Liu, Y., Ma, Y. Q., Xu, J. N., Chen, Y. C., Xie, J., et al. (2017). Apolipoproteins adsorption and brain-targeting evaluation of baicalin nanocrystals modified by combination of Tween80 and TPGS. *Colloids Surf., B*, **160**, 619–627.

176. Sowndhararajan, K., Deepa, P., Kim, M., Park, S. J., Kim, S. (2018). Neuroprotective and cognitive enhancement potentials of baicalin: a review. *Brain Sci.*, **8**, 24.

177. Chai, Z. L., Ran, D. N., Lu, L. W., Zhan, C. Y., Ruan, H. T., et al. (2019). Ligand-modified cell membrane enables the targeted delivery of drug nanocrystals to glioma. *ACS Nano*, **13**, 5591–5601.

178. Mitragotri, S., Burke, P. A., Langer, R. (2014). Overcoming the challenges in administering biopharmaceuticals: formulation and delivery strategies. *Nat. Rev. Drug Discovery*, **13**, 655–672.

179. Khan, A. R., Liu, M. R., Khan, M. W., Zhai, G. X. (2017). Progress in brain targeting drug delivery system by nasal route. *J. Control. Release*, **268**, 364–389.

180. Wu, H. B., Hu, K. L., Jiang, X. G. (2008). From nose to brain: understanding transport capacity and transport rate of drugs. *Expert Opin. Drug Deliv.*, **5**, 1159–1168.

181. Erdo, F., Bors, L. A., Farkas, D., Bajza, A., Gizurarson, S. (2018). Evaluation of intranasal delivery route of drug administration for brain targeting. *Brain Res. Bull.*, **143**, 155–170.

182. Mistry, A., Stolnik, S., Illum, L. (2009). Nanoparticles for direct nose-to-brain delivery of drugs. *Int. J. Pharm.*, **379**, 146–157.

183. Sonvico, F., Clementino, A., Buttini, F., Colombo, G., Pescina, S., et al. (2018). Surface-modified nanocarriers for nose-to-brain delivery: from bioadhesion to targeting. *Pharmaceutics*, **10**, 1–34.

184. Arora, P., Sharma, S., Garg, S. (2002). Permeability issues in nasal drug delivery. *Drug Discov. Today*, **7**, 967–975.

185. Pailla, S. R., S. Talluri, Rangaraj, N., Ramavath, R., Challa, V. S., et al. (2019). Intranasal Zotepine Nanosuspension: intended for improved brain distribution in rats. *DARU J. Pharm. Sci.*, **27**, 541–556.

Chapter 8

Lipid Nanocarriers for Oligonucleotide Delivery to the Brain

Andreia F. Jorge,[a] Santiago Grijalvo,[b] Alberto Pais[a] and Ramón Eritja[b]

[a]*Coimbra Chemistry Centre (CQC), Department of Chemistry, University of Coimbra, Rua Larga, 3004-535 Coimbra, Portugal*

[b]*Institute for Advanced Chemistry of Catalonia (IQAC-CSIC), Jordi Girona 18-26, E-08034 Barcelona, Spain. Networking Center on Bioengineering, Biomaterials and Nanomedicine (CIBER-BBN), Jordi Girona 18-26, E-08034 Barcelona, Spain*

andreiaj@qui.uc.pt

The number of patients with brain pathologies is increasing worldwide as a consequence of the modern living style and a growing percentage of the elderly population. Developments in the design of drugs are needed to cope with this demanding social situation. Several promising approaches based in the knowledge of the human genome are actively pursued. In this chapter, we review recent developments in the use of synthetic oligonucleotides to control gene expression in neuronal cells and the potential formulations to reach the brain. This includes the description of the most common modifications for oligonucleotides to increase their stability in

Nanoparticles for Brain Drug Delivery
Edited by Carla Vitorino, Andreia Jorge and Alberto Pais

ISBN 978-981-4877-31-2 (Hardcover), 978-1-003-11932-6 (eBook)
www.jennystanford.com

physiological media and the use of lipid nanocarriers for enhancing brain delivery.

8.1 Introduction

Brain pathologies affect a large number of individuals and have devastating repercussions in global health. The population ageing is expected to increase the incidence of brain diseases in the forthcoming years. Nevertheless, for most of such diseases, curative and disease-modifying treatment options are still scarce.

In the past years, significant discoveries have unveiled important functional information about the human genome, opening a new era for neurological conditions research and ultimately for the development of therapies to prevent the onset or slow disease progression and ideally repair normal brain function. The aetiology of most neurological disorders is multifunctional in nature, that is, results from the interplay of genetic and environmental risk factors [1]. Genetic defects have been proven to play a central role in brain disorders and may provide alternative routes to identify new targets to ameliorate the treatment of these pathologies [2, 3].

The translation of these insights into clinical research has put in evidence the value of therapeutic oligonucleotides (ODNs) to address with high specificity targets otherwise inaccessible for conventional drugs. In this context, RNA-based therapeutics provide a new therapeutic paradigm in the treatment of brain diseases, enabling us to downregulate and upregulate gene expression, to modulate messenger RNA (mRNA) splicing, to target trinucleotide repeat regions or long noncoding RNAs (ncRNAs) and to edit the genome by using the CRISPR-Cas9 tool [4–7]. RNA inhibition strategies for brain disorders aiming at downregulating a pathological gene are currently widely exploited in clinical trials, while strategies for the upregulation of RNA are still in a preclinical stage [8]. Two decades after the first application of ODNs in living mammalian brain [9], the therapeutic merits of these drugs have been recently recognised by the US Food and Drug Administration (FDA) after approving the commercial use of eteplirsen, Exondys 51™ (Serepta Therapeutics, Cambridge, USA) in 2016 and nusinersen, Spinraza™ (Biogen, Cambridge, USA) in 2017 for a defined subset of Duchenne muscular dystrophy (DMD) and for spinal muscular atrophy, respectively.

At a molecular level, negatively charged ODNs face a number of obstacles, especially if their faith is to transverse the protective barriers of the brain, the blood–brain barrier (BBB) or the blood–spinal cord barrier (BSCB). After intravenous injection, the large majority of ODNs is not able to cross the BBB and is readily degraded under physiological conditions. Owing to this, brain drug delivery remains one of the most challenging and attractive areas of research. So far multiple routes of administration have been exploited for central nervous system (CNS) gene delivery, including intranasal, intracarotid, intravitreal, intrathecal and intramuscular. However, neither of these routes has proved to be an effective gold standard, whereas their selection is dependent on pondering between associated risks and efficacy. For instance, intrathecal injection has demonstrated promising results in delivering antisense oligonucleotides (ASOs) in mice and nonhuman primates [10], yet there are concerns about potential neurotoxic effects [11]. At the same time, a great deal of attention has been dedicated to develop smart vehicles, either nonviral- or viral-based systems, with higher propensity to cross the BBB mainly through systemic, intranasal or oral administration [12], as well as devise potent ODN chemistries [13, 14]. Chemical modifications largely improved the overall pharmacological properties of ODNs. Viral vector-mediated gene delivery has emerged as a promising approach to target the brain, which is considered immune-privileged [15, 16]. However, safety concerns were posed about the use of viral vectors. Within nonviral approaches, lipid-based nanoparticles and ODN-lipid conjugates are at forefront of the developing field of nonviral vectors for ODN delivery, being the most clinically advanced materials of their class.

This chapter summarises the state of lipid-based technology applied to ODN delivery in the brain and emphasises how recent advances in this field position ODNs to be a relevant contributor to advanced therapeutics. A brief introduction will be firstly made to establish the main differences and opportunities provided by ASOs, RNA interference (RNAi) and steric blocking ODNs, all of them operating by an antisense mechanism. A general description of aptamers will be also made to highlight their potential application in diagnosis, targeting and therapeutic activity in brain conditions. Additionally, antiproliferative ODNs will be succinctly introduced due to their promising application in the treatment of CNS disorders.

8.2 Oligonucleotide-Based Therapeutics

8.2.1 Antisense Oligonucleotides

One of the most exciting nucleic acid–based therapeutics used for downregulating gene expression is the ASO. In the late 1970s, Paul Zamecnick in a seminal work demonstrated that synthetic ASOs could be used therapeutically to inhibit protein translation [17]. ASOs are chemically modified single-stranded DNA (ssDNA) molecules, typically 12–30 nucleotides (nt) in length, which specifically bind to endogenous target mRNA by Watson–Crick base-pairing rules [18]. Following these rules, complementary base pairs are held together via specific hydrogen-bonding interactions and strengthened by the hydrophobic interactions arisen from purine–pyrimidine shape complementarity and base stacking. The chemical modification of ASOs is a requisite to guarantee stability in physiological conditions and to increase their potency and specificity to silence the mRNA target [19]. The most remarkable advance made towards the use of ASOs as therapeutic agents was the introduction of the phosphorothioate (PS) backbone modification, disclosed in 1970, which largely extends the half-lives of ASOs in serum and facilitates cellular uptake [20]. Equally relevant was the introduction of 2′-O-methyl (2′-O-Me; Fig. 8.1) modified ODNs which dramatically increased the resistance of ASOs to nucleases [21].

Once internalised, ASOs modulate target mRNA activity through two main mechanisms: (i) ribonuclease H (RNAse H)-dependent mechanism [22] and (ii) nondegradative steric blocking mechanisms [23]. In the degradative mechanism, RNAse H enzyme binds to the mRNA–ASO heteroduplex through a binding domain inserted on the N terminus of the protein and catalyses the cleavage of the mRNA strand. In humans, the specific enzyme recruited is RNAse H1, and it is ubiquitously found in the nucleus, mitochondria and cytoplasm [22]. The cleaved debris of mRNA is then processed by the typical cellular degradation pathways, while the intact DNA is again available to hybridise with an additional target mRNA [24]. Endonuclease-mediated degradation is particularly attractive for the treatment of neurological diseases in which the aetiology is known to be dependent on protein dysregulation or accumulation. The high number of preclinical and clinical studies which employ

ASOs designed for RNAse activation validates the interest in the field [25, 26]. However, since RNAse-H is a required mediator, it should be considered a rate-limiting step for ASO activity. As alternative to the use of the catalytic activity of endonucleases, ASOs with intrinsic enzymatic activity can be synthetically designed, as, for instance, DNAzymes or ribozymes [27]. The number of modifications on the ASO backbone may also interfere in their activity. The triggered mechanism(s) by which ASOs exert their antisense activity are thus dependent on ASO chemistry and design. RNase H–mediated ODNs often include internucleotide linkage modifications such as PS, phosphonoacetate (PACE), and boranophosphate [28–30] (Fig. 8.1). Sugar modifications are generally considered incompatible with RNase H–mediated gene silencing. However, they can be implemented in a 'gapmer' design, where the unmodified central DNA core guarantees high affinity to RNAse H, while their overhangs can be successfully protected with 2′-O-Me, 2′-O-(2-methoxyethyl) (2′-MOE), bicyclic locked nucleic acid (LNA) and 2′-deoxy-2′-fluoro-β-D-arabino (2′-F-ANA) sugar modifications [31–33] (Fig. 8.1). Gapmers modified with 2′-MOE are currently tested clinically for the treatment of amyotrophic lateral sclerosis (ALS) [34].

In the nondegradative steric blocking mechanisms, the binding of ASOs to pre-mRNA and mRNA creates steric hindrance, which blocks the access of the ribosomal machinery and therefore inhibits translation, without mRNA direct degradation. In addition, ASOs can selectively interfere in the intermediary processing steps of RNA metabolism to redirect splicing or prevent translation by modifying 5′ cap or polyadenylation site [23]. The design of splice-switching ASOs has received much attention due to their ability to originate a steric block to the binding of splicing factors to the pre-mRNA (e.g. RNA-binding proteins or components of the spliceosome) and block RNA sequences required for splicing, as small nuclear RNA [35]. This strategy beneficially suits the treatment of diseases with a known splicing defect, since rationally designed ASOs permit either to induce exon exclusion or exon inclusion, as it is the mechanism of eteplirsen and nusinersen, respectively, both recently approved ASOs for neurological disorders. In this particular strategy, modification of ASOs with phosphorodiamidate morpholino oligomers (PMOs; Fig. 8.1) activates splice-switching and steric blocking mechanisms, while enhancing cell uptake due to their neutral charge [36]. Tricyclo-DNA (tc-DNA; Fig. 8.1) is a new class of conformationally constrained ODNs with remarkable ability to promote exon skipping, which enables to re-establish the levels of dystrophin in a mouse model of DMD upon systemic delivery [37, 38]. In addition, other modifications, including 2′-O-Me, 2′-MOE, LNA not in a gapmer design and peptide nucleic acid (PNA; Fig. 8.1), activate the nondegradative mechanisms [39].

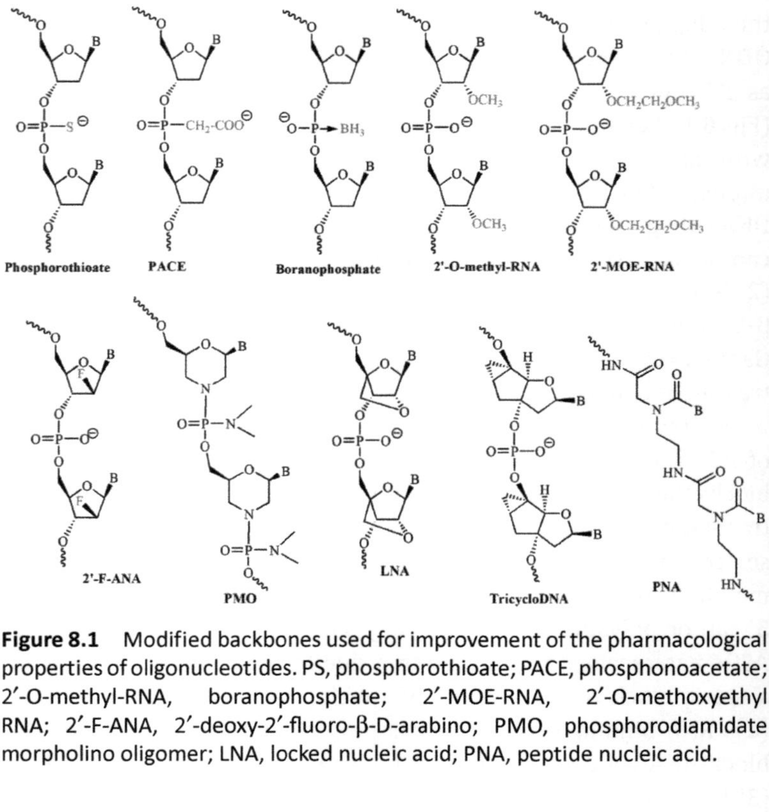

Figure 8.1 Modified backbones used for improvement of the pharmacological properties of oligonucleotides. PS, phosphorothioate; PACE, phosphonoacetate; 2′-O-methyl-RNA, boranophosphate; 2′-MOE-RNA, 2′-O-methoxyethyl RNA; 2′-F-ANA, 2′-deoxy-2′-fluoro-β-D-arabino; PMO, phosphorodiamidate morpholino oligomer; LNA, locked nucleic acid; PNA, peptide nucleic acid.

8.2.2 RNA Interference

The RNAi pathway was firstly identified by Mello and Fire [40], and it is a natural regulatory process whereby small-sized double-stranded RNAs (dsRNAs) downregulate gene expression. These endogenous ncRNAs are active regulators of gene expression acting at a posttranscriptional level and are commonly classified into three main subclasses in animals: (i) small interfering RNA (siRNA), (ii) microRNA (miRNA) and (iii) Piwi-interacting RNA (piRNA). Endogenously, siRNA are diced from longer RNA transcripts by an enzyme known as Dicer [41] to generate an ODN 21–23 nt in length, while miRNAs are processed from longer hairpin transcripts by the consecutive action of two RNase III proteins, Drosha and Dicer [42], to end up with a ~22 nt length. After breakdown, siRNA and miRNA are loaded into the RNA-induced silencing complex (RISC) in a double-stranded conformation. This complex is composed by Dicer, Argonaute2 (Ago2) and transactivation response RNA-binding (TRBP) proteins [43, 44]. In the case of siRNA, a process deemed RISC maturation triggers the release of the sense strand, whereas the antisense strand is paired to a complementary mRNA. The perfect match between antisense siRNA and mRNA results in an endonucleolytic cleavage of the target mRNA promoted by the slicing effector Ago2 of the RNAi process [45]. Conversely, complementary between the seed region of one strand of the hairpin duplex of miRNA (positions 2–8 from the 5′ miRNA) with the 3′ untranslated region (3′ UTR) of the target mRNA is the only prerequisite to silence the expression of the target genes through mechanisms of translation repression and mRNA destabilisation [46]. Fully complementarity between miRNA and mRNA activates a process of degradation of the mRNA, while a partial complementarity induces translational inhibition.

RNAi-based therapeutics involve the delivery of synthetic small RNA duplexes, as, for instance, siRNA, artificial miRNA and small hairpin RNA (shRNA), into a determined target cell to produce the gene-silencing effect. Ago2-mediated mechanisms, as RNase-H-dependent ones, may be modulated by the design of chemically modified ODNs [47–49]. The first siRNA-based approved drug, Patisiran (Alnylam Pharmaceuticals, Cambridge, MA, USA), was developed to treat patients with polyneuropathy caused by hereditary transthyretin-mediated amyloidosis (hATTR) in adults, by exploiting the use of lipid nanoparticles to deliver the drug directly into the liver [50, 51].

8.2.3 Anti-miRNA oligonucleotides

The brain possesses the widest range of miRNA expression among all human tissues, and some of them are exclusively expressed in this organ. These ncRNAs control brain development and were identified as important biomarkers in the pathogenesis of brain disorders. The misregulation of miRNAs has proved to be associated with a number of human conditions, including cancer, neurodegenerative diseases and autoimmune diseases [52, 53]. The use of synthetic miRNA emerged as an attractive tool to regulate the expression of endogenous miRNA. miRNA-based therapeutics may be divided into two strategies: miRNA mimics (agonist, dsRNA), used to restore the suppressed miRNA level, and inhibitors of endogenous miRNA (antagonist, single-stranded RNA [ssRNA]), known as antimiRs, with potential to downregulate overactive miRNA expression [54]. AntimiRs, as ASOs, are ssRNAs fully complementary to mature miRNA which degrades or represses miRNA translation mediated by Argonaute-containing miRNA-induced silencing complex (miRISC).

Modifications at the 2′ position of the sugar moiety, such as 2′-O-Me, 2′-MOE and 2′-fluoro, and also insertions of LNA (Fig. 8.1) have demonstrated to be useful for enhancing the pharmacokinetic properties, while they do not interfere with miRISC loading [48, 55–58]. PS, PNA modifications or PMO oligomers (Fig. 8.1) were also developed for antimiRs [59–61]. New antimiRs targeting different miRNAs are currently being tested mostly at a preclinical level. The ability to specifically design these molecules to target disease-causing miRNAs combined with the advances in the chemistry of ODNs made the application of this technology feasible in vivo. For instance, an antimiR targeting miR-21, including modifications of 2′-O-MOE, convincingly demonstrated the ability to downregulate miR-21 of glioma in mice, reducing their migratory and invasion abilities [62]. Likewise, the administration of miR-380-5p antagonist efficiently reduces the tumour size in an orthotopic mouse model of neuroblastoma [63]. The therapeutic potential of miR-155 antagonist was also validated for the treatment of ALS in model superoxide dismutase 1 (SOD1) transgenic mice [64].

8.2.4 Aptamers

Aptamers are nontoxic and non-immunogenic ssDNA or ssRNA ODNs, having a length of 40–100 nt, which specifically bind with high affinity to target molecules, including small organic molecules, amino acids, proteins, antibodies, cells, bacteria and organs, via shape recognition [65–70]. Their structures are rigorously selected and optimised via a procedure known as systematic evolution of ligands by exponential enrichment (SELEX) [71]. Variations of the SELEX procedure have enabled us to design artificial aptamers with special properties, as brain-penetrating aptamers [72]. By injecting into the mice a library of 2′-F-modified RNA aptamers, the authors identified aptamers with ability to attach brain capillary endothelia and traverse into the parenchyma. As it occurs for the aforementioned therapeutics, if not chemically modified aptamers are highly susceptible to degradation in physiological media [73]. The incorporation of modifications such as 2′-F or 2′-O-methyl are among the most common and demonstrated to enhance plasma stability and circulating half-life.

Despite the uncertainties regarding the physiopathology of neurodegenerative diseases, it is generally accepted that there is an accumulation of misfolded proteins at the origin of the pathology. As a therapeutic approach, aptamers may be used to prevent the aggregation of these misfolded proteins. In this context, several DNA and RNA aptamers have been developed to interrupt the accumulation of pathogenic proteins, such as amyloid-β [74, 75], α-Syn [76], mutant Huntingtin [77, 78] and myelin [79] involved in Alzheimer's disease, Parkinson's disease, Huntington's disease and multiple sclerosis (MS), respectively. For instance, the administration of a 40 nt antimyelin DNA aptamers induced remyelination of CNS lesions in mice infected by Theiler´s virus model of MS [79]. Other therapeutic aptamers were employed as remyelination agents [80, 81].

The application of these chimeras has proven to be also valuable in the treatment, diagnosis and imaging of brain tumours [82–85]. In this field, unique properties of aptamers have been exploited to detect tumour initiating cells by targeting the glycoprotein CD133 [69] or to distinguish glioblastoma multiforme (GBM) cells (U118-MG) from astroglial cells (SVGp12) [86]. Likewise, their high affinity to membrane receptors overexpressed in tumours may inhibit the signalling of, for instance, tyrosine kinase (Axl) receptors or growth factor receptor β(PDGFRβ), thus regulating tumour cell proliferation and migration [87, 88]. As an alternative, cell type–specific aptamers may be conjugated with therapeutic moieties, for example, siRNA, microRNA, anti-miR or antiproliferative agents, alone or coupled with nanoparticles for targeted delivery in tumour cells, thereby reducing unwanted off-target effects [89–92].

8.2.5 Antiproliferative Oligonucleotides

The antitumoural action of the decamer FdU_{10} composed by 10 monomers of 5-fluoro-2′-deoxyuridine monophosphate (FdU) has been demonstrated in in vivo preclinical models of acute myeloid leukaemia [93], acute lymphocytic leukaemia [94], prostate cancer [95] and GBM [96]. Once internalised, the metabolites of the polymeric fluoropyrimidine drug bind covalently to the nucleotide-binding site of thymidylate synthase (TS), inhibiting in this way the synthesis of deoxythymidine monophosphate (dTMP) and, consequently, triggering an apoptosis mechanism called 'thymineless cell death' [97]. FdU_{10} has displayed minimal penetrance of the BBB, but through intracerebral administration, it has been demonstrated to be safe and efficient in reducing tumour progression [96]. Histological analyses revealed almost complete suppression of tumours in a GBM mouse orthotopic xenograft model. Of note, recently DNA nanoassemblies were designed to hide in scaffold polymeric fluoropyrimidine strands, representing a promising approach for cancer therapy [98, 99].

8.3 Lipid-Based Nanocarriers for Brain Delivery

8.3.1 Oligonucleotide–Lipid Conjugates

The clinical success of therapeutic ODNs in the CNS depends on their efficient and safe delivery to neuronal cells. Naked single-stranded ASOs, contrarily to double-stranded siRNAs, are able to enter into cells through gymnosis when administered in saline solution [100]. The gymnotic uptake poses great convenience in the delivery of ASOs, yet this strategy requires cost-prohibitive concentrations to reach an adequate efficacy. As an alternative, different approaches were appraised for increasing siRNA uptake, including either (i) the use of ssRNAs, these being still active for the RNAi pathway [101], or (ii) the conjugation of dsRNAs with hydrophobic modifications. The conjugation of lipophilic or amphiphilic molecules confers a hydrophobic character to ODNs, thereby facilitating the interaction of negatively charged ODNs with hydrophobic cell membranes. These moieties can be synthetically incorporated in three different positions in the ODN chain: (i) in the 3′-end by using a solid support holding the selected lipid, (ii) in the 5′-end by introducing a hydrophobic phosphoramidite and (iii) within the ODN sequence, where one nucleosidic building block bears itself the hydrophobic moiety. Nevertheless, the modification at the 5′-end is the most suitable to incorporate the lipid. In the case of siRNAs and miRNAs, due to steric reasons, the conjugation is usually introduced in the 3′- or 5′-overhangs of the sense strand since the antisense one is incorporated into RISC. Either presynthetic or postsynthetic approaches may be used to engineer the hybrid lipid–ODN conjugates. These two chemical routes have been reviewed in detail elsewhere [102].

Cholesterol (chol) is one of the most common lipophilic moieties employed to modulate the delivery of ODNs. ASOs were the first ODNs tested with chol analogues [103, 104]. In these experimental works, the ability of the lipophilic conjugates to enhance the biodistribution and pharmacokinetics of chemically modified ASOs was demonstrated compared to their unconjugated counterpart. The uptake mechanism of such conjugates in hepatic cells was further proved to be receptor-mediated, binding specifically to scavenger receptors type A1/AII and galactose receptors, while facilitating the association with lactosylated-low-density lipoprotein (LDL) particles [105]. The nature of the linker and the location of chol along the ODN chain were also recognised as key factors for changing the liver tropism and toxicity [105]. These insights were soon adapted to modulate siRNA delivery. Soutschek et al. in a seminal work demonstrated that chol–siRNA conjugates, connected via a pyrrolidine linker (Fig. 8.2), downregulate an endogenous gene encoding apolipoprotein B (ApoB) after intravenous injection in mice, in the two major sites for ApoB production, in the liver and in the jejunum [106]. Chol–siRNA conjugates, presumably due to their affinity to serum protein, conferred prolonged circulation time compared to naked siRNA. Other studies further confirmed the crucial role of endogenous lipoprotein particles, lipoprotein receptors and transmembrane proteins to provide an efficient and selective delivery of chol–siRNA conjugates [107, 108]. It is worth mentioning that the association of lipid–siRNA conjugates to high-density lipoprotein (HDL) leads to a selective uptake by mouse brain capillary endothelial cells, the major functional component of the BBB, but not to neurons or glia [108].

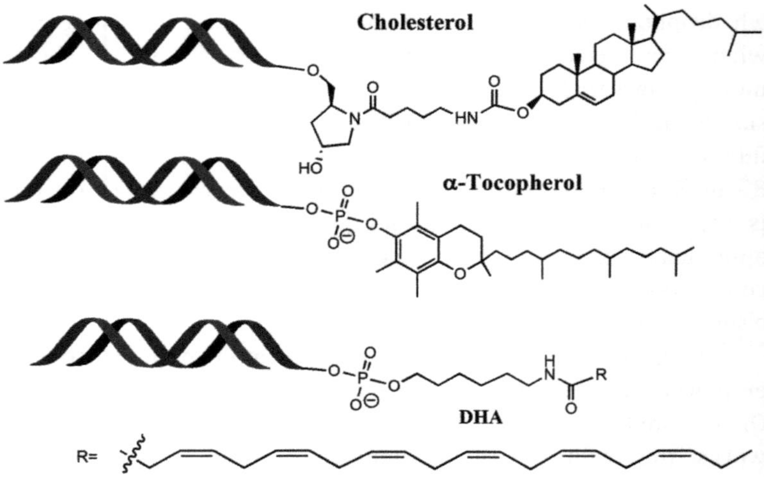

Figure 8.2 Lipid–oligonucleotide conjugates used for delivery of siRNAs in the brain: cholesterol, α-tocopherol and docosahexaenoic acid (DHA).

To assess the CNS, DiFiglia et al. tested chol-conjugated siRNAs (21 nt) with PS-modified overhangs administered through intrastriatal injection in mice to target mutant huntingtin (*Htt*) [109]. Results showed that a single administration of chol–siRNA conjugates into the striatum was well tolerated and led to a reduction of mutant Htt protein. The amelioration of motor behaviours and neuropathology symptoms confirmed the positive effect of gene silencing in the reduction of striatal neuronal dysfunction. Later, Chen et al. demonstrated that the conjugation of siRNA to chol with a cleavable disulphide linker increased the silencing potency upon intraparenchymal (CNS) infusion [110]. For the same purpose, Khvorova and colleagues have performed a library of 94 chemically modified siRNAs, conjugated to tetraethylene glycol cholesterol (teg-Chol), targeting the human huntingtin (*HTT*) mRNA in primary neurons and in the mouse brain [111]. The most potent chol-modified siRNA (HTT10150) displayed great ability to enhance cell uptake while promoting a specific and potent long-term modulation of gene expression in primary neurons in vitro. In addition, HTT10150 exhibited highly efficient cell uptake after injected intrastriatally in wild-type FVB/NJ mice, being mainly retained around the site of injection, and reduced *Htt* mRNA levels in a dose-dependent fashion, with up to 77% of silencing at the highest dose, displaying minimal cytotoxicity or immune activation. In a recent work, the same authors proposed the use of chol–siRNA conjugates to silence gene expression in orthotopic brain tumours [112]. Chol–siRNAs, modified with 2′-O-methyl and 2′-fluoro nucleotides, were found to infiltrate brain tumours after a single intratumoural injection, inducing potent and durable silencing of tumour-specific reporter genes.

Apart from chol, other hydrophobic moieties, such as docosahexaenoic acid (DHA; Fig. 8.2), have been conjugated to siRNAs to facilitate CNS delivery [113, 114]. DHA is a long-chain omega-3 fatty acid with a remarkable role on growth and development of the brain [115]. The DHA moiety was conjugated to the 3′-end of the siRNA sense strand through an amino linker. The resultant DHA–siRNA conjugate was designed to targeting *Htt* and CyclophilinB (*Ppib)* mRNAs, and its action was compared with a chol–siRNA conjugate [113]. Results evidenced that the hydrophobicity of the lipidic moieties dictates the distribution of the siRNA around the site of injection, where DHA–siRNA conjugates were found to distribute more broadly than chol–siRNA conjugates to both the ipsilateral striatum and cortex. A maximal *Htt* mRNA knockdown of 70%–80% was observed after administration of 25 μg of DHA–siRNA conjugates, this effect being still persistent for 4 weeks after a single injection with a lower concentration of the conjugate. Comparable levels of gene silencing were detected for *Ppib* mRNA (~80%). In terms of neuronal toxicity, chol–siRNA conjugates induced a significant loss of brain matter at doses above 25 μg, whereas DHA–siRNA conjugates did not trigger an innate immune response or neuronal toxicity over 20-fold above the successful dose. In a follow-up work, the same authors hypothesised whether the use of a structure resembling the endogenously esterified DHA bioconjugate, as phosphocholine–DHA (PC–DHA), could enhance siRNA activity [114]. However, PC–DHA–siRNA did not outperform DHA–siRNA conjugates and revealed an increment in neuronal toxicity and astrogliosis.

The natural isomer of the lipophilic vitamin E, α-tocopherol, has also emerged as a successful vector for siRNA delivery in the mouse liver and brain [116, 117]. HDL plays a key role in mediating the cellular delivery of α-tocopherol in different tissues, including the brain, promoting lipid uptake via scavenger receptor class B, type I (SR-B1) [118, 119]. Therefore, the combination of HDL as a second carrier of the α-tocopherol–siRNA conjugate (Fig. 8.2) enables the specific knockdown of β-site amyloid precursor protein cleaving enzyme 1 (*BACE1*) mRNA [117]. Variations in the design of 13-mer LNA/DNA gapmer modified with α-tocopherol have also been carried out to test the influence of this lipidic moiety in the delivery of ASOs [120]. In this report, it was shown that the direct conjugation of α-tocopherol to 13-mer LNA/DNA gapmer reduces drastically the silencing effect in the mouse liver, mainly due to sterical impediments hampering ASO activity. However, when using the same LNA/DNA gapmer (HDO) and its complementary strand (sRNA), and conjugating this latter with α-tocopherol at the 5′-end, there exists an increment in the binding of α-tocopherol-HDO with serum lipoproteins, thus increasing their transport into the cells and enhancing the silencing activity of the gapmer by 20-fold (compared with parent unmodified HDO) when targeted to the liver [121]. In a proof-of-concept study, α-tocopherol–HDO conjugates were administrated intravenously in mice to reduce the expression of the organic anion transporter 3 (*OAT3*) gene in brain microvascular endothelial cells, the major component of the BBB [122]. Results indicate the ability of α-tocopherol–HDO conjugates to silence OAT3 at the gene and protein levels, thus modulating the protein function at the BBB.

8.4 Vesicular Systems: Liposomes and Niosomes

Lipid spherical vesicles, such as liposomes, were first introduced in 1965, and since then they have been at the forefront of drug delivery science. The encapsulation of ODNs in liposomes is a valuable strategy used to keep these therapeutic molecules intact and biologically active after administration. Cationic liposomes due to the multiple positively charged groups disposed in their surface are the most frequently used nonviral entities to complex negatively charged nucleic acids. The conventional methods of preparation of liposome–ODN complexes result from the direct mixing of cationic liposomes and anionic ODNs or through rehydration of a thin-layer lipid film with ODN aqueous solutions.

Liposomes typically are composed by (i) cationic lipids, such as chol, dioleolyphosphatidylethanolamine (DOPE), dioleoyldimethylammoniumpropane (DODAP), phosphatidylcholine (PC) and unsaturated fatty acids; (ii) neutral lipids, also referred to as helper lipids; and (iii) polyethylene glycol (PEG) lipids or polysaccharides, to form a protective hydrophilic layer on the surface of liposomes and increase colloidal stability [123]. The structural features of the constitutive lipids, such as the nature and structure of head groups, length of the hydrophobic chains and the number of unsaturated alkyl chains, are also determinant to modulate the success of their transfection. Many researchers have developed libraries of newly synthesised lipid compounds to gain a better understanding of the parameters required for rationally designed, highly efficient candidates [124, 125]. To increase the efficiency in the delivery of small-molecule drugs and nucleic acids, liposomes have been properly designed with specific components which tend to respond to certain stimuli such as pH, heat, magnetic fields or light among others [126]. Extensive research has been reported with the preparation of pH-responsive liposomes as drug delivery systems. This strategy has gained increased attention due to existing differences in the pH between certain tissues and other cellular compartments. In addition, tumour tissues display ~0.5–1.0 pH values lower when compared to pH exhibited by normal tissues [127]. In this sense, liposomes made up of phosphatidylethanolamine (PE) and some derivatives like DOPE have been widely used for delivering small molecules and macromolecules. To increase long-lived circulation rates, these particles have been further modified with PEG and many other derivatives [128].

These attractive platforms, which are stable at physiological pH, are able to destabilise in acid environments, thus favouring endocytic pathways. In this regard, a recent research article reported by Liu et al. described the use of ionisable liposomes under low pH and hypoxia conditions in order to transfect glioma cells [129]. Results showed that liposomes containing malate dehydrogenase were able to interact with a siRNA targeting Polo-like kinase-1 (siPLK1). This liposomal formulation was able to promote siRNA uptake and inhibit PLK1 protein expression, showing a reduction of tumour growth in animal models after systemic administration.

The ideal liposome for brain delivery should present less than 100 nm in diameter, be shielded with PEG, have an overall neutral or negative surface charge and, importantly, incorporate a targeting ligand to facilitate specific cellular targeting [130]. Receptor-mediated transcytosis is the most relevant transport mechanism used by liposomes to reach the brain, and due to this cell-penetrating peptides have demonstrated great ability to transport cargo into cells. Dual targeting has become an efficient strategy to circumvent receptor saturation and to efficiently target cancerous cells [131]. Recently, Rodrigues et al. combined transferrin (Tf) receptor and penetratin (Pen) on the surface of liposomes to improve the delivery of plasmid β-galactosidase into the brain [132]. This strategy demonstrated great ability to accumulate in the brain and transfect neurons while significantly induced gene expression in vivo.

Stable nucleic acid lipid particles (SNALPs) were first developed in 2001 by Semple and colleagues and are considered an evolution of the cationic liposomes for delivering nucleic acids. Driven by this initial proposal, a lipid formulation composed of DODAP/disaturated-phosphatidylcholine (DSPC)/chol/C16 mPEG2000 was devised to encapsulate LNA-modified anti-miR-21 or siRNA followed by postinsertion of micelles functionalised with chlorotoxin (CTX) to bind selectively to glioma cells. The assembled SNALPs displayed high encapsulation yields attributed to the complexation of ODNs with positive charged DODAP, a net surface charge close to neutrality and small sizes (<180 nm). Study outcomes described an increased cellular association and internalisation of CTX-targeted SNALPs by tumour cells, while sparing normal cells, increased tumour suppressor expression and caspase activity and a reduction in tumour cell proliferation [133]. The CTX-functionalised SNALPs with miR-21 were shown to accumulate preferentially within brain tumours and induce miR-21 silencing and decreased the tumour cell proliferation and tumour size, while showing no signs of systemic immunogenicity [134]. The same authors have used the same strategy to address Machado–Joseph disease (MJD) to deliver siRNA designed to target the *ataxin-3* gene in neuronal cells. Initially, siRNA was encapsulated inside ceramide-PEGylated liposomes constituted by DODAP, DSPC and chol. In a second step, the resultant liposomes were involved by micelles made of DSPE–PEG functionalised with rabies virus glycoprotein–derived peptide RVG-r9. The intravenous administration of these SNALPs targeting neurons resulted in a significant knockdown of mutant *ataxin-3* expression and aggregate formation [135].

Niosomes are another important class of vesicular systems similar to liposomes in which the phospholipids are substituted by non-ionic surfactants. This simple variation not only reduces the cost of production and potential toxicity but also increases the storage stability. A complete description of niosomes, including their methods of preparation, drug administration routes and applications, is well detailed in good reviews [136]. Recently, a cationic niosome formulation was prepared based on mixing DOTMA, non-ionic surfactant Polysorbate 60 and Lycopene, a natural carotenoid with antioxidant properties, via reverse-phase emulsification evaporation for delivering nucleic acids into the brain [137]. Experiments with niosomes encapsulating the pCMS conjugated to enhanced green fluorescent protein (pCMS-EGFP) plasmid revealed transfection efficiencies of ~17% without cytotoxic effects. In vivo experiments performed by direct intracranial administration revealed good capacity of niosomes to transfect neuroglia and cells in blood vessel walls.

The same authors also found promising in vitro and in vivo delivery efficiencies when cationic niosomes made up of a modified amino lipid containing two saturated lipid tails of 14 atoms of carbons were used to transfect the same pCMS-EGFP plasmid [138]. These positive results allowed the authors to chemically modify such amino lipid with two pendent polar groups like a triglycine peptide and a dimethylaminoethyl residues [139]. The resultant synthetic amino lipids produced niosomes in the presence of polysorbate 80 and squalene as a helper lipid. Interestingly, transfection efficiencies strongly relied not only on the niosome chemical composition but also on DNA/cationic lipid ratios. In this sense, cationic niosomes containing dimethylaminoethyl polar tails exhibited greater transfection efficiencies in vivo and higher protein expression levels than other formulations tested after brain administration.

8.5 Natural Vesicular Systems: Exosomes

Exosomes are extracellular vesicles actively secreted by almost all cell types, with a defined size of ~40–100 nm. These natural vesicles recently emerged as a novel lipid carrier for the delivery of lipids, nucleic acids or proteins with advantageous features as they may interact with cells via natural pathways. Despite cellular mechanisms being still poorly understood, exosomes have demonstrated unique properties to interact with brain endothelial cells and exhibit brain tropism and BBB tropism. Resembling the cell plasma membrane, the specialised exosomal membrane contains a great number of raft-lipids, ceramides, sphingolipids, chol and glycerophospholipids [140].

The concept of using exosomes as carriers of siRNA into the brain was previously reported by Alvarez-Erviti et al. [141]. In this work, the authors injected intravenously purified RVG peptide–targeted exosomes loaded with exogenous glyceraldehyde 3-phosphate dehydrogenase (GAPDH) siRNA through electroporation in mice. Results have shown a potent silencing activity, up to 60% of mRNA and 62% of protein knockdown of BACE1, a therapeutic target in Alzheimer´s disease. Since this seminal work, other studies have been carried out on the role of exosomes in brain tumour and neurological disorders [142]. One of the most explored strategies to achieve BBB crossing is to engineer targeting ligands into exosomal membrane. The encapsulation of a hydrophobic modified siRNA was also recently tested, showing a statistically significant knockdown of *HTT* mRNA of ~35% [143]. Despite these encouraging results many hurdles must still be overcome to achieve a wider clinical application such as optimisation of the methods of purification and gene loading, selection of exosomes donor cells, minimisation of toxicity and enhancement of their pharmacokinetic properties.

8.6 Solid Lipid-Based Nanocarriers

In the past two decades solid lipid nanoparticles (SLNs) have proved to be a valuable candidate for ODN delivery in the brain. SLNs claim several advantages over other proposed lipid-based carriers, including a well-defined size and high encapsulation capacity, biocompatibility, control over drug and gene release, prevention of reticuloendothelial system uptake and rapid renal filtration, great storage stability, feasibility for lyophilisation and sterilisation and high-scale production and reproducibility [144, 145]. And interestingly, SLNs favour the penetration of the BBB and increase the bioavailability of drugs in the brain [146]. SLNs are generally composed of solid lipids at both room temperature and body temperature, such as fatty acids, glycerides or waxes, while nanostructured lipid carriers (NLCs) are generated from a blend of solid and liquid lipids, such as oils. In what regards ODN complexation, solid lipid-based nanoparticles may incorporate positive entities to confer them an overall positive charge which electrostatically interact with negatively charged nucleic acids. Or, as an alternative, to further improve the protection to ODNs, neutral lipid nanoparticles can be employed to encapsulate preneutralised ODNs. The variety of techniques employed to produce nanoparticles are well documented elsewhere, as well as the pros and cons involved in siRNA loading into SLNs [147].

SLNs composed of cholesteryl oleate, glyceryl triolate, DOPE, chol and DC-chol were prepared by solvent emulsification-evaporation to conjugate electrostatically PEGylated–siRNA as a carrier system to downregulate c-Met expression levels in glioblastoma [148]. The conjugation of PEG proved to prevent nonspecific protein interaction, thus enhancing the stability of siRNA/SLN complexes in serum and prolonging their circulation in physiological fluids [149]. The results revealed an enhanced accumulation of siRNA/SLN complexes in a U-87MG xenograft tumour model and a significant inhibition of c-Met expression at tumour tissue without inducing toxicity in mice. As alternative production methodologies SLNs can also be used to encapsulate nucleic acids in their lipophilic core rather than complex them into the surface. Lobovkina el al. proposed to use a hydrophobic ion-pairing strategy to encapsulate siRNA in an SLN composed of lecithin and DSPE-PEG after its prior neutralisation with a cationic lipid (DOTAP) [150]. The intradermal injection of the developed siRNA/SLN in mice demonstrated a sustained release of siRNA over a period of 10–13 days. Following a different procedure, siRNA was encapsulated in polymeric and SLNs via a modified solvent emulsification evaporation method, producing an encapsulation efficiency of ~50%. The functionalisation of the resultant nanoparticles with a peptide-binding transferrin receptor increased their interaction with brain endothelial cells up to threefold when compared to the nonmodified ones [151]. SLNs prepared using Witepsol E85 solid triglycerides through a solvent emulsification-evaporation method based on the water-oil-water (w/o/w) double-emulsion technique were used to encapsulate siRNA targeting the *BACE1* gene relevant in the treatment of Alzheimer's disease. The optimal molar ratio between *BACE1* siRNA and a cell-penetrating peptide RVG-9R was firstly elucidated and thereafter the siRNA/RVG-9R complex encapsulated in the core of SLNs. Positively charged SLNs were obtained after coating with chitosan, which increased their mucoadhesiveness and prolonged their residence time in the nasal cavity [151].

SLNs have been exploited also in the treatment of brain tumours for co-delivering therapeutic ODNs and chemotherapeutic drugs. Taking advantage of their ability to encapsulate hydrophobic and hydrophilic entities, Chen et al. encapsulated temozolomide (TMZ) and DNA in NLCs and evaluated their therapeutic efficacy in U87MG cells [152]. In vitro transfection and in vivo antitumour growth efficiencies of TMZ/DNA/NLCs were inspected in tumour-bearing BALB/c nude mice. After 15 days of administration, TMZ/DNA/NLCs exhibited tumour inhibition rates of 69% and 21% compared to controls (saline solution).

8.7 Conclusions

Hitherto, research efforts have barely scratched the surface in terms of the insight which human genetic information can generate. This information will provide the potential to tackle targets now deemed 'undruggable'. The insights obtained so far have fuelled the interest in exploiting multiple options available for chemically modified therapeutic ODNs to induce targeted protein degradation in brain tissues. However, selective barriers which protect the brain along with the rapid degradation of ODNs in biological fluids make the delivery of therapeutic entities a hard task to achieve. Given these obstacles, it is remarkable the progress made in the development of lipid-based systems, yet there is still a need for more efficient delivery strategies of this type.

Acknowledgements

The authors acknowledge the financial support provided by CIBER-BBN an initiative funded by the VI National R+D+I Plan 2008–2011, Iniciativa Ingenio 2010, Consolider Program and the Instituto de Salud Carlos III with assistance from the European Regional Development and ICTS NANBIOSIS (Oligonucleotide synthesis platform U29). The IQAC group is supported by the Spanish Ministerio de Ciencia e Innovación (CTQ2017-84415-R) and Generalitat de Catalunya (2017SGR114). The CQC is supported by the FCT through the projects Pest-OE-QUI/UI0313/2014 and POCI-01-0145-FEDER-007630. A.F.J. acknowledges Fundação para a Ciência e Tecnologia (FCT), Portugal, for financial support regarding postdoctoral grant SFRH/BPD/104544/2014.

References

1. Orsini, A., Zara, F., Striano, P. (2018). Recent advances in epilepsy genetics. *Neurosci. Lett.*, **667**, 4–9.
2. Brooks, P., Cheng, T.-F., Cooper, L. (2008). Do all of the neurologic diseases in patients with DNA repair gene mutations result from the accumulation of DNA damage? *DNA Repair*, **7**(6), 834–848.
3. McKinnon, P. J. (2009). DNA repair deficiency and neurological disease. *Nat. Rev. Neurosci.*, **10**(2), 100.
4. Li, L., Matsui, M., Corey, D. R. (2016). Activating frataxin expression by repeat-targeted nucleic acids. *Nat. Commun.*, **7**, 10606.
5. Tabebordbar, M., et al. (2016). In vivo gene editing in dystrophic mouse muscle and muscle stem cells. *Science*, **351**(6271), 407–411.
6. Nelson, C. E., et al. (2016). In vivo genome editing improves muscle function in a mouse model of Duchenne muscular dystrophy. *Science*, **351**(6271), 403–407.
7. Lee, Y., Rio, D. C. (2015). Mechanisms and regulation of alternative pre-mRNA splicing. *Annu. Rev. Biochem.*, **84**, 291–323.
8. Gustincich, S., Zucchelli, S., Mallamaci, A. (2017). The Yin and Yang of nucleic acid-based therapy in the brain. *Prog. Neurobiol.*, **155**, 194–211.
9. Chiasson, B. J., et al. (1992). Antisense oligonucleotide eliminates in vivo expression of c-fos in mammalian brain. *Eur. J. Pharmacol. Mol. Pharmacol.*, **227**(4), 451–453.

10. Rigo, F., et al. (2014). Pharmacology of a central nervous system delivered 2′-O-methoxyethyl–modified survival of motor neuron splicing oligonucleotide in mice and nonhuman primates. *J. Pharmacol. Exp. Ther.*, **350**(1), 46–55.
11. Samaranch, L., et al. (2014). AAV9-mediated expression of a non-self protein in nonhuman primate central nervous system triggers widespread neuroinflammation driven by antigen-presenting cell transduction. *Mol. Ther.*, **22**(2), 329–337.
12. Alam, M. I., et al. (2010). Strategy for effective brain drug delivery. *Eur. J. Pharm. Sci.*, **40**(5), 385–403.
13. Khvorova, A., Watts, J. K. (2017). The chemical evolution of oligonucleotide therapies of clinical utility. *Nat. Biotechnol.*, **35**(3), 238.
14. Deleavey, G. F., Damha, M. J. (2012). Designing chemically modified oligonucleotides for targeted gene silencing. *Chem. Biol.*, **19**(8), 937–954.
15. Choudhury, S. R., et al. (2017). Viral vectors for therapy of neurologic diseases. *Neuropharmacology*, **120**, 63–80.
16. Davidson, B. L., Breakefield, X. O. (2003). Viral vectors for gene delivery to the nervous system. *Nat. Rev. Neurosci.*, **4**(5), 353.
17. Stephenson, M. L., Zamecnik, P. C. (1978). Inhibition of Rous sarcoma viral RNA translation by a specific oligodeoxyribonucleotide. *Proc. Natl. Acad. Sci.*, **75**(1), 285–288.
18. Dias, N., Stein, C. (2002). Antisense oligonucleotides: basic concepts and mechanisms. *Mol. Cancer Ther.*, **1**(5), 347–355.
19. Kurreck, J. (2003). Antisense technologies: improvement through novel chemical modifications. *Eur. J. Biochem.*, **270**(8), 1628–1644.
20. Eckstein, F. (1970). Nucleoside phosphorothioates. *J. Am. Chem. Soc.*, **92**(15), 4718–4723.
21. Shibahara, S., et al. (1989). Inhibition of human immunodeficiency virus (HIV-1) replication by synthetic oligo-RNA derivatives. *Nucleic Acids Res.*, **17**(1), 239–252.
22. Wu, H., et al. (2004). Determination of the role of the human RNase H1 in the pharmacology of DNA-like antisense drugs. *J. Biol. Chem.*, **279**(17), 17181–17189.
23. Bennett, C. F., Swayze, E. E. (2010). RNA targeting therapeutics: molecular mechanisms of antisense oligonucleotides as a therapeutic platform. *Annu. Rev. Pharmacol. Toxicol.*, **50**, 259–293.

24. Cerritelli, S. M., R. J. Crouch, (2009). Ribonuclease H: the enzymes in eukaryotes. *FEBS J.*, **276**(6), 1494–1505.
25. Rinaldi, C., Wood, M. J. (2018). Antisense oligonucleotides: the next frontier for treatment of neurological disorders. *Nat. Rev. Neurol.*, **14**(1), 9.
26. Bennett, C. F., et al. (2017). Pharmacology of antisense drugs. *Annu. Rev. Pharmacol. Toxicol.*, **57**, 81–105.
27. Breaker, R. R., Joyce, G. F. (1994). A DNA enzyme that cleaves RNA. *Chem. Biol.*, **1**(4), 223–229.
28. Sheehan, D., et al. (2003). Biochemical properties of phosphonoacetate and thiophosphonoacetate oligodeoxyribonucleotides. *Nucleic Acids Res.*, **31**(14), 4109–4118.
29. Rait, V. K., Shaw, B. R. (1999). Boranophosphates support the RNase H cleavage of polyribonucleotides. *Antisense Nucleic Acid Drug Dev.*, **9**(1), 53–60.
30. Agrawal, S., Kandimalla, E. R. (2000). Antisense therapeutics: is it as simple as complementary base recognition? *Mol. Med. Today*, **6**(2), 72–81.
31. Manoharan, M. (1999). 2′-Carbohydrate modifications in antisense oligonucleotide therapy: importance of conformation, configuration and conjugation. *Biochim. Biophys. Acta, Gene Struct. Expression*, **1489**(1), 117–130.
32. Ng, E. W., et al. (2006). Pegaptanib, a targeted anti-VEGF aptamer for ocular vascular disease. *Nat. Rev. Drug Discovery*, **5**(2), 123.
33. Wilds, C. J., Damha, M. J. (2000). 2′-Deoxy-2′-fluoro-β-D-arabinonucleosides and oligonucleotides (2′ F-ANA): synthesis and physicochemical studies. *Nucleic Acids Res.*, **28**(18), 3625–3635.
34. Miller, T. M., et al. (2013). An antisense oligonucleotide against SOD1 delivered intrathecally for patients with SOD1 familial amyotrophic lateral sclerosis: a phase 1, randomised, first-in-man study. *Lancet Neurol.*, **12**(5), 435–442.
35. Havens, M. A., Hastings, M. L. (2016). Splice-switching antisense oligonucleotides as therapeutic drugs. *Nucleic Acids Res.*, **44**(14), 6549–6563.
36. Summerton, J. (1999). Morpholino antisense oligomers: the case for an RNase H-independent structural type. *Biochim. Biophys. Acta, Gene Struct. Expression*, **1489**(1), 141–158.
37. Goyenvalle, A., et al. (2015). Functional correction in mouse models of muscular dystrophy using exon-skipping tricyclo-DNA oligomers. *Nat. Med.*, **21**(3), 270.

38. Relizani, K., et al. (2017). Efficacy and safety profile of tricyclo-DNA antisense oligonucleotides in Duchenne muscular dystrophy mouse model. *Mol. Ther. Nucleic Acids*, **8**, 144–157.
39. Schoch, K. M., Miller, T. M. (2017). Antisense oligonucleotides: translation from mouse models to human neurodegenerative diseases. *Neuron*, **94**(6), 1056–1070.
40. Fire, A., et al. (1998). Potent and specific genetic interference by double-stranded RNA in Caenorhabditis elegans. *Nature*, **391**(6669), 806.
41. Elbashir, S. M., et al. (2001). Duplexes of 21-nucleotide RNAs mediate RNA interference in cultured mammalian cells. *Nature*, **411**(6836), 494.
42. Ha, M., V. N. Kim, (2014). Regulation of microRNA biogenesis. *Nat. Rev. Mol. Cell Biol.*, **15**(8), 509.
43. Wilson, R. C., et al. (2015). Dicer-TRBP complex formation ensures accurate mammalian microRNA biogenesis. *Mol. Cell*, **57**(3), 397–407.
44. Schirle, N. T., MacRae, I. J. (2012). The crystal structure of human Argonaute2. *Science*, **336**(6084), 1037–1040.
45. Wilson, R. C., Doudna, J. A. (2013). Molecular mechanisms of RNA interference. *Annu. Rev. Biophys.*, **42**, 217–239.
46. Huntzinger, E., Izaurralde, E. (2011). Gene silencing by microRNAs: contributions of translational repression and mRNA decay. *Nat. Rev. Genet.*, **12**(2), 99.
47. Kenski, D. M., et al. (2012). SiRNA-optimized modifications for enhanced in vivo activity. *Mol. Ther. Nucleic Acids*, **1**, e5.
48. Davis, S., et al. (2006). Improved targeting of miRNA with antisense oligonucleotides. *Nucleic Acids Res.*, **34**(8), 2294–2304.
49. Lam, J. K., et al. (2015). SiRNA versus miRNA as therapeutics for gene silencing. *Mol. Ther. Nucleic Acids*, **4**, e252.
50. Coelho, T., et al. (2013). Safety and efficacy of RNAi therapy for transthyretin amyloidosis. *N. Engl. J. Med.*, **369**(9), 819–829.
51. Suhr, O. B., et al. (2015). Efficacy and safety of patisiran for familial amyloidotic polyneuropathy: a phase II multi-dose study. *Orphanet J. Rare Dis.*, **10**(1), 109.
52. Zhang, B., et al. (2007). MicroRNAs as oncogenes and tumor suppressors. *Dev. Biol.*, **302**(1), 1–12.
53. Kumar, M. S., et al. (2007). Impaired microRNA processing enhances cellular transformation and tumorigenesis. *Nat. Genet.*, **39**(5), 673.

54. Van Rooij, E., Kauppinen, S. (2014). Development of microRNA therapeutics is coming of age. *EMBO Mol. Med.*, **6**(7), 851–864.

55. Davis, S., et al. (2008). Potent inhibition of microRNA in vivo without degradation. *Nucleic Acids Res.*, **37**(1), 70–77.

56. Elmén, J., et al. (2008). LNA-mediated microRNA silencing in non-human primates. *Nature*, **452**(7189), 896.

57. Elmen, J., et al. (2007). Antagonism of microRNA-122 in mice by systemically administered LNA-antimiR leads to up-regulation of a large set of predicted target mRNAs in the liver. *Nucleic Acids Res.*, **36**(4), 1153–1162.

58. Esau, C., et al. (2006). MiR-122 regulation of lipid metabolism revealed by in vivo antisense targeting. *Cell Metab.*, **3**(2), 87–98.

59. Lennox, K. A., Behlke, M. A. (2010). A direct comparison of anti-microRNA oligonucleotide potency. *Pharm. Res.*, **27**(9), 1788–1799.

60. Kloosterman, W. P., et al. (2007). Targeted inhibition of miRNA maturation with morpholinos reveals a role for miR-375 in pancreatic islet development. *PLoS Biol.*, **5**(8), e203.

61. Fabani, M. M., Gait, M. J. (2008). MiR-122 targeting with LNA/2′-O-methyl oligonucleotide mixmers, peptide nucleic acids (PNA), and PNA–peptide conjugates. *RNA*, **14**(2), 336–346.

62. Gabriely, G., et al. (2008). MicroRNA 21 promotes glioma invasion by targeting matrix metalloproteinase regulators. *Mol. Cell. Biol.*, **28**(17), 5369–5380.

63. Swarbrick, A., et al. (2010). MiR-380-5p represses p53 to control cellular survival and is associated with poor outcome in MYCN-amplified neuroblastoma. *Nat. Med.*, **16**(10), 1134.

64. Butovsky, O., et al. (2015). Targeting mi R-155 restores abnormal microglia and attenuates disease in SOD 1 mice. *Ann. Neurol.*, **77**(1), 75–99.

65. Tuerk, C., Gold, L. (1990). Systematic evolution of ligands by exponential enrichment: RNA ligands to bacteriophage T4 DNA polymerase. *Science*, **249**(4968), 505–510.

66. Colas, P., et al. (1996). Genetic selection of peptide aptamers that recognize and inhibit cyclin-dependent kinase 2. *Nature*, **380**(6574), 548.

67. Ellington, A. D., Szostak, J. W. (1990). In vitro selection of RNA molecules that bind specific ligands. *Nature*, **346**(6287), 818.

68. Shaltiel-Karyo, R., et al. (2010). Inhibiting α-synuclein oligomerization by stable cell-penetrating β-synuclein fragments recovers phenotype of Parkinson's disease model flies. *PLoS One*, **5**(11), e13863.
69. Shigdar, S., et al. (2013). RNA aptamers targeting cancer stem cell marker CD133. *Cancer Lett.*, **330**(1), 84–95.
70. Vuyisich, M., Beal, P. A. (2002). Controlling protein activity with ligand-regulated RNA aptamers. *Chem. Biol.*, **9**(8), 907–913.
71. Yang, Y., et al. (2007). Advances in SELEX and application of aptamers in the central nervous system. *Biomol. Eng.*, **24**(6), 583–592.
72. Cheng, C., et al. (2013). In vivo SELEX for Identification of Brain-penetrating Aptamers. *Mol. Ther. Nucleic Acids*, **2**, e67.
73. Ni, S., et al. (2017). Chemical modifications of nucleic acid aptamers for therapeutic purposes. *Int. J. Mol. Sci.*, **18**(8), 1683.
74. Liang, H., et al. (2015). Inhibition of BACE1 activity by a DNA aptamer in an Alzheimer's disease cell model. *PLoS One*, **10**(10), e0140733.
75. Rentmeister, A., et al. (2006). RNA aptamers selectively modulate protein recruitment to the cytoplasmic domain of β-secretase BACE1 in vitro. *RNA*, **12**(9), 1650–1660.
76. Tsukakoshi, K., et al. (2012). Selection of DNA aptamers that recognize α-synuclein oligomers using a competitive screening method. *Anal. Chem.*, **84**(13), 5542–5547.
77. Skogen, M., et al. (2006). Short G-rich oligonucleotides as a potential therapeutic for Huntington's disease. *BMC Neurosci.*, **7**, 65.
78. Shin, B., et al. (2018). Novel DNA aptamers that bind to mutant huntingtin and modify its activity. *Mol. Ther. Nucleic Acids*, **11**, 416–428.
79. Nastasijevic, B., et al. (2012). Remyelination induced by a DNA aptamer in a mouse model of multiple sclerosis. *PLoS One*, **7**(6), e39595.
80. Smestad, J., Maher III, L. J. (2012). Ion-dependent conformational switching by a DNA aptamer that induces remyelination in a mouse model of multiple sclerosis. *Nucleic Acids Res.*, **41**(2), 1329–1342.
81. Rozenblum, G. T., Kaufman, T., Vitullo, A. D. (2014). Myelin basic protein and a multiple sclerosis-related MBP-peptide bind to oligonucleotides. *Mol. Ther. Nucleic Acids*, **3**, e192.
82. Chandola, C., et al. (2016). Application of aptamers in diagnostics, drug-delivery and imaging. *J. Biosci.*, **41**(3), 535–561.
83. Sriramoju, B., et al. (2015). Aptamer-targeted oligonucleotide theranostics: a smarter approach for brain delivery and the treatment of neurological diseases. *Curr. Top. Med. Chem.*, **15**(12), 1115–1124.

84. Gijs, M., et al. (2016). Aptamers as radiopharmaceuticals for nuclear imaging and therapy. *Nucl. Med. Biol.*, **43**(4), 253–271.

85. Hays, E., Duan, W., Shigdar, S. (2017). Aptamers and glioblastoma: their potential use for imaging and therapeutic applications. *Int. J. Mol. Sci.*, **18**(12), 2576.

86. Kang, D., et al. (2012). Selection of DNA aptamers against glioblastoma cells with high affinity and specificity. *PLoS One*, **7**(10), e42731.

87. Cerchia, L., et al. (2012). Targeting Axl with an high-affinity inhibitory aptamer. *Mol. Ther.*, **20**(12), 2291–2303.

88. Camorani, S., et al. (2014). Inhibition of receptor signaling and of glioblastoma-derived tumor growth by a novel PDGFRβ aptamer. *Mol. Ther.*, **22**(4), 828–841.

89. Huang, Y. F., et al. (2009). Molecular assembly of an aptamer–drug conjugate for targeted drug delivery to tumor cells. *ChemBioChem*, **10**(5), 862–868.

90. Li, X., Zhao, Q., Qiu, L. (2013). Smart ligand: aptamer-mediated targeted delivery of chemotherapeutic drugs and siRNA for cancer therapy. *J. Control. Release*, **171**(2), 152–162.

91. Sun, H., et al. (2014). Oligonucleotide aptamers: new tools for targeted cancer therapy. *Mol. Ther. Nucleic Acids*, **3**, e182.

92. Kruspe, S., Giangrande, P. (2017). Aptamer-siRNA chimeras: discovery, progress, and future prospects. *Biomedicines*, **5**(3), 45.

93. Pardee, T. S., et al. (2012). Unique dual targeting of thymidylate synthase and topoisomerase1 by FdUMP [10] results in high efficacy against AML and low toxicity. *Blood*, **119**(15), 3561–3570.

94. Pardee, T. S., et al. (2014). The poison oligonucleotide F10 is highly effective against acute lymphoblastic leukemia while sparing normal hematopoietic cells. *Oncotarget*, **5**(12), 4170.

95. Gmeiner, W. H., et al. (2014). F10 inhibits growth of PC3 xenografts and enhances the effects of radiation therapy. *J. Clin. Oncol. Res.*, **2**(4), 1028.

96. Gmeiner, W. H., et al. (2014). Selective anti-tumor activity of the novel fluoropyrimidine polymer F10 towards G48a orthotopic GBM tumors. *J. Neuro-Oncol.*, **116**(3), 447–454.

97. Goulian, M., et al. (1986). Mechanism of thymineless death, in *Purine and Pyrimidine Metabolism in Man V*. Springer, New York, pp. 89–95.

98. Mou, Q., et al. (2017). DNA trojan horses: self-assembled floxuridine-containing DNA polyhedra for cancer therapy. *Angew. Chem.*, **129**(41), 12702–12706.

99. Jorge, A., et al. (2018). DNA-based nanoscaffolds as vehicles for 5-fluoro-2′-deoxyuridine oligomers in colorectal cancer therapy. *Nanoscale*, **10**(15), 7238–7249.
100. Stein, C., et al. (2009). Efficient gene silencing by delivery of locked nucleic acid antisense oligonucleotides, unassisted by transfection reagents. *Nucleic Acids Res.*, **38**(1), e3.
101. Lima, W. F., et al. (2012). Single-stranded siRNAs activate RNAi in animals. *Cell*, **150**(5), 883–894.
102. Raouane, M., et al. (2012). Lipid conjugated oligonucleotides: a useful strategy for delivery. *Bioconjugate Chem.*, **23**(6), 1091–1104.
103. Crooke, S. T., et al. (1996). Pharmacokinetic properties of several novel oligonucleotide analogs in mice. *J. Pharmacol. Exp. Ther.*, **277**(2), 923–937.
104. Bijsterbosch, M. K., et al. (2000). Modulation of plasma protein binding and in vivo liver cell uptake of phosphorothioate oligodeoxynucleotides by cholesterol conjugation. *Nucleic Acids Res.*, **28**(14), 2717–2725.
105. Wada, S., et al. (2016). Evaluation of the effects of chemically different linkers on hepatic accumulations, cell tropism and gene silencing ability of cholesterol-conjugated antisense oligonucleotides. *J. Control. Release*, **226**, 57–65.
106. Soutschek, J., et al. (2004). Therapeutic silencing of an endogenous gene by systemic administration of modified siRNAs. *Nature*, **432**(7014), 173.
107. Wolfrum, C., et al. (2007). Mechanisms and optimization of in vivo delivery of lipophilic siRNAs. *Nat. Biotechnol.*, **25**(10), 1149.
108. Kuwahara, H., et al. (2011). Efficient in vivo delivery of siRNA into brain capillary endothelial cells along with endogenous lipoprotein. *Mol. Ther.*, **19**(12), 2213–2221.
109. DiFiglia, M., et al. (2007). Therapeutic silencing of mutant huntingtin with siRNA attenuates striatal and cortical neuropathology and behavioral deficits. *Proc. Natl. Acad. Sci.*, **104**(43), 17204–17209.
110. Chen, Q., et al. (2010). Lipophilic siRNAs mediate efficient gene silencing in oligodendrocytes with direct CNS delivery. *J. Control. Release*, **144**(2), 227–232.
111. Alterman, J. F., et al. (2015). Hydrophobically modified siRNAs silence huntingtin mRNA in primary neurons and mouse brain. *Mol. Ther. Nucleic Acids*, **4**, e266.
112. Osborn, M. F., et al. (2018). Efficient gene silencing in brain tumors with hydrophobically modified siRNAs. *Mol. Cancer Ther.*, **17**(6), 1251–1258.

113. Nikan, M., et al. (2016). Docosahexaenoic acid conjugation enhances distribution and safety of siRNA upon local administration in mouse brain. *Mol. Ther. Nucleic Acids*, **5**, e344.

114. Nikan, M., et al. (2017). Synthesis and evaluation of parenchymal retention and efficacy of a metabolically stable O-phosphocholine-N-docosahexaenoyl-l-serine siRNA conjugate in mouse brain. *Bioconjugate Chem.*, **28**(6), 1758–1766.

115. Kawakita, E., Hashimoto, M., Shido, O. (2006). Docosahexaenoic acid promotes neurogenesis in vitro and in vivo. *Neuroscience*, **139**(3), 991–997.

116. Nishina, K., et al. (2008). Efficient in vivo delivery of siRNA to the liver by conjugation of α-tocopherol. *Mol. Ther.*, **16**(4), 734–740.

117. Uno, Y., et al. (2010). High-density lipoprotein facilitates in vivo delivery of α-tocopherol–conjugated short-interfering RNA to the brain. *Hum. Gene Ther.*, **22**(6), 711–719.

118. Balazs, Z., et al. (2004). Uptake and transport of high-density lipoprotein (HDL) and HDL-associated α-tocopherol by an in vitro blood–brain barrier model. *J. Neurochem.*, **89**(4), 939–950.

119. Mardones, P., et al. (2002). α-Tocopherol metabolism is abnormal in scavenger receptor class B type I (SR-BI)-deficient mice. *J. Nutr.*, **132**(3), 443–449.

120. Nishina, T., et al. (2015). Chimeric antisense oligonucleotide conjugated to α-tocopherol. *Mol. Ther. Nucleic Acids*, **4**, e220.

121. Nishina, K., et al. (2015). DNA/RNA heteroduplex oligonucleotide for highly efficient gene silencing. *Nat. Commun.*, **6**, 7969.

122. Kuwahara, H., et al. (2018). Modulation of blood-brain barrier function by a heteroduplex oligonucleotide in vivo. *Sci. Rep.*, **8**(1), 4377.

123. Suk, J. S., et al. (2016). PEGylation as a strategy for improving nanoparticle-based drug and gene delivery. *Adv. Drug Deliv. Rev.*, **99**, 28–51.

124. Love, K. T., et al. (2010). Lipid-like materials for low-dose, in vivo gene silencing. *Proc. Natl. Acad. Sci.*, **107**(5), 1864–1869.

125. Akinc, A., et al. (2008). A combinatorial library of lipid-like materials for delivery of RNAi therapeutics. *Nat. Biotechnol.*, **26**(5), 561.

126. Lee, Y., Thompson, D. (2017). Stimuli-responsive liposomes for drug delivery. *Wiley Interdiscip. Rev. Nanomed. Nanobiotechnol.*, **9**(5), e1450.

127. Shaikh, R. P., et al. (2010). A review of multi-responsive membranous systems for rate-modulated drug delivery. *AAPS PharmSciTech*, **11**(1), 441–459.

128. Simões, S., et al. (2004). On the formulation of pH-sensitive liposomes with long circulation times. *Adv. Drug Deliv. Rev.*, **56**(7), 947–965.

129. Liu, H.-M., et al. (2017). Hypoxia-responsive ionizable liposome delivery siRNA for glioma therapy. *Int. J. Nanomed.*, **12**, 1065.

130. MacKay, J. A., Deen, D. F., Szoka Jr, F. C. (2005). Distribution in brain of liposomes after convection enhanced delivery; modulation by particle charge, particle diameter, and presence of steric coating. *Brain Res.*, **1035**(2), 139–153.

131. Gao, H. (2017). Perspectives on dual targeting delivery systems for brain tumors. *J. Neuroimmune Pharmacol.*, **12**(1), 6–16.

132. dos Santos Rodrigues, B., et al. (2018). Dual functionalized liposome-mediated gene delivery across triple co-culture blood brain barrier model and specific in vivo neuronal transfection. *J. Control. Release*, **286**, 264–278.

133. Costa, P. M., et al. (2013). Tumor-targeted chlorotoxin-coupled nanoparticles for nucleic acid delivery to glioblastoma cells: a promising system for glioblastoma treatment. *Mol. Ther. Nucleic Acids*, **2**, e100.

134. Costa, P. M., et al. (2015). MiRNA-21 silencing mediated by tumor-targeted nanoparticles combined with sunitinib: a new multimodal gene therapy approach for glioblastoma. *J. Control. Release*, **207**, 31–39.

135. Conceição, M., et al. (2016). Intravenous administration of brain-targeted stable nucleic acid lipid particles alleviates Machado-Joseph disease neurological phenotype. *Biomaterials*, **82**, 124–137.

136. Grijalvo, S., et al. (2019). Cationic niosomes as non-viral vehicles for nucleic acids: challenges and opportunities in gene delivery. *Pharmaceutics*, **11**(2), 50.

137. Mashal, M., et al. (2018). Non-viral vectors based on cationic niosomes as efficient gene delivery vehicles to central nervous system cells into the brain. *Int. J. Pharm.*, **552**(1–2), 48–55.

138. Puras, G., et al. (2014). A novel cationic niosome formulation for gene delivery to the retina. *J. Control. Release*, **174**, 27–36.

139. Ojeda, E., et al. (2016). The influence of the polar head-group of synthetic cationic lipids on the transfection efficiency mediated by niosomes in rat retina and brain. *Biomaterials*, **77**, 267–279.

140. Simons, M., Raposo, G. (2009). Exosomes–vesicular carriers for intercellular communication. *Curr. Opin. Cell Biol.*, **21**(4), 575–581.

141. Alvarez-Erviti, L., et al. (2011). Delivery of siRNA to the mouse brain by systemic injection of targeted exosomes. *Nat. Biotechnol.*, **29**(4), 341.

142. Ciregia, F., Urbani, A., Palmisano, G. (2017). Extracellular vesicles in brain tumors and neurodegenerative diseases. *Front. Mol. Neurosci.*, **10**, 276.

143. Didiot, M.-C., et al. (2016). Exosome-mediated delivery of hydrophobically modified siRNA for Huntingtin mRNA silencing. *Mol. Ther.*, **24**(10), 1836–1847.

144. Dolatabadi, J. E. N., Omidi, Y. (2016). Solid lipid-based nanocarriers as efficient targeted drug and gene delivery systems. *TrAC Trends Anal. Chem.*, **77**, 100–108.

145. Müller, R. H., Maèder, K., Gohla, S. (2000). Solid lipid nanoparticles (SLN) for controlled drug delivery: a review of the state of the art. *Eur. J. Pharm. Biopharm.*, **50**(1), 161–177.

146. Blasi, P., et al. (2007). Solid lipid nanoparticles for targeted brain drug delivery. *Adv. Drug Deliv. Rev.*, **59**(6), 454–477.

147. Jorge, A., Pais, A., Vitorino, C. (2020). Targeted siRNA delivery using lipid nanoparticles, in *Drug Delivery Systems, Methods in Molecular Biology*, Jain, K. K., ed., Springer, pp. 259–283.

148. Jin, J., et al. (2011). In vivo specific delivery of c-Met siRNA to glioblastoma using cationic solid lipid nanoparticles. *Bioconjugate Chem.*, **22**(12), 2568–2572.

149. Kim, H. R., et al. (2008). Cationic solid lipid nanoparticles reconstituted from low density lipoprotein components for delivery of siRNA. *Mol. Pharmaceutics*, **5**(4), 622–631.

150. Lobovkina, T., et al. (2011). In vivo sustained release of siRNA from solid lipid nanoparticles. *ACS Nano*, **5**(12), 9977–9983.

151. Gomes, M. J., et al. (2017). Tailoring lipid and polymeric nanoparticles as siRNA carriers towards the blood-brain barrier–from targeting to safe administration. *J. Neuroimmune Pharmacol.*, **12**(1), 107–119.

152. Chen, Z., et al. (2016). Nanostructured lipid carriers based temozolomide and gene co-encapsulated nanomedicine for gliomatosis cerebri combination therapy. *Drug Deliv.*, **23**(4), 1369–1373.

Chapter 9

Carriers for Nucleic Acid Delivery to the Brain

Sören Reinhard[a] and Ernst Wagner[a,b]
[a]*Department of Pharmacy, Pharmaceutical Biotechnology, Center of Nanoscience (CeNS), Ludwig-Maximilians-Universität, Butenandtstr. 5-13, 81377 Munich, Germany*
[b]*Nanosystems Initiative Munich (NIM), Schellingstr. 4, 80799 Munich, Germany*
reinhard.soeren@gmail.com

As the prevalence and understanding of central nervous system (CNS)-related diseases increases, therapeutic nucleic acids offer great opportunities for their treatment. However, the efficient delivery of nucleic acids to the brain is limited by the blood–brain barrier (BBB). Although viral vectors have been widely used for clinical gene delivery, nonviral nucleic acid delivery systems have lower safety concerns, are easier to manufacture and enable the delivery of all types of nucleic acid cargoes, including chemically modified nucleic acids. This book chapter focuses on nonviral nucleic acid vehicles and the barriers to their delivery to the CNS. Systemic injection and

Nanoparticles for Brain Drug Delivery
Edited by Carla Vitorino, Andreia Jorge and Alberto Pais

ISBN 978-981-4877-31-2 (Hardcover), 978-1-003-11932-6 (eBook)
www.jennystanford.com

intracranial routes of administration with their specific barriers are discussed. Ligands for receptor- and carrier-mediated transport to the CNS are presented in the context of vehicles and strategies which have been successfully used to overcome delivery barriers in vivo. A guided and transient BBB disruption by sonoporation is discussed as an option to increase brain delivery with minimal side effects. Another focus of this book chapter is the nucleic acid delivery to glioma, one of the most devastating neurological diseases. BBB impairment in late states of glioma provides improved conditions for the delivery of therapeutics. The presented delivery strategies summarise the efforts made to overcome the barriers to nonviral delivery of therapeutic nucleic acids to the CNS and may provide guidelines for the development of novel gene delivery vectors for clinical use.

9.1 Introduction

The increasing prevalence of central nervous system (CNS)-related diseases urgently requires the development of biological drugs such as proteins, antibodies, peptides or nucleic acids which can cross the blood–brain barrier (BBB) [1, 2]. The transfer of therapeutic genes and oligonucleotides offers great opportunities for the treatment of serious neurological diseases such as Alzheimer's disease, amyotrophic lateral sclerosis, multiple sclerosis and Parkinson's disease. Despite the enormous potential of therapeutic nucleic acids, minimal BBB transport is the main reason that only 1.8% of all gene therapy clinical trials worldwide address neurological disorders [3]. Efficient delivery of therapeutic agents to the brain is limited by the BBB consisting of endothelial cells along with astrocytes, pericytes and the basal lamina at the plasma membrane of the capillary of the brain parenchyma [4]. Large nucleic acids, either free or formulated as nanoparticles, lack the requirements for free diffusion into the brain (molecular weight <400 Da, <8 hydrogen bonds). Therefore, such therapeutics need to be designed to exploit carrier-mediated transport (CMT) or receptor-mediated transport (RMT) systems or need to undergo adsorptive-mediated transcytosis (AMT) [5, 6].

9.2 Nonviral Nucleic Acid Carriers

Free nucleic acids cannot use any of the above-mentioned CMT, RMT or AMT pathways, which is why they must be formulated with suitable carriers for brain delivery. Viral vectors such as adenoviruses or adeno-associated viruses found wide application for clinical gene delivery. However, nonviral nucleic acid delivery systems have lower safety concerns, are easier to manufacture and allow for delivery of all types of nucleic acid cargoes, such as chemically modified mRNA or small interfering RNA (siRNA), which induce gene silencing by RNA interference (RNAi) [7]. The first siRNA drug, Patisiran, a liposomal liver-targeted formulation of siRNA for the treatment of hereditary ATTR amyloidosis, has obtained market approval by the US Food and Drug Administration (FDA) in August 2018 [8].

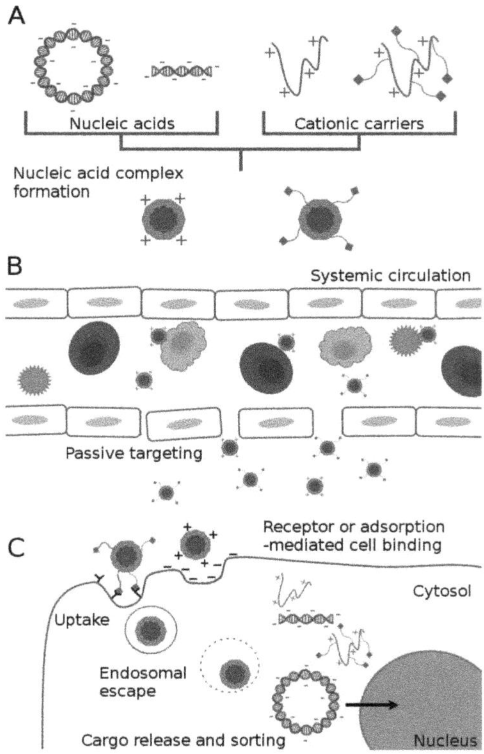

Figure 9.1 Barriers in the delivery of therapeutic nucleic acids. (A) Formation of stable complexes, (B) avoidance of rapid clearance and unspecific interactions with blood components, (C) cellular entry, endosomal escape and cargo release.

In addition to the BBB hurdle for brain delivery, there are general critical challenges in delivery of nucleic acids via synthetic vehicles: Extracellular requirements include (i) stability through stable complex formation and shielding to avoid rapid disintegration, clearance and nonspecific interactions and (ii) specific target cell binding and uptake. Intracellular challenges include (iii) efficient endosomal escape and (iv) liberation of the cargo in the cytosol in case of siRNA [9] or the nucleus in case of DNA [10, 11] (Fig. 9.1). Noncovalent complexation and encapsulation into multifunctional and bioresponsive carrier nanoparticles is a strategy which can address all steps of the delivery process. Nonviral nucleic acid formulations include lipid-based nanoparticles such as liposomal encapsulations or nucleic acid complexes with cationic liposomes, termed 'lipoplexes', or polymer-based nanosystems, including polymerosomes, polymer micelles, hydrogels and complexes of nucleic acids with cationic polymers such as polyethylenimine (PEI), termed 'polyplexes' [12, 13]. Condensation of polyanionic nucleic acids by entropy-driven electrostatic interaction with cationic carriers is necessary to prevent degradation, neutralise negative charges and reduce the size of large nucleic acids such as plasmid DNA (pDNA) [14, 15]. The binding to the nucleic acid should be reversible so that the therapeutic cargo is well available after reaching the target site. However, the sole complexation with cationic carriers can cause binding of positively charged nanoparticles to serum proteins, activation of the innate immune system [16, 17], self-aggregation or aggregation of blood cells [18]. Such unspecific interactions can be circumvented by shielding of positive charges by hydrophilic polymers such as polyethylene glycol (PEG) [19–21], *N*-(2-hydroxypropyl) methacrylamide (pHPMA) [22, 23], hydroxyethyl starch (HES) [24], hyaluronic acid [25], poly(2-oxazoline) [26] or polysarcosine [27]. Extending the circulation time of nanoparticles with hydrophilic shielding domains increases the time which therapeutics can interact with target cells. Specific uptake into target cells can be achieved by exposing a broad spectrum of ligands [28] from small chemical compounds such as vitamins and drugs [29, 30], carbohydrates [31], peptides [32], proteins [33–35], antibodies [36, 37] and aptamers [38] on the surface of the nanoparticles. Targeting ligands and shielding agents may be incorporated either directly to the nucleic acid (preconjugation) or subsequent to nucleic acid core nanoparticle formation (Fig. 9.2) [27, 39–42].

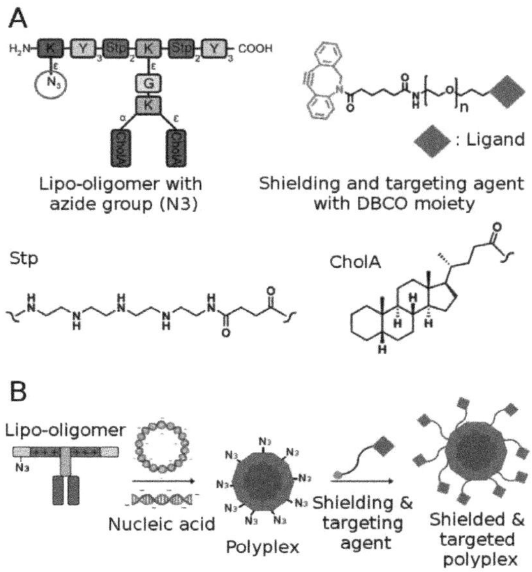

Figure 9.2 (A) Schematic illustration of a sequence-defined t-shape lipo-oligomer and a DBCO-shielding and DBCO-targeting agent. Units of the oligomer: Y, tyrosine; K, lysine; G, glycine; Stp, succinoyltetraethylene-pentamine; CholA, 5b-cholanic acid. (B) Targeted nucleic acid nanoparticles prepared by click modification of azide-containing lipo-oligomer core nanoparticles with DBCO-shielding and DBCO-targeting agents [42].

9.3 Brain-Targeted Nucleic Acid Delivery

Besides the efforts to achieve brain delivery by crossing of the BBB after systemic injection, transcranial delivery strategies aim to bypass the BBB by intracerebral implantation, intracerebroventricular infusion and convection-enhanced diffusion. However, intracranial injections rely on the diffusion of therapeutic agents in the brain parenchyma, which decreases with the square of diffusion distance and usually limits the applicability of such approaches to localised targets [43]. Microvessels in the brain are only 40 μm apart and account for about 95% of the total area of the barriers between blood and brain [44, 45]. Consequently, complete and near-instantaneous distribution throughout the CNS is achieved as soon as a therapeutic substance or formulation crosses the BBB.

9.3.1 Transport across the Blood–Brain Barrier

A fundamental issue of brain delivery is the optimal size of nanoparticles, regardless of their decoration with targeting ligands. The biodistribution of polystyrene nanoparticles between 25 and 500 nm showed a strong correlation to nanoparticle size with the highest accumulation of 25 and 50 nm particles in the brain tissue 3 hours after intravenous (i.v.) injection into rats [46]. Similar results were found after i.v. injection of gold nanoparticles of 15, 50, 100 and 200 nm size in mice. Highest gold concentrations of 15 and 50 nm nanoparticles in the brain after 24 hours revealed that the smaller sized particles are better able to pass the BBB [47].

9.3.1.1 Protein ligands

Targeting the transferrin receptor (TfR) at the BBB with Transferrin (Tf) or monoclonal antibodies (mAb) against the TfR (TfRmAb) is a common strategy for brain delivery via RMT [48]. After binding the TfR, nanoparticles should be internalised at the luminal side of the brain endothelium and eventually be transcytosed and released at the opposite basal surface. The Tf content (avidity) on the nanoparticle surface plays a critical role in the fate of the nanoparticles after uptake in brain capillary endothelial cells (BCECs). Systemic administration of TF-decorated gold nanoparticles showed that nanoparticles with large amounts of Tf remained strongly attached to BCECs, whereas those with less Tf are capable of both interacting with TfR on the luminal side of the BBB and detaching from TfR on the abluminal side [49]. An alternative favorable measure presents the labile Tf linkage to nanocarriers which reverses during the transcytosis process [50]. Tf-decoration of pDNA complexes with polyamidoamine (PAMAM) dendrimers via a PEG linker showed a 2.25-fold higher brain uptake compared with PEGylated nanoparticles alone [51]. TfRmAbs were used for TfR-targeting of 85 nm PEGylated immunoliposomes with pDNA encoding tyrosine hydroxylase in a rat model of Parkinson's disease, demonstrating the possibility to normalise brain enzyme activity by i.v. administration of nonviral gene vectors [52]. The activity of the lysosomal enzyme beta-glucuronidase in murine brains deficient of the protein was >10-fold increased after delivery of the encoding pDNA in TfRmAb-decorated liposomes [53]. The adsorption of certain plasma proteins such as apolipoprotein E

(ApoE) and apolipoprotein B (ApoB) is an alternative to the covalent attachment of protein ligands to the nanoparticle surface. Poly(butyl cyanoacrylate) nanoparticles coated with polysorbate 80 adsorb ApoE and ApoB and enable the brain delivery of a number of drugs via low-density lipoprotein (LDL) receptor interaction which are unable to cross the BBB in free form [54, 55].

9.3.1.2 Peptide ligands

Although large protein ligands such as Tf or antibodies were used successfully for brain delivery, their large size and charge can destabilise nanoparticles and thereby limit their biodistribution in vivo [41]. Smaller peptide ligands are an alternative to protein ligands, especially since display techniques such as messenger RNA (mRNA) or phage display enable the screening of large peptide libraries for binding to target receptors and cells (Table 9.1) [56–58]. Among the most commonly used peptide ligands for BBB transfer is rabies virus glycoprotein (RVG), a 29-amino-acid peptide which binds the nicotinic acetylcholine receptor. RVG bound to a nucleic acid–binding oligo-arginine residue was used for siRNA brain delivery after systemic administration [59]. Since then, nucleic acid formulations for BBB transfer included RVG-decorated PAMAM dendrimers [60], liposomes [61], chitosan nanoparticles [62], poly(mannitol-co-PEI) complexes [63] and exosomes [64], but overall results were not convincing. Other peptide ligands for brain delivery of nucleic acids or nanoparticles include angiopep-2 for LRP-1 binding [65], chlorotoxin, which specifically binds glioma cells and matrix metalloproteinase-2 (MMP-2) [66], EPRNEEK binding the laminin receptor [67], a leptin-derived peptide binding the leptin receptor [68], g7 which promotes brain delivery via AMT [69] or the TfR-binding peptide THR [70]. Small peptide ligands must be presented on the nanoparticle surface to be available for target receptor or cell interaction. In addition, the protease stability of peptides is a major concern when decorated nanoparticles are systemically administered in vivo, as rapid degradation of the ligands results in a loss of targeting capability. The *retro-enantio* approach inverts the peptide sequence, and L-amino acids are replaced by D-amino acids, resulting in protease-resistant analogues which retain the binding ability of the parent peptide. The TfR binding peptide THR has been converted into the fully protease-resistant

Table 9.1 Peptide ligands and carrier systems used for targeted nanoparticle delivery into the brain and glioma

Peptide ligand	Receptor	Carrier system	Key findings in vivo	Reference
		Brain targeting		
RVG29	nAChR	DNA/PAMAM-PEG	Brain accumulation, gene expression	[60]
		siRNA/Liposomes	Brain delivery	[61]
		siRNA/Chitosan-PEG	Brain accumulation	[62]
		siRNA/Poly(mannitol-co-PEI)	Brain delivery, gene KD	[63]
		siRNA/Exosomes	Brain delivery, gene KD	[64]
Angiopep-2	LRP-1	DNA/PAMAM-PEG	Brain accumulation, gene expression	[65]
Leptin30	LeptinR	DNA/DGL-PEG	Brain delivery, gene expression	[68]
g7	– (AMT)	PLGA	BBB-crossing, brain delivery	[69]
THR	TfR	AuNPs	Brain delivery	[70]
retro-enantio THR		QDots	BBB-crossing, brain delivery	[71]
Mini-Ap4	– (KCa channel?)	AuNPs, GFP, QDots	Brain delivery	[73]

Peptide ligand	Receptor	Carrier system	Key findings in vivo	Reference
		Glioma targeting		
Chlorotoxin	– (MMP-2)	siRNA/Liposomes	Internalisation into glioma	[66]
		anti-miR-21/Liposomes	Tumour growth inhibition, prolonged mouse survival	[115]
EPRNEEK	LamininR	DNA/DGL-PEG	Tumour growth inhibition, prolonged mouse survival	[67]
Angiopep-2	LRP-1	siRNA/Oligoaminoamides	Glioma penetration, gene KD	[101]
		siRNA/PLGA NPs + Doxorubicin	Prolonged mouse survival, induction of apoptosis	[116]
		siRNA/Liposomes	Tumour growth inhibition	[120]
I_6P_7	IL6R	DNA/Oligoaminoamides	Prolonged mouse survival, induction of apoptosis	[102]
retro-enantio CendR peptide	Neuropilin-1	DNA/PEI-PEG	Prolonged mouse survival	[104]
T7	TfR	siRNA/DGL-PEG	Tumour growth inhibition, prolonged mouse survival	[117]
		siRNA/Liposomes	Prolonged mouse survival	[118]

PAMAM, polyamidoamine; PEI, polyethylenimine; KD, knockdown; DGL, dendrigraft poly-L-lysine; AMT, adsorptive-mediated transcytosis; PLGA, poly(lactic-*co*-glycolic acid).

THR *retro-enantio* peptide, which acts as a BBB shuttle for the CNS delivery of a variety of cargoes. [71]. Cyclisation and substitution of natural amino acids by nonnatural residues are further strategies to optimise peptide ligands for systemic brain delivery, as shown for the LDL receptor–binding peptide-22 [72] or the cyclic bee venom–derived peptide MiniAp-4 [73].

9.3.1.3 Carrier-mediated transport

Endogenous transport systems of the cerebral vasculature include carrier-mediated transporters such as glucose and amino acid carriers [6]. Such transporters are selective for their small endogenous ligands and usually cannot be exploited for the transport of large nanoparticles. However, glucose transporter-1 (GLUT1), which is highly expressed in BCECs, is an attractive target for brain delivery by glucose-decorated nanoparticles. A recent study shows that glycemic control enables the transport of glucosylated nanocarriers through BBB crossing into the brain [31]. Polyion complex (PIC) micelles were modified with noncharged PEG shells and Gluc(6), a glucose molecule attached via the C6 hydroxyl group. Nanoparticles with surface glucose densities of 10%, 25% and 50% Gluc(6) were tested for brain uptake in vivo after systemic injection. In free-feeding mice, none of the Gluc(6) decorated PIC micelles showed enhanced brain accumulation compared to the PEGylated control. Glycemic control was introduced by one-day fasting prior to nanoparticle injection because it was reported that low blood glucose levels facilitate GLUT1 localisation on the luminal plasma membrane in BCECs and increase GLUT1 synthesis at the gene expression level. A 20 wt% glucose solution was intraperitoneally administered 30 min after the micelle injection to elevate blood glucose concentration, which is speculated to induce internalisation and translocation of GLUT1 and bound micelles to the BCEC abluminal plasma membrane. The density of Gluc(6) on the nanoparticle surface played a crucial role in the brain accumulation, as extensive distribution throughout the brain parenchyma was observed for only 25% Gluc(6) micelles. Micelles with 50% glucose stayed in and/or around the BCECs probably due to their lower dissociation constant to GLUT1 because of the high surface glucose density [31]. This study shows that not only the design of nanoparticles, but also the control of endogenous biological processes and parameters can influence the success of delivery strategies into the brain.

9.3.2 Blood–Brain Barrier Disruption

Despite the enormous surface area of cerebral vessels, the highly complex and restrictive physiological structure of the BBB makes it the biggest bottleneck in brain delivery. Therefore, methods were developed which combine systemic application of nucleic acid formulations with temporary disruption of the BBB. Injection of hypertonic solutions of mannitol before administration of therapeutics is a way to widen tight junctions by shrinking of BCECs [74] and was shown to significantly enhance the distribution of RVG-decorated miRNA-PEI complexes throughout the brain [75]. More recent approaches involve the administration of gas-filled microbubbles which temporarily disrupt and permeabilise the BBB by producing micropores upon activation by ultrasound, a process called sonoporation [76, 77]. Sonoporation has been used to improve the delivery of anti-Huntingtin siRNA [78], DNA complexed with cationic polymer-decorated microbubbles [79] and folate-conjugated microbubbles [80] and DNA encapsulated in liposomes [81] or polyplexes [82] upon co-administration with microbubbles. Most approaches use MRI-guided focused ultrasound which targets the ultrasound to a specific point with contrast agent microbubbles to minimise side effects [83].

9.3.3 Intracranial Delivery

Intracranial injection into the cerebral parenchyma or cerebrospinal fluid (CSF) initially avoids systemic circulation and brings therapeutics close to the target side. Therapeutics injected into the CSF face the much less restrictive single-layer barrier of epithelial cells with gap-junctions between the CSF and the brain tissue [84]. However, the much smaller barrier surface compared to the BBB, constant turnover of CSF into the blood and limited diffusion within the brain parenchyma limit intracranial approaches [85, 86]. Still, the antisense oligonucleotide Nusinersen (Spinraza) gained FDA approval in 2016 for the treatment of spinal muscular atrophy and is administered by intrathecal injection into the CSF for the delivery of a therapeutic gene to neural stem cells [87]. Intraventricularly administered cationic liposomes and organically modified silica nanoparticles were used to successfully deliver siRNA [88] and pDNA [89] to neuronal cells in vivo. Luciferase encoding pDNA encapsulated in liposomes showed luciferase activity throughout the brain after injection in the cisterna magna of rats, but not after direct injection into the parenchyma [90]. Injection of luciferase expressing mRNA incorporated in polyplex nanomicelles into the cisterna magna of mice resulted in protein expression in the CSF for almost a week [91]. Biodegradable arginine ester of PAMAM dendrimers were used to deliver siRNA in the post-ischaemic brain by injection into the cortex of rats [92]. Tf-decorated siRNA-containing liposomes showed extensive local distribution and gene silencing after stereotactic administration into the striatum [93]. Silencing of the transcription factor c-Jun by RNA interference significantly decreased both cell death following glutamate-induced excitotoxic damage in primary neuronal cultures and neuronal death and inflammation following kainic acid-mediated lesions in the mouse hippocampus [94, 95]. Continuous injections of siRNA against toxic Huntingtin protein into the brain parenchyma were performed with osmotic pumps [96] and convection-enhanced delivery [97].

9.4 Glioma-Targeted Nucleic Acid Delivery

Glioma-bearing patients, despite aggressive treatment, including surgical removal of the primary tumour mass and subsequent chemo- and radiotherapy, have a particularly poor prognosis with only 14 months median survival and a 2-year survival rate of 3%–5% [98, 99]. This results in the urgent need for the development of new therapeutic approaches. Notably, in late stages of glioma development, the BBB is impaired by formation of fenestrations, altered thickness of the basal lamina and tight junction disruption [100]. This, on the one hand, leads to serious symptoms of the disease, but on the other hand facilitates the delivery of therapeutics due to the less restrictive physiology of the BBB.

Sequence-defined oligoaminoamide oligomers were used for receptor-mediated delivery of siRNA [101] and pDNA [102] into glioma in vivo after systemic injection. For siRNA delivery, an untargeted lipo-oligomer was mixed with a PEGylated oligomer containing an angiopep-2 ligand targeting the LRP-1 receptor, which is overexpressed both on the surface of BCECs and glioma cells [101]. A similar cascade-targeting strategy was used for the delivery of therapeutic pDNA. Here, a nontargeted oligomer was mixed with a PEGylated oligomer containing the heptapeptide I_6P_7, which binds the interleukin 6 receptor (IL6R). IL6R expression was detected both on the tumour BBB and in various brain tumours such as glioblastoma (Fig. 9.3). Targeted delivery of pDNA encoding inhibitor of growth 4 (pING4) significantly prolonged the survival time of orthotopic U87 glioma-bearing mice [102]. Reporter gene expression was found in the brains of U87 glioblastoma-bearing mice after intracranial injection of pDNA polyplexes formed with bioreducibly linked (cRGDyK)-PEG-ss-PEI. The Arg-Gly-Asp (RGD) sequence binds integrin receptors which are highly expressed in glioma cells, while the cyclic RGD peptide cRGDyK is known to increase the affinity and selectivity of the receptor by providing conformational restraint [32, 103]. PEG–PEI polyplexes carrying the therapeutic gene *pORF-hTRAIL* were targeted with a protease-resistant *retro-enantio* C-end rule (CendR) peptide-binding neuropilin-1, which plays an important role in tumour angiogenesis, growth and metastasis [104]. Intravenous injection of the polyplexes significantly prolonged the survival time of intracranial U87 glioma-bearing mice from 25 to 30 days. Epidermal growth factor receptor (EGFR)-targeted intratumoural delivery of the synthetic antiproliferative double-stranded RNA polyinosine-cytosine (poly IC) formulated with PEI-PEG-EGF [105–107] induced the complete regression of intracranial tumours in mice, with no obvious adverse toxic effects on normal brain tissue [105]. Several preclinical studies explore the delivery of siRNAs to target genes involved in gliomagenesis, tumour progression and therapy resistance of glial tumours [99]. Tumour growth inhibition and prolonged survival of animals was found after both local application [108–114] and systemic injection [115–120] of siRNA nanoparticles (Table 9.1). Another potentially promising target for glioma-directed delivery of therapeutics is the proangiogenic apelin receptor (APLNR) and its cognate ligand apelin, which play a central role in controlling glioblastoma vascularisation [121]. Apelin and APLNR were found to be dramatically upregulated in glioblastoma-associated microvascular proliferations, but not in the healthy brain [122].

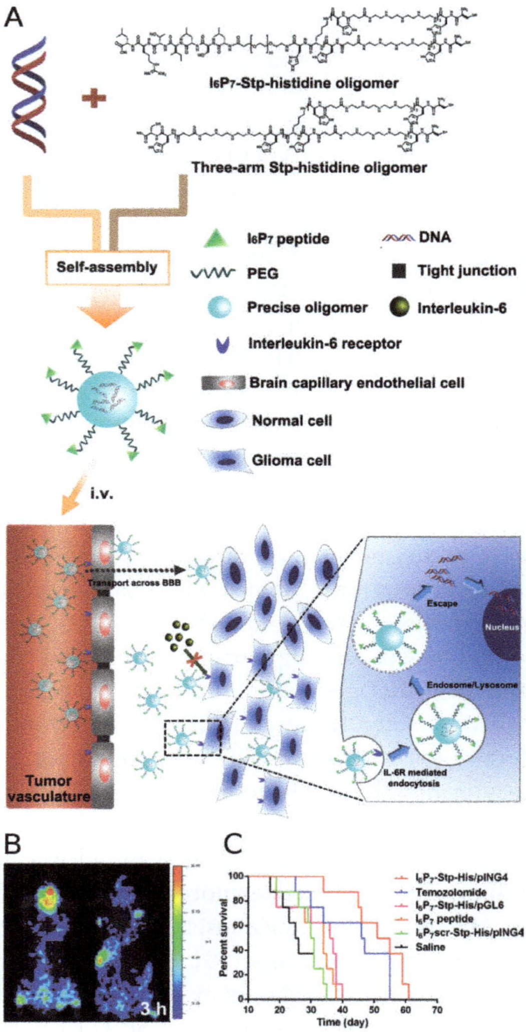

Figure 9.3 (A) Interleukin 6 receptor cascade–targeted pING4 DNA polyplexes for glioma therapy. Nontargeted three-arm oligomer containing ionisable histidins and succinoyltetraethylene-pentamine (Stp) units was mixed with a PEGylated oligomer containing the heptapeptide I_6P_7, which binds the interleukin 6 receptor. (B) In vivo fluorescent images of glioma-bearing mice 3 hours after intravenous administration of I_6P_7-Stp-His/DNA (left) and I_6P_7scr-Stp-His/DNA (right). (C) Kaplan–Meier survival curves of glioma-bearing mice after different treatments. Reprinted from Ref. [102], Copyright (2017), with permission from Elsevier.

9.5 Conclusions

Despite the large number of patients with CNS disorders and the urgent need to develop new biological medicines, there are only a few pharmaceutical companies which have program for brain-targeted drug delivery, and only 1.8% of all gene therapy clinical trials address neurological disorders [3, 43]. Major hurdles to the development of new therapeutic approaches for neurological disorders are the highly restrictive physiology of the BBB and the poor diffusion of therapeutic agents in the brain parenchyma after local injection. However, major advances in the design of nucleic acids and viral and nonviral carriers for their delivery have allowed the engineering of nucleic acid formulations to overcome plenty of the challenges of brain delivery. Each administration route has advantages and disadvantages and some specific obstacles. Damage to the brain vasculature or healthy brain tissue must be avoided in any case, since side effects can be particularly serious here. Although mainly viral vectors are used for clinical gene delivery, nonviral nucleic acid delivery systems are becoming more popular because of lower safety concerns, ease of preparation and the ability to deliver all types of nucleic acids [7]. Virus-inspired bioresponsive design of nucleic acid nanoparticles improves their transfection efficiency [123]. New shielding and targeting strategies are being developed to prevent premature degradation of nucleic acids and increase their uptake and distribution throughout the CNS, especially since display technologies allow for the screening of large ligand libraries [56–58]. It should be noted that complex multicomponent systems can complicate the manufacturing, reproducibility and upscaling and thus delay the approval and translation of nucleic acid therapeutics into the clinic. A successful example, however, is the market approval of the first siRNA lipid nanoparticle Patisiran by the US FDA in August 2018, which should further accelerate the development and clinical application of nonviral nucleic acid formulations [8].

Apart from addressing challenges in nucleic acid delivery, the identification and selection of promising therapeutic genes or target genes for RNAi is of utmost importance and may include individualised therapies due to the recent tremendous progress in molecular profiling of patients [99]. Stability, specificity and immunogenicity of therapeutic nucleic acids can be optimised with advanced chemical modifications [124].

New techniques such as localised microbubble-mediated sonoporation of the BBB with minimal side effects will further improve the brain delivery of nucleic acid formulations and pave the way for clinical evaluation of gene therapeutics for CNS disorders in the coming years.

Acknowledgements

This work was supported by German Research Foundation (DFG) Excellence Cluster Nanosystems Initiative Munich (NIM) and the DFG-NSFC Joint Sino-German Research project 410149116.

References

1. Peluffo, H., Unzueta, U., Negro-Demontel, M. L., Xu, Z., Vaquez, E., Ferrer-Miralles, N., Villaverde, A. (2015). BBB-targeting, protein-based nanomedicines for drug and nucleic acid delivery to the CNS. *Biotechnol. Adv.*, **33**, 277–287.
2. Tan, J. Y., Sellers, D. L., Pham, B., Pun, S. H., Horner, P. J. (2016). Non-viral nucleic acid delivery strategies to the central nervous system. *Front. Mol. Neurosci.*, **9**, 108.
3. Ginn, S. L., Amaya, A. K., Alexander, I. E., Edelstein, M., Abedi, M. R. (2018). Gene therapy clinical trials worldwide to 2017: an update. *J. Gene Med.*, **20**, e3015.
4. Pardridge, W. M. (2016). CSF, blood-brain barrier, and brain drug delivery. *Expert Opin. Drug Deliv.*, **13**, 963–975.
5. Herve, F., Ghinea, N., Scherrmann, J. M. (2008). CNS delivery via adsorptive transcytosis. *AAPS J.*, **10**, 455–472.
6. Pardridge, W. M. (2012). Drug transport across the blood-brain barrier. *J. Cereb. Blood Flow Metab.*, **32**, 1959–1972.
7. Burke, P. A., Pun, S. H., Reineke, T. M. (2013). Advancing polymeric delivery systems amidst a nucleic acid therapy renaissance. *ACS Macro Lett.*, **2**, 928–934.
8. Adams, D., Gonzalez-Duarte, A., O'Riordan, W. D., Yang, C. C., Ueda, M., Kristen, A. V., Tournev, I., Schmidt, H. H., Coelho, T., Berk, J. L., Lin, K. P., Vita, G., Attarian, S., Plante-Bordeneuve, V., Mezei, M. M., Campistol, J. M., Buades, J., Brannagan, 3rd, T. H., Kim, B. J., Oh, J., Parman, Y., Sekijima, Y., Hawkins, P. N., Solomon, S. D., Polydefkis, M., Dyck, P. J., Gandhi, P. J., Goyal, S., Chen, J., Strahs, A. L., Nochur, S. V., Sweetser, M. T.,

Garg, P. P., Vaishnaw, A. K., Gollob, J. A., Suhr, O. B. (2018). Patisiran, an RNAi therapeutic, for hereditary transthyretin amyloidosis. *N. Engl. J. Med.*, **379**, 11–21.

9. Reinhard, S., Wagner, E. (2017). How to tackle the challenge of siRNA delivery with sequence-defined oligoamino amides. *Macromol. Biosci.*, **17**.
10. Brunner, S., Sauer, T., Carotta, S., Cotten, M., Saltik, M., Wagner, E. (2000). Cell cycle dependence of gene transfer by lipoplex, polyplex and recombinant adenovirus. *Gene Ther.*, **7**, 401–407.
11. Levacic, A. K., Morys, S., Kempter, S., Lächelt, U., Wagner, E. (2017). Minicircle versus plasmid DNA delivery by receptor-targeted polyplexes. *Hum. Gene Ther.*, **28**, 862–874.
12. Felgner, P. L., Barenholz, Y., Behr, J. P., Cheng, S. H., Cullis, P., Huang, L., Jessee, J. A., Seymour, L., Szoka, F., Thierry, A. R., Wagner, E., Wu, G. (1997). Nomenclature for synthetic gene delivery systems. *Hum. Gene Ther.*, **8**, 511–512.
13. Lächelt, U., Wagner, E. (2015). Nucleic acid therapeutics using polyplexes: a journey of 50 years (and beyond). *Chem. Rev.*, **115**, 11043–11078.
14. Bloomfield, V. A. (1991). Condensation of DNA by multivalent cations: considerations on mechanism. *Biopolymers*, **31**, 1471–1481.
15. Wagner, E., Cotten, M., Foisner, R., Birnstiel, M. L. (1991). Transferrin-polycation-DNA complexes: the effect of polycations on the structure of the complex and DNA delivery to cells. *Proc. Natl. Acad. Sci. U. S. A.*, **88**, 4255–4259.
16. Plank, C., Mechtler, K., Szoka, Jr., F. C., Wagner, E. (1996). Activation of the complement system by synthetic DNA complexes: a potential barrier for intravenous gene delivery. *Hum. Gene Ther.*, **7**, 1437–1446.
17. Merkel, O. M., Urbanics, R., Bedocs, P., Rozsnyay, Z., Rosivall, L., Toth, M., Kissel, T., Szebeni, J. (2011). In vitro and in vivo complement activation and related anaphylactic effects associated with polyethylenimine and polyethylenimine-graft-poly(ethylene glycol) block copolymers. *Biomaterials*, **32**, 4936–4942.
18. Chollet, P., Favrot, M. C., Hurbin, A., Coll, J. L. (2002). Side-effects of a systemic injection of linear polyethylenimine-DNA complexes. *J. Gene Med.*, **4**, 84–91.
19. Ogris, M., Brunner, S., Schuller, S., Kircheis, R., Wagner, E. (1999). PEGylated DNA/transferrin-PEI complexes: reduced interaction with blood components, extended circulation in blood and potential for systemic gene delivery. *Gene Ther.*, **6**, 595–605.

20. Meyer, M., Dohmen, C., Philipp, A., Kiener, D., Maiwald, G., Scheu, C., Ogris, M., Wagner, E. (2009). Synthesis and biological evaluation of a bioresponsive and endosomolytic siRNA-polymer conjugate. *Mol. Pharm.*, **6**, 752–762.

21. Dirisala, A., Osada, K., Chen, Q., Tockary, T. A., Machitani, K., Osawa, S., Liu, X., Ishii, T., Miyata, K., Oba, M., Uchida, S., Itaka, K., Kataoka, K. (2014). Optimized rod length of polyplex micelles for maximizing transfection efficiency and their performance in systemic gene therapy against stroma-rich pancreatic tumors. *Biomaterials*, **35**, 5359–5368.

22. Johnson, R. N., Chu, D. S., Shi, J., Schellinger, J. G., Carlson, P. M., Pun, S. H. (2011). HPMA-oligolysine copolymers for gene delivery: optimization of peptide length and polymer molecular weight. *J. Control. Release*, **155**, 303–311.

23. Laga, R., Carlisle, R., Tangney, M., Ulbrich, K., Seymour, L. W. (2012). Polymer coatings for delivery of nucleic acid therapeutics. *J. Control. Release*, **161**, 537–553.

24. Noga, M., Edinger, D., Rödl, W., Wagner, E., Winter, G., Besheer, A. (2012). Controlled shielding and deshielding of gene delivery polyplexes using hydroxyethyl starch (HES) and alpha-amylase. *J. Control. Release*, **159**, 92–103.

25. Guter, M., Breunig, M. (2017). Hyaluronan as a promising excipient for ocular drug delivery. *Eur. J. Pharm. Biopharm.*, **113**, 34–49.

26. Manzenrieder, F., Luxenhofer, R., Retzlaff, M., Jordan, R., Finn, M. G. (2011). Stabilization of virus-like particles with poly(2-oxazoline)s. *Angew. Chem. Int. Ed. Engl.*, **50**, 2601–2605.

27. Klein, P. M., Klinker, K., Zhang, W., Kern, S., Kessel, E., Wagner, E., Barz, M. (2018). Efficient shielding of polyplexes using heterotelechelic polysarcosines. *Polymers*, **10**, 689.

28. Ogris, M., Wagner, E. (2011). To be targeted: is the magic bullet concept a viable option for synthetic nucleic acid therapeutics? *Hum. Gene Ther.*, **22**, 799–807.

29. Dohmen, C., Edinger, D., Fröhlich, T., Schreiner, L., Lächelt, U., Troiber, C., Rädler, J., Hadwiger, P., Vornlocher, H. P., Wagner, E. (2012). Nanosized multifunctional polyplexes for receptor-mediated siRNA delivery. *ACS Nano*, **6**, 5198–5208.

30. Lee, D. J., Kessel, E., Edinger, D., He, D., Klein, P. M., Voith von Voithenberg, L., Lamb, D. C., Lächelt, U., Lehto, T., Wagner, E. (2016). Dual antitumoral potency of EG5 siRNA nanoplexes armed with cytotoxic bifunctional glutamyl-methotrexate targeting ligand. *Biomaterials*, **77**, 98–110.

31. Anraku, Y., Kuwahara, H., Fukusato, Y., Mizoguchi, A., Ishii, T., Nitta, K., Matsumoto, Y., Toh, K., Miyata, K., Uchida, S., Nishina, K., Osada, K., Itaka, K., Nishiyama, N., Mizusawa, H., Yamasoba, T., Yokota, T., Kataoka, K. (2017). Glycaemic control boosts glucosylated nanocarrier crossing the BBB into the brain. *Nat. Commun.*, **8**, 1001.

32. Martin, I., Dohmen, C., Mas-Moruno, C., Troiber, C., Kos, P., Schaffert, D., Lächelt, U., Teixido, M., Gunther, M., Kessler, H., Giralt, E., Wagner, E. (2012). Solid-phase-assisted synthesis of targeting peptide-PEG-oligo(ethane amino)amides for receptor-mediated gene delivery. *Org. Biomol. Chem.*, **10**, 3258–3268.

33. Zenke, M., Steinlein, P., Wagner, E., Cotten, M., Beug, H., Birnstiel, M. L. (1990). Receptor-mediated endocytosis of transferrin-polycation conjugates: an efficient way to introduce DNA into hematopoietic cells. *Proc. Natl. Acad. Sci. U. S. A.*, **87**, 3655–3659.

34. Bellocq, N. C., Pun, S. H., Jensen, G. S., Davis, M. E. (2003). Transferrin-containing, cyclodextrin polymer-based particles for tumor-targeted gene delivery. *Bioconjugate Chem.*, **14**, 1122–1132.

35. Zhang, W., Rödl, W., He, D., Döblinger, M., Lächelt, U., Wagner, E. (2015). Combination of sequence-defined oligoaminoamides with transferrin-polycation conjugates for receptor-targeted gene delivery. *J. Gene Med.*, **17**, 161–172.

36. Buschle, M., Cotten, M., Kirlappos, H., Mechtler, K., Schaffner, G., Zauner, W., Birnstiel, M. L., Wagner, E. (1995). Receptor-mediated gene transfer into human T lymphocytes via binding of DNA/CD3 antibody particles to the CD3 T cell receptor complex. *Hum. Gene Ther.*, **6**, 753–761.

37. Gu, J., Al-Bayati, K., Ho, E. A. (2017). Development of antibody-modified chitosan nanoparticles for the targeted delivery of siRNA across the blood-brain barrier as a strategy for inhibiting HIV replication in astrocytes. *Drug Deliv. Transl. Res.*, **7**, 497–506.

38. Saw, P. E., Zhang, A., Nie, Y., Zhang, L., Xu, Y., Xu, X. (2018). Tumor-associated fibronectin targeted liposomal nanoplatform for cyclophilin A siRNA delivery and targeted malignant glioblastoma therapy. *Front. Pharmacol.*, **9**, 1194.

39. Blessing, T., Kursa, M., Holzhauser, R., Kircheis, R., Wagner, E. (2001). Different strategies for formation of pegylated EGF-conjugated PEI/DNA complexes for targeted gene delivery. *Bioconjugate Chem.*, **12**, 529–537.

40. Müller, K., Klein, P. M., Heissig, P., Roidl, A., Wagner, E. (2016). EGF receptor targeted lipo-oligocation polyplexes for antitumoral siRNA and miRNA delivery. *Nanotechnology*, **27**, 464001.

41. Zhang, W., Müller, K., Kessel, E., Reinhard, S., He, D., Klein, P. M., Höhn, M., Rödl, W., Kempter, S., Wagner, E. (2016). Targeted siRNA delivery using a lipo-oligoaminoamide nanocore with an influenza peptide and transferrin shell. *Adv. Healthcare Mater.*, **5**, 1493–1504.
42. Klein, P. M., Kern, S., Lee, D. J., Schmaus, J., Höhn, M., Gorges, J., Kazmaier, U., Wagner, E. (2018). Folate receptor-directed orthogonal click-functionalization of siRNA lipopolyplexes for tumor cell killing in vivo. *Biomaterials*, **178**, 630–642.
43. Pardridge, W. M. (2005). The blood-brain barrier: bottleneck in brain drug development. *NeuroRx*, **2**, 3–14.
44. Kabanov, A. V., Gendelman, H. E. (2007). Nanomedicine in the diagnosis and therapy of neurodegenerative disorders. *Prog. Polym. Sci.*, **32**, 1054–1082.
45. Pardridge, W. M. (2015). Targeted delivery of protein and gene medicines through the blood-brain barrier. *Clin. Pharmacol. Ther.*, **97**, 347–361.
46. Kulkarni, S. A., Feng, S. S. (2013). Effects of particle size and surface modification on cellular uptake and biodistribution of polymeric nanoparticles for drug delivery. *Pharm. Res.*, **30**, 2512–2522.
47. Sonavane, G., Tomoda, K., Makino, K. (2008). Biodistribution of colloidal gold nanoparticles after intravenous administration: effect of particle size. *Colloids Surf., B*, **66**, 274–280.
48. Paterson, J., Webster, C. I. (2016). Exploiting transferrin receptor for delivering drugs across the blood-brain barrier. *Drug Discov. Today Technol.*, **20**, 49–52.
49. Wiley, D. T., Webster, P., Gale, A., Davis, M. E. (2013). Transcytosis and brain uptake of transferrin-containing nanoparticles by tuning avidity to transferrin receptor. *Proc. Natl. Acad. Sci. U.S.A.*, **110**, 8662–8667.
50. Clark, A. J., Davis, M. E. (2015). Increased brain uptake of targeted nanoparticles by adding an acid-cleavable linkage between transferrin and the nanoparticle core. *Proc. Natl. Acad. Sci. U.S.A.*, **112**, 12486–12491.
51. Huang, R. Q., Qu, Y. H., Ke, W. L., Zhu, J. H., Pei, Y. Y., Jiang, C. (2007). Efficient gene delivery targeted to the brain using a transferrin-conjugated polyethyleneglycol-modified polyamidoamine dendrimer. *FASEB J.*, **21**, 1117–1125.
52. Zhang, Y., Calon, F., Zhu, C., Boado, R. J., Pardridge, W. M. (2003). Intravenous nonviral gene therapy causes normalization of striatal tyrosine hydroxylase and reversal of motor impairment in experimental parkinsonism. *Hum. Gene Ther.*, **14**, 1–12.

53. Zhang, Y., Wang, Y., Boado, R. J., Pardridge, W. M. (2008). Lysosomal enzyme replacement of the brain with intravenous non-viral gene transfer. *Pharm. Res.*, **25**, 400–406.

54. Kreuter, J., Shamenkov, D., Petrov, V., Ramge, P., Cychutek, K., Koch-Brandt, C., Alyautdin, R. (2002). Apolipoprotein-mediated transport of nanoparticle-bound drugs across the blood-brain barrier. *J. Drug Targeting*, **10**, 317–325.

55. Kreuter, J., Ramge, P., Petrov, V., Hamm, S., Gelperina, S. E., Engelhardt, B., Alyautdin, R., von Briesen, H., Begley, D. J. (2003). Direct evidence that polysorbate-80-coated poly(butylcyanoacrylate) nanoparticles deliver drugs to the CNS via specific mechanisms requiring prior binding of drug to the nanoparticles. *Pharm. Res.*, **20**, 409–416.

56. van Rooy, I., Cakir-Tascioglu, S., Couraud, P. O., Romero, I. A., Weksler, B., Storm, G., Hennink, W. E., Schiffelers, R. M., Mastrobattista, E. (2010). Identification of peptide ligands for targeting to the blood-brain barrier. *Pharm. Res.*, **27**, 673–682.

57. Bakhshinejad, B., Karimi, M., Khalaj-Kondori, M. (2015). Phage display: development of nanocarriers for targeted drug delivery to the brain. *Neural Regener. Res.*, **10**, 862–865.

58. Huang, Y., Wiedmann, M. M., Suga, H. (2019). RNA display methods for the discovery of bioactive macrocycles. *Chem. Rev.*, **119**, 10360–10391.

59. Kumar, P., Wu, H., McBride, J. L., Jung, K. E., Kim, M. H., Davidson, B. L., Lee, S. K., Shankar, P., Manjunath, N. (2007). Transvascular delivery of small interfering RNA to the central nervous system. *Nature*, **448**, 39–43.

60. Liu, Y., Huang, R., Han, L., Ke, W., Shao, K., Ye, L., Lou, J., Jiang, C. (2009). Brain-targeting gene delivery and cellular internalization mechanisms for modified rabies virus glycoprotein RVG29 nanoparticles. *Biomaterials*, **30**, 4195–4202.

61. Pulford, B., Reim, N., Bell, A., Veatch, J., Forster, G., Bender, H., Meyerett, C., Hafeman, S., Michel, B., Johnson, T., Wyckoff, A. C., Miele, G., Julius, C., Kranich, J., Schenkel, A., Dow, S., Zabel, M. D. (2010). Liposome-siRNA-peptide complexes cross the blood-brain barrier and significantly decrease PrP on neuronal cells and PrP in infected cell cultures. *PLoS One*, **5**, e11085.

62. Gao, Y., Wang, Z. Y., Zhang, J., Zhang, Y., Huo, H., Wang, T., Jiang, T., Wang, S. (2014). RVG-peptide-linked trimethylated chitosan for delivery of siRNA to the brain. *Biomacromolecules*, **15**, 1010–1018.

63. Park, T. E., Singh, B., Li, H., Lee, J. Y., Kang, S. K., Choi, Y. J., Cho, C. S. (2015). Enhanced BBB permeability of osmotically active poly(mannitol-co-PEI) modified with rabies virus glycoprotein via selective stimulation of caveolar endocytosis for RNAi therapeutics in Alzheimer's disease. *Biomaterials*, **38**, 61–71.

64. Alvarez-Erviti, L., Seow, Y., Yin, H., Betts, C., Lakhal, S., Wood, M. J. (2011). Delivery of siRNA to the mouse brain by systemic injection of targeted exosomes. *Nat. Biotechnol.*, **29**, 341–345.

65. Ke, W., Shao, K., Huang, R., Han, L., Liu, Y., Li, J., Kuang, Y., Ye, L., Lou, J., Jiang, C. (2009). Gene delivery targeted to the brain using an Angiopep-conjugated polyethyleneglycol-modified polyamidoamine dendrimer. *Biomaterials*, **30**, 6976–6985.

66. Costa, P. M., Cardoso, A. L., Mendonca, L. S., Serani, A., Custodia, C., Conceicao, M., Simoes, S., Moreira, J. N., Pereira de Almeida, L., Pedroso de Lima, M. C. (2013). Tumor-targeted chlorotoxin-coupled nanoparticles for nucleic acid delivery to glioblastoma cells: a promising system for glioblastoma treatment. *Mol. Ther. Nucleic Acids*, **2**, e100.

67. Liu, Y., He, X., Kuang, Y., An, S., Wang, C., Guo, Y., Ma, H., Lou, J., Jiang, C. (2014). A bacteria deriving peptide modified dendrigraft poly-l-lysines (DGL) self-assembling nanoplatform for targeted gene delivery. *Mol. Pharm.*, **11**, 3330–3341.

68. Liu, Y., Li, J., Shao, K., Huang, R., Ye, L., Lou, J., Jiang, C. (2010). A leptin derived 30-amino-acid peptide modified pegylated poly-L-lysine dendrigraft for brain targeted gene delivery. *Biomaterials*, **31**, 5246–5257.

69. Costantino, L., Gandolfi, F., Tosi, G., Rivasi, F., Vandelli, M. A., Forni, F. (2005). Peptide-derivatized biodegradable nanoparticles able to cross the blood-brain barrier. *J. Control. Release*, **108**, 84–96.

70. Prades, R., Guerrero, S., Araya, E., Molina, C., Salas, E., Zurita, E., Selva, J., Egea, G., Lopez-Iglesias, C., Teixido, M., Kogan, M. J., Giralt, E. (2012). Delivery of gold nanoparticles to the brain by conjugation with a peptide that recognizes the transferrin receptor. *Biomaterials*, **33**, 7194–7205.

71. Prades, R., Oller-Salvia, B., Schwarzmaier, S. M., Selva, J., Moros, M., Balbi, M., Grazu, V., de La Fuente, J. M., Egea, G., Plesnila, N., Teixido, M., Giralt, E. (2015). Applying the retro-enantio approach to obtain a peptide capable of overcoming the blood-brain barrier. *Angew. Chem. Int. Ed. Engl.*, **54**, 3967–3972.

72. Malcor, J. D., Payrot, N., David, M., Faucon, A., Abouzid, K., Jacquot, G., Floquet, N., Debarbieux, F., Rougon, G., Martinez, J., Khrestchatisky, M., Vlieghe, P., Lisowski, V. (2012). Chemical optimization of new ligands of the low-density lipoprotein receptor as potential vectors for central nervous system targeting. *J. Med. Chem.*, **55**, 2227–2241.
73. Oller-Salvia, B., Sanchez-Navarro, M., Ciudad, S., Guiu, M., Arranz-Gibert, P., Garcia, C., Gomis, R. R., Cecchelli, R., Garcia, J., Giralt, E., Teixido, M. (2016). MiniAp-4: a venom-inspired peptidomimetic for brain delivery. *Angew. Chem. Int. Ed. Engl.*, **55**, 572–575.
74. Rapoport, S. I. (2001). Advances in osmotic opening of the blood-brain barrier to enhance CNS chemotherapy. *Expert Opin. Investig. Drugs*, **10**, 1809–1818.
75. Hwang, D. W., Son, S., Jang, J., Youn, H., Lee, S., Lee, D., Lee, Y. S., Jeong, J. M., Kim, W. J., Lee, D. S. (2011). A brain-targeted rabies virus glycoprotein-disulfide linked PEI nanocarrier for delivery of neurogenic microRNA. *Biomaterials*, **32**, 4968–4975.
76. Meairs, S., Alonso, A. (2007). Ultrasound, microbubbles and the blood-brain barrier. *Prog. Biophys. Mol. Biol.*, **93**, 354–362.
77. Rychak, J. J., Klibanov, A. L. (2014). Nucleic acid delivery with microbubbles and ultrasound. *Adv. Drug Deliv. Rev.*, **72**, 82–93.
78. Burgess, A., Huang, Y., Querbes, W., Sah, D. W., Hynynen, K. (2012). Focused ultrasound for targeted delivery of siRNA and efficient knockdown of Htt expression. *J. Control. Release*, **163**, 125–129.
79. Huang, Q., Deng, J., Wang, F., Chen, S., Liu, Y., Wang, Z., Wang, Z., Cheng, Y. (2012). Targeted gene delivery to the mouse brain by MRI-guided focused ultrasound-induced blood-brain barrier disruption. *Exp. Neurol.*, **233**, 350–356.
80. Fan, C. H., Chang, E. L., Ting, C. Y., Lin, Y. C., Liao, E. C., Huang, C. Y., Chang, Y. C., Chan, H. L., Wei, K. C., Yeh, C. K. (2016). Folate-conjugated gene-carrying microbubbles with focused ultrasound for concurrent blood-brain barrier opening and local gene delivery. *Biomaterials*, **106**, 46–57.
81. Lin, C. Y., Hsieh, H. Y., Pitt, W. G., Huang, C. Y., Tseng, I. C., Yeh, C. K., Wei, K. C., Liu, H. L. (2015). Focused ultrasound-induced blood-brain barrier opening for non-viral, non-invasive, and targeted gene delivery. *J. Control. Release*, **212**, 1–9.
82. Mead, B. P., Mastorakos, P., Suk, J. S., Klibanov, A. L., Hanes, J., Price, R. J. (2016). Targeted gene transfer to the brain via the delivery of brain-penetrating DNA nanoparticles with focused ultrasound. *J. Control. Release*, **223**, 109–117.

83. Hynynen, K., McDannold, N., Vykhodtseva, N., Jolesz, F. A. (2001). Noninvasive MR imaging-guided focal opening of the blood-brain barrier in rabbits. *Radiology*, **220**, 640–646.

84. de Boer, A. G., Gaillard, P. J. (2007). Drug targeting to the brain. *Annu. Rev. Pharmacol. Toxicol.*, **47**, 323–355.

85. Wang, D., Wu, L. P. (2017). Nanomaterials for delivery of nucleic acid to the central nervous system (CNS). *Mater. Sci. Eng., C*, **70**, 1039–1046.

86. Pardridge, W. M. (2011). Drug transport in brain via the cerebrospinal fluid. *Fluids Barriers CNS*, **8**, 7.

87. Stein, C. A., Castanotto, D. (2017). FDA-approved oligonucleotide therapies in 2017. *Mol. Ther.*, **25**, 1069–1075.

88. Zou, S., Scarfo, K., Nantz, M. H., Hecker, J. G. (2010). Lipid-mediated delivery of RNA is more efficient than delivery of DNA in non-dividing cells. *Int. J. Pharm.*, **389**, 232–243.

89. Bharali, D. J., Klejbor, I., Stachowiak, E. K., Dutta, P., Roy, I., Kaur, N., Bergey, E. J., Prasad, P. N., Stachowiak, M. K. (2005). Organically modified silica nanoparticles: a nonviral vector for in vivo gene delivery and expression in the brain. *Proc. Natl. Acad. Sci. U.S.A.*, **102**, 11539–11544.

90. Hauck, E. S., Zou, S., Scarfo, K., Nantz, M. H., Hecker, J. G. (2008). Whole animal in vivo imaging after transient, nonviral gene delivery to the rat central nervous system. *Mol. Ther.*, **16**, 1857–1864.

91. Uchida, S., Itaka, K., Uchida, H., Hayakawa, K., Ogata, T., Ishii, T., Fukushima, S., Osada, K., Kataoka, K. (2013). In vivo messenger RNA introduction into the central nervous system using polyplex nanomicelle. *PLoS One*, **8**, e56220.

92. Kim, I. D., Lim, C. M., Kim, J. B., Nam, H. Y., Nam, K., Kim, S. W., Park, J. S., Lee, J. K. (2010). Neuroprotection by biodegradable PAMAM ester (e-PAM-R)-mediated HMGB1 siRNA delivery in primary cortical cultures and in the postischemic brain. *J. Control. Release*, **142**, 422–430.

93. Cardoso, A. L., Simoes, S., de Almeida, L. P., Plesnila, N., Pedroso de Lima, M. C., Wagner, E., Culmsee, C. (2008). Tf-lipoplexes for neuronal siRNA delivery: a promising system to mediate gene silencing in the CNS. *J. Control. Release*, **132**, 113–123.

94. Cardoso, A. L., Simoes, S., de Almeida, L. P., Pelisek, J., Culmsee, C., Wagner, E., Pedroso de Lima, M. C. (2007). siRNA delivery by a transferrin-associated lipid-based vector: a non-viral strategy to mediate gene silencing. *J. Gene Med.*, **9**, 170–183.

95. Cardoso, A. L., Costa, P., de Almeida, L. P., Simoes, S., Plesnila, N., Culmsee, C., Wagner, E., de Lima, M. C. (2010). Tf-lipoplex-mediated c-Jun silencing improves neuronal survival following excitotoxic damage in vivo. *J. Control. Release*, **142**, 392–403.

96. Godinho, B. M., Ogier, J. R., Darcy, R., O'Driscoll, C. M., Cryan, J. F. (2013). Self-assembling modified beta-cyclodextrin nanoparticles as neuronal siRNA delivery vectors: focus on Huntington's disease. *Mol. Pharm.*, **10**, 640–649.

97. Stiles, D. K., Zhang, Z., Ge, P., Nelson, B., Grondin, R., Ai, Y., Hardy, P., Nelson, P. T., Guzaev, A. P., Butt, M. T., Charisse, K., Kosovrasti, V., Tchangov, L., Meys, M., Maier, M., Nechev, L., Manoharan, M., Kaemmerer, W. F., Gwost, D., Stewart, G. R., Gash, D. M., Sah, D. W. (2012). Widespread suppression of huntingtin with convection-enhanced delivery of siRNA. *Exp. Neurol.*, **233**, 463–471.

98. Adamson, C., Kanu, O. O., Mehta, A. I., Di, C., Lin, N., Mattox, A. K., Bigner, D. D. (2009). Glioblastoma multiforme: a review of where we have been and where we are going. *Expert Opin. Investig. Drugs*, **18**, 1061–1083.

99. Aigner, A., Kogel, D. (2018). Nanoparticle/siRNA-based therapy strategies in glioma: which nanoparticles, which siRNAs? *Nanomedicine (London)*, **13**, 89–103.

100. Dubois, L. G., Campanati, L., Righy, C., D'Andrea-Meira, I., Spohr, T. C., Porto-Carreiro, I., Pereira, C. M., Balca-Silva, J., Kahn, S. A., DosSantos, M. F., Oliveira Mde, A., Ximenes-da-Silva, A., Lopes, M. C., Faveret, E., Gasparetto, E. L., Moura-Neto, V. (2014). Gliomas and the vascular fragility of the blood brain barrier. *Front. Cell Neurosci.*, **8**, 418.

101. An, S., He, D., Wagner, E., Jiang, C. (2015). Peptide-like polymers exerting effective glioma-targeted siRNA delivery and release for therapeutic application. *Small*, **11**, 5142–5150.

102. Wang, S. Reinhard, S., Li, C., Qian, M., Jiang, H., Du, Y., Lächelt, U., Lu, W., Wagner, E., Huang, R. (2017). Antitumoral cascade-targeting ligand for IL-6 receptor-mediated gene delivery to glioma. *Mol. Ther.*, **25**, 1556–1566.

103. Erbacher, P., Remy, J. S., Behr, J. P. (1999). Gene transfer with synthetic virus-like particles via the integrin-mediated endocytosis pathway. *Gene Ther.*, **6**, 138–145.

104. Wang, J., Lei, Y., Xie, C., Lu, W., Wagner, E., Xie, Z., Gao, J., Zhang, X., Yan, Z., Liu, M. (2014). Retro-inverso CendR peptide-mediated polyethyleneimine for intracranial glioblastoma-targeting gene therapy. *Bioconjugate Chem.*, **25**, 414–423.

105. Shir, A., Ogris, M., Wagner, E., Levitzki, A. (2006). EGF receptor-targeted synthetic double-stranded RNA eliminates glioblastoma, breast cancer, and adenocarcinoma tumors in mice. *PLoS Med.*, **3**, e6.
106. Shir, A., Ogris, M., Rödl, W., Wagner, E., Levitzki, A. (2011). EGFR-homing dsRNA activates cancer-targeted immune response and eliminates disseminated EGFR-overexpressing tumors in mice. *Clin. Cancer Res.*, **17**, 1033–1043.
107. Schaffert, D., Kiss, M., Rödl, W., Shir, A., Levitzki, A., Ogris, M., Wagner, E. (2011). Poly(I:C)-mediated tumor growth suppression in EGF-receptor overexpressing tumors using EGF-polyethylene glycol-linear polyethylenimine as carrier. *Pharm. Res.*, **28**, 731–741.
108. Kato, T., Natsume, A., Toda, H., Iwamizu, H., Sugita, T., Hachisu, R., Watanabe, R., Yuki, K., Motomura, K., Bankiewicz, K., Wakabayashi, T. (2010). Efficient delivery of liposome-mediated MGMT-siRNA reinforces the cytotoxity of temozolomide in GBM-initiating cells. *Gene Ther.*, **17**, 1363–1371.
109. Hendruschk, S., Wiedemuth, R., Aigner, A., Topfer, K., Cartellieri, M., Martin, D., Kirsch, M., Ikonomidou, C., Schackert, G., Temme, A. (2011). RNA interference targeting survivin exerts antitumoral effects in vitro and in established glioma xenografts in vivo. *Neuro Oncol.*, **13**, 1074–1089.
110. Cohen, Z. R., Ramishetti, S., Peshes-Yaloz, N., Goldsmith, M., Wohl, A., Zibly, Z., Peer, D. (2015). Localized RNAi therapeutics of chemoresistant grade IV glioma using hyaluronan-grafted lipid-based nanoparticles. *ACS Nano*, **9**, 1581–1591.
111. Danhier, F., Messaoudi, K., Lemaire, L., Benoit, J. P., Lagarce, F. (2015). Combined anti-Galectin-1 and anti-EGFR siRNA-loaded chitosan-lipid nanocapsules decrease temozolomide resistance in glioblastoma: in vivo evaluation. *Int. J. Pharm.*, **481**, 154–161.
112. Van Woensel, M., Mathivet, T., Wauthoz, N., Rosiere, R., Garg, A. D., Agostinis, P., Mathieu, V., Kiss, R., Lefranc, F., Boon, L., Belmans, J., Van Gool, S. W., Gerhardt, H., Amighi, K., De Vleeschouwer, S. (2017). Sensitization of glioblastoma tumor micro-environment to chemo- and immunotherapy by Galectin-1 intranasal knock-down strategy. *Sci. Rep.*, **7**, 1217.
113. Yu, D., Khan, O. F., Suva, M. L., Dong, B., Panek, W. K., Xiao, T., Wu, M., Han, Y., Ahmed, A. U., Balyasnikova, I. V., Zhang, H. F., Sun, C., Langer, R., Anderson, D. G., Lesniak, M. S. (2017). Multiplexed RNAi therapy against brain tumor-initiating cells via lipopolymeric nanoparticle infusion delays glioblastoma progression. *Proc. Natl. Acad. Sci. U.S.A.*, **114**, E6147–E6156.

114. Peng, Y., Huang, J., Xiao, H., Wu, T., Shuai, X. (2018). Codelivery of temozolomide and siRNA with polymeric nanocarrier for effective glioma treatment. *Int. J. Nanomed.*, **13**, 3467–3480.

115. Costa, P. M., Cardoso, A. L., Custodia, C., Cunha, P., Pereira de Almeida, L., Pedroso de Lima, M. C. (2015). MiRNA-21 silencing mediated by tumor-targeted nanoparticles combined with sunitinib: a new multimodal gene therapy approach for glioblastoma. *J. Control. Release*, **207**, 31–39.

116. Wang, L., Hao, Y., Li, H., Zhao, Y., Meng, D., Li, D., Shi, J., Zhang, H., Zhang, Z., Zhang, Y. (2015). Co-delivery of doxorubicin and siRNA for glioma therapy by a brain targeting system: angiopep-2-modified poly(lactic-co-glycolic acid) nanoparticles. *J. Drug Targeting*, **23**, 832–846.

117. Kuang, Y., Jiang, X., Zhang, Y., Lu, Y., Ma, H., Guo, Y., Zhang, Y., An, S., Li, J., Liu, L., Wu, Y., Liang, J., Jiang, C. (2016). Dual functional peptide-driven nanoparticles for highly efficient glioma-targeting and drug codelivery. *Mol. Pharm.*, **13**, 1599–1607.

118. Wei, L., Guo, X. Y., Yang, T., Yu, M. Z., Chen, D. W., Wang, J. C. (2016). Brain tumor-targeted therapy by systemic delivery of siRNA with transferrin receptor-mediated core-shell nanoparticles. *Int. J. Pharm.*, **510**, 394–405.

119. Cai, W., Lv, W., Feng, Y., Yang, H., Zhang, Y., Yang, G., Duan, Y., Wang, J. (2018). The therapeutic effect in gliomas of nanobubbles carrying siRNA combined with ultrasound-targeted destruction. *Int. J. Nanomed.*, **13**, 6791–6807.

120. Yuan, Z., Zhao, L., Zhang, Y., Li, S., Pan, B., Hua, L., Wang, Z., Ye, C., Lu, J., Yu, R., Liu, H. (2018). Inhibition of glioma growth by a GOLPH3 siRNA-loaded cationic liposomes. *J. Neurooncol.*, **140**, 249–260.

121. Kalin, R. E., Kretz, M. P., Meyer, A. M., Kispert, A., Heppner, F. L., Brandli, A. W. (2007). Paracrine and autocrine mechanisms of apelin signaling govern embryonic and tumor angiogenesis. *Dev. Biol.*, **305**, 599–614.

122. Mastrella, G., Hou, M., Li, M., Stoecklein, V. M., Zdouc, N., Volmar, M. N. M., Miletic, H., Reinhard, S., Herold-Mende, C. C., Kleber, S., Eisenhut, K., Gargiulo, G., Synowitz, M., Vescovi, A. L., Harter, P. N., Penninger, J. M., Wagner, E., Mittelbronn, M., Bjerkvig, R., Hambardzumyan, D., Schuller, U., Tonn, J. C., Radke, J., Glass, R., Kalin, R. E. (2019). Targeting APLN/APLNR improves anti-angiogenic efficiency and blunts pro-invasive side effects of VEGFA/VEGFR2-blockade in glioblastoma. *Cancer Res.*, 79(9), 2298–2313.

123. Hager, S., Wagner, E. (2018). Bioresponsive polyplexes - chemically programmed for nucleic acid delivery. *Expert Opin. Drug Deliv.*, **15**, 1067–1083.

124. Grünweller, A., Hartmann, R. K. (2016). Chemical modification of nucleic acids as a key technology for the development of RNA-based therapeutics. *Pharmazie*, **71**, 8–16.

Chapter 10

Advances in Nanotheranostics with Plasmonic and Magnetic Nanoparticles

Sérgio R. S. Veloso,[a] Paula M. T. Ferreira,[b] J. A. Martins,[b] Paulo J. G. Coutinho[a] and Elisabete M. S. Castanheira[a]
[a]*Centre of Physics (CFUM), University of Minho, Campus de Gualtar, 4710-057 Braga, Portugal*
[b]*Centre of Chemistry (CQUM), University of Minho, Campus de Gualtar, 4710-057 Braga, Portugal*
ecoutinho@fisica.uminho.pt

Brain drug delivery remains a challenge for nanomedicine owing to a large variety of difficulties, ranging from the blood–brain barrier hindering most of chemotherapeutic drugs to the essential and delicate anatomical structures surrounding the target blocking a proper detection/monitoring of the disease. Magnetic and plasmonic nanoparticles have provided a means for the development of nanotheranostic agents, through an improvement of contrast of modern imaging techniques and the exploration of adjuvant therapies, magnetic hyperthermia and photothermia. Hereby, an overview on the current brain delivery difficulties, concepts and strategies is undertaken (Sections 10.1 and 10.2), followed by a

Nanoparticles for Brain Drug Delivery
Edited by Carla Vitorino, Andreia Jorge and Alberto Pais

ISBN 978-981-4877-31-2 (Hardcover), 978-1-003-11932-6 (eBook)
www.jennystanford.com

brief introduction to plasmonic (Section 10.2.1) and magnetic nanoparticles (Section 10.2.3), and the respective applications as theranostic agents are critically discussed. Magnetoliposomes (Section 10.2.5) are further discussed as a recent nanosystem for enhancing both therapeutic and diagnostic modalities and extending the applicability of theranostic agents to other diseases.

10.1 Nanomedicine in Brain Therapy

Since the introduction of the nanotechnology concept, the different matter properties at the nanoscale, that is, at dimensions between 1 and 100 nm, have been extensively revolutionising the current technological, industrial and medical paradigm [1, 2].

Nanomaterials went from simple structural substituents to complex multifunctional materials capable of drug delivery, stimulating cell differentiation, transmitting information and providing better contrast agents [3–6], apart from inspiring a greener economy owing to the development of new energetic, electronic and depollution technologies [7].

The future highly depends on the mastery of materials, and nowadays it is possible to converge materials science with biology, due to the recent advancements on the synthesis, manipulation and visualisation of materials at the nanoscale. Naturally, the requirements of materials for application in humans led to an increasing trend in the development of biocompatible nanoparticles, thus appearing nanomedicine as a new area of nanotechnology, which seek to solve modern problems. Cancer is currently one of the leading causes of mortality worldwide, which is continuously rising every year and becoming an increasing problem in low-income countries [8, 9]. Such is associated with not only the economic transition induced changes in social, economic and cultural relations but also the adoption of unhealthy lifestyles of the high-income countries, such as tobacco, physical inactivity and excess body weight [9–11].

Considering the difficulty of early stage detection and the proximity to anatomical structures responsible for essential functions, malignant glioma therapy is currently imposed as one of the greatest challenges [12, 13], which worsens owing to peritumoural oedema, not providing a precise discrimination of tumour margins [14], and the blood–brain barrier (BBB) hindering most of the chemotherapeutic drugs from reaching the tumour [15, 16]. From the different glioma varieties, glioblastoma multiforme (GBM) is the most aggressive malignancy of the central nervous system (CNS), with an incidence rate of about 3.19 per 100.000 people per annum and a median survival less than 2 years [17, 18], where only 5% survive longer than 5 years. This type of glioma is associated with an extensive infiltration, a strong vascular proliferation and a complex genetic expression, including additions in chromosomes 7 and 19, losses in chromosomes 10 and 13, gene amplifications and mutations, changes in mitotic and cellular activity, significant angiogenesis and necrosis [18, 19]. Hereby, brain tumour is a challenge for surgical, chemotherapeutic and radiotherapeutic conventional methods, which produce various side effects, such as resistance to therapy, devastating neurologic deterioration and the emergence of therapy-resistant populations [12].

Neurodegenerative diseases such as multiple sclerosis have been showing a larger impact on society, affecting already about 1 million people worldwide [20]. Multiple sclerosis is a disease of the CNS associated with the demyelination and axonal loss, which leads to visual problems, muscle weakness and difficulty in coordination and speech, and whose treatment is highly hindered by the BBB and other side effects [20, 21].

Besides the challenging trespassing of the BBB, conventional methods of drug administration possess other limitations, such as a lack of specificity towards neoplastic tissues, a lack of selectivity in the mechanism of action and the high concentration required, which is associated with low-molecular-weight drugs' high pharmacokinetic volume of distribution or their low therapeutic index, which might lead to toxicity and dose-dependent side effects [8]. Moreover, drugs require a proper size, surface composition, charge and aqueous solubility to reduce undesired effects such as the possibility of local toxicity or embolisation of the blood vessels due to aggregation [8]. Hereby, nanomedicine has provided an alternative to conventional chemotherapy by incorporation of drugs into nanoparticles due to increasing drug stability and solubility, reducing systemic clearance, improving the specificity by active (e.g. surface functionalisation) or passive (e.g. via enhanced permeability and retention [EPR] effect) targeting, allowing synergistic therapy through drug delivery combined with other localised therapeutic strategies (Fig. 10.1) [8, 19, 22, 23], such as magnetic or photoinduced hyperthermia. Furthermore, the combination with plasmonic and magnetic nanoparticles has the potentiality of theranostics, that is, the combined diagnostic and therapeutic capabilities in a single agent [24].

Therefore, this chapter is divided into an initial overview on theranostics, the current advances and main strategies using nanoparticles and the recent plasmonic/magnetic generation nanosystems (magnetoliposomes) to brain drug delivery for cancer and neurodegenerative diseases therapy.

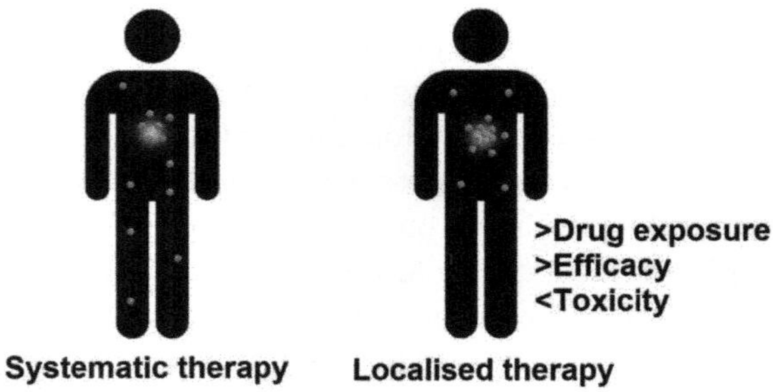

Figure 10.1 Schematic illustration of localised delivery associated benefits compared to conventional chemotherapeutic approaches. Adapted from Ref. [20], MDPI (Basel), 2018 (available under open access).

10.2 Nanotheranostics: Concepts and Strategies

Over the past years, the term 'nanotheranostics' has acquired a firm position as an alternative to conventional medicine, where the diagnostic and therapeutic capabilities are combined in a single agent by employing nanomedicine materials and methods [24, 25]. The nanomaterials can be peptide or synthetic polymers, dendrimers, micelles, liposomes, inorganic nanoparticles or carbon nanotubes, which are conceived to attain a sustained, controlled and targeted delivery of the theranostic agents. These are adsorbed, conjugated, entrapped or encapsulated into the nanosystem and simultaneously used for diagnosis and therapy at cellular and molecular level (Fig. 10.2) [19, 26].

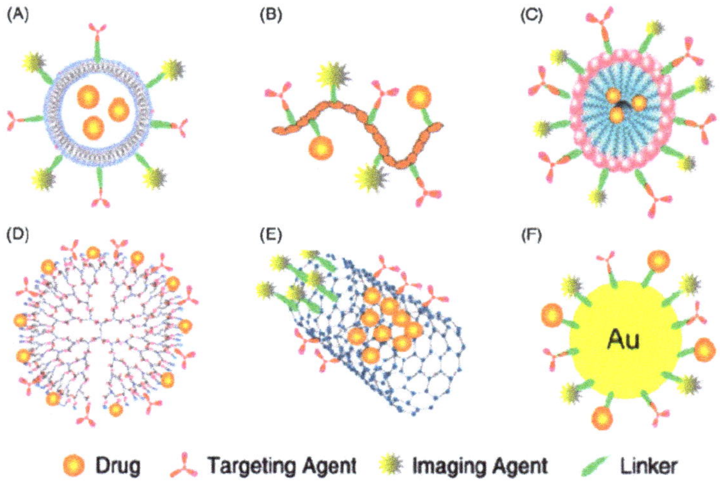

Figure 10.2 Schematic representation of nanomaterials used as theranostic agents, which include (A) liposomes, (B) polymer conjugates, (C) micelles, (D) dendrimers, (E) carbon nanotubes and (F) metallic nanoparticles. Reprinted from Ref. [8] with permission from Taylor & Francis, 2016 (http://www.informaworld.com).

The theranostic systems include therapeutic agents which can be detected by imaging techniques, such as optical imaging, nuclear magnetic resonance imaging (MRI), positron emission tomography (PET) or single-photon emission computed tomography (SPECT), which leads to the reclassification of these therapeutic agents as theranostic agents [26]. By combining diagnostic and therapeutic capabilities in a single agent, precision and personalised medicine are sought as current objectives to follow in real time the patient's progress and response to therapeutic drugs [19]. However, certain parameters have to be considered in the design of the theranostic system, mainly the specific accumulation in the desired tissue; the selective and controlled delivery of an effective therapeutic action; biocompatibility and biodegradability; sensitive diagnosis, which will allow an imaging before, after and during the treatment regimen; surface hydrophobicity to avoid aggregation, opsonisation or nonspecific binding to other entities; and the zeta potential, which should be in the range of ±10 mV, to promote a longer circulation lifetime [19, 24–26].

Considering the required sensitivity and the unspecificity issues associated with conventional contrast agents, MRI is highly interesting as imaging technique for diagnosis, owing to its high anatomical resolution with unlimited tissue depth and soft tissue contrast [27, 28]. Other commonly used imaging techniques include computed tomography (CT) and PET. However, the former has lower resolution than MRI, and the latter has little use for diagnosis of GBM, as the brain exhibits a higher glucose uptake compared to other organs [19].

Magnetic nanoparticles have been playing a particular important role as bionanosystem because they can work as T_2 contrast agents, offer the possibility of exploring the EPR effect to passively accumulate in the tumour, and allow to further conceptualise and tailor the physicochemical properties to actively direct to it, making magnetic nanoparticles ideal to monitor diseases and detect injuries or deficiencies [27–30].

Moreover, the magnetic nanoparticle contrast can be enhanced by combination with other materials, exploring the proton spin dephasing (T_2 relaxation) mechanisms: motional averaging regime (MAR), visit-limited regime (VLR) or static dephasing regime (SDR) [30]. In the MAR, the relaxation rates are proportional to the particle size, as the distance between particles is smaller than the one travelled by the proton. The proton is subjected to different magnetic environments which might refocus it when an opposite polarity is found and, thus, full proton dephasing is not achieved and the overall relaxation rate is retarded [30]. The VLR occurs at a critical size where the proton can be fully dephased in a single encounter if it spends enough time in a full dephasing zone defined around the nanoparticle, which makes the process also dependent on the distance to the particle [30]. In the SDR, the proton is subjected to a constant magnetic environment due to the interparticle distance being longer than the distance travelled by the proton, when the particles are large enough. Such regimes can be explored in the design of bionanosystems. For example, in magnetoliposomes the hydrophobic coating might hinder the protons from entering the dephasing zone; thus the relaxation rates of the MAR and VLR will be reduced. However, in magnetogels, the hydrogel network will enhance the MAR relaxation rate and reduce the relaxation rate for particles in the VLR, due to the reduction of water self-diffusion and proton exchange between the inner and outer coating environments [31].

When developing theranostic agents to brain delivery, some aspects related with the BBB and the blood–cerebrospinal fluid barrier (BCSFB) should be considered. The former is formed by tight junctions of capillary endothelial cells and different perivascular cells, such as pericytes, astrocytes microglial cells and smooth muscle cells, while the latter results from tight junctions between the choroid plexus cells which encompass the microvascular endothelium [19, 20]. Besides these junctions limiting the paracellular diffusion of small and lipid-soluble molecules, the associated high trans-endothelial electrical resistance, adenosine triphosphate (ATP)-binding cassette transporters and p-glycoproteins synergistically contribute to the efflux of most drugs from the cell [15, 17–19]. The strategies to overcome this obstacle include the presence of surface ligands such as insulin, lactoferrin or transferrin, which allow the transfer of macromolecules through receptor-mediator mechanisms, while the presence of cationic entities (e.g. albumin) allows crossing the barriers through receptor-mediated absorptive endocytosis [21]. Apart from the possibility of exploring the BBB leakiness under disease conditions, the nanosystem can be designed to co-deliver the drug and a BBB permeability enhancer, to improve the drug penetration by transiently opening the BBB, for example, by decreasing expression or function of proteins required for BBB integrity through the use of compounds such as cereport, regadenoson or borneol [22].

Moreover, the nanosystem can be tailored with multitargeting functionalities to synergistically enhance adsorptive and receptor-mediated transcytosis and the proportion of cells labelled with the theranostic entity without harming normal cells [32]. Currently, there is a wide variety of active targeting strategies which make use of ligand- or antibody-mediated targeting whose receptors are overexpressed in cancer cells. A peptide ligand commonly used is the peptide sequence arginine-glycine-aspartic acid (RGD) which binds to $\alpha_v\beta_3$ integrins, mediating migration in neovascular tumour endothelial cells. Combined with targeting vascular endothelial growth factor receptor (VEGFR), it can also be an interesting functionality allowing a reduction of neovascularisation and thus promoting tumour cell death, due to the lack of oxygen and nutrients, but also providing selective delivery of the nanosystem to angiogenic blood vessels [8]. Also, an usually used vitamin is folic acid (vitamin B9) whose receptor is overexpressed in a variety of cancer tissues, including brain tissue [8, 33]. The interest in folate is associated with its stability to temperature and pH, with its non-immunogenic character, apart from retaining the ability to bind after conjugation with drugs or theranostic agents [33]. Another interesting target is the transferrin receptor, a type II receptor which resides on the outer cell membrane, where transferrin is efficiently internalised by receptor-mediated endocytosis in a clathrin-/dynamin-dependent manner, which could be useful for delivery of the theranostic agent or, alternatively, blocked to induce cancer cell death [34]. Hereby, the following section is focused on the discussion of the current strategies and advances of nanosystems using plasmonic- and/or magnetic-based multifunctional theranostic agents.

10.2.1 Plasmonic Nanoparticles

Metals such as gold and silver have been of great importance in our lives since antiquity. For example, gold salts were used in Chinese traditional medicine for the treatment of rheumatoid arthritis [35, 36]. Indeed, gold has been one of the most interesting materials for biomedical applications, mainly in the development of nanoparticles owing to its unique optical and physical properties [35–38]. Besides the aspects in common with other nanoparticles, which include the optoelectronic properties dependence on size and shape and the high surface-to-volume ratio, gold nanoparticles (GNPs) are highly advantageous due to the easy surface functionalisation, possible synthesisable shapes (Fig. 10.3), biocompatibility, low toxicity and the surface plasmon resonance (SPR) phenomenon, which have contributed for the use of GNPs in several biomedical applications [35–37].

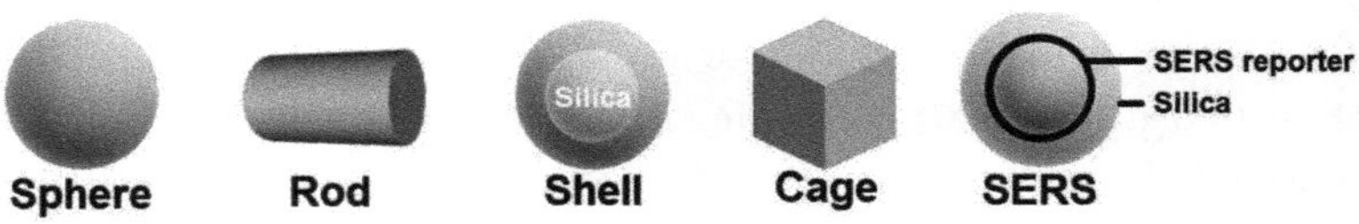

Figure 10.3 Examples of possible gold-based nanoparticles.

The SPR consists of an externally applied electric field–induced collective motion of the conductive electrons in relation to the crystal lattice, where a depolarising electric field acts as a restoring force (Fig. 10.4) but also behaves as a damped oscillator through interactions between electrons and the environment/vicinity [37]. However, such effect is hindered for particles smaller than 2 nm, owing to the quantisation energy of the electronic levels becoming high enough.

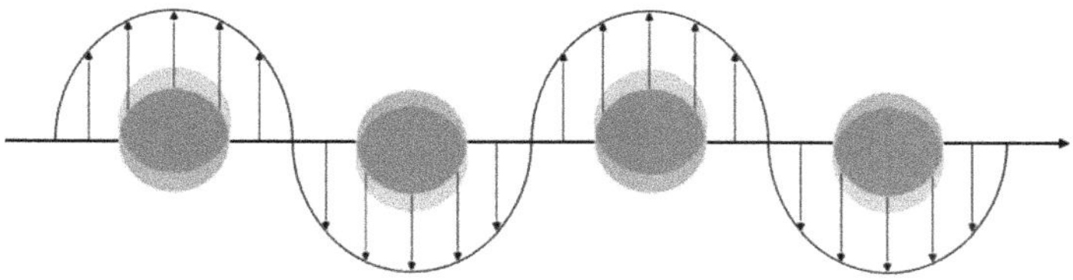

Figure 10.4 Schematic representation of the collective motion of conductive electrons induced though the incidence of electromagnetic radiation.

Moreover, the SPR is dependent on both particle size and environment (particularly on the dielectric constant), which can be explored in the development of sensors where the bonding of molecules or their proximity to the nanoparticle surface will modify the SPR frequency [37]. Apart from the environment, the plasmon band is sensible to the type of ligand (donor or withdrawing ligand), core charge, temperature, shape and aggregation, the latter inducing effects such as bathochromic shift and bandwidth widening owing to the interparticle plasmonic coupling [37]. The nanoparticles can also induce fluorescence quenching due to Förster resonance energy transfer or modulated photoinduced electron transfer [37]. Hereby, plasmonic nanoparticles, mainly the gold-based ones, have found application in different technological areas such as biosensors, clinic chemistry methods, immunologic assays, photothermolysis of tumour cells, detection and control of microorganisms, transport of drugs and monitorisation of biological cells [35, 39–41].

Besides SPR enhancement of the local electromagnetic field, which is useful for optical imaging, the plasmonic nanoparticles high absorption cross section (typically, for sizes below 20 nm) allows conversion of the absorbed light into heat through nonradiative processes, due to the fast phase loss of the coherently excited electrons [40, 42]. According to the heat content, the surrounding environment can be heated through phonon–phonon relaxation while the lattice cools off, which can be achieved by using continuous wave lasers, or the lattice heating is enough to lead to particle melting or ablation by using high-intensity laser pulses (Fig. 10.5), which can then be used to induce cell damage through hyperthermia, coagulation and evaporation [42, 43].

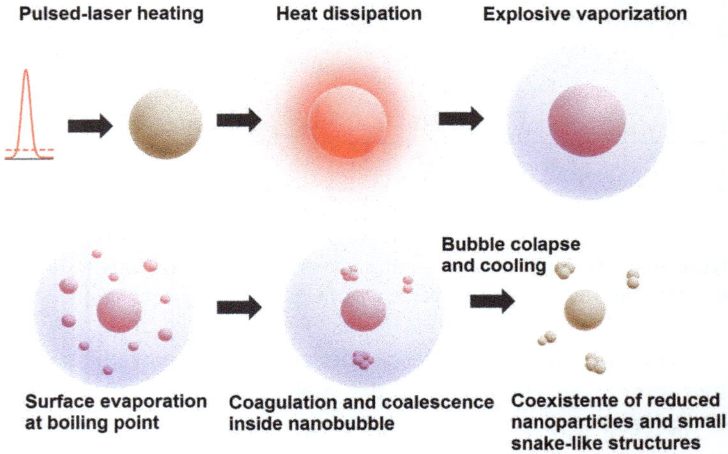

Figure 10.5 Schematic representation of nanoparticle size reduction induced by the incidence of nanosecond-pulsed-laser irradiation.

The use of plasmonic nanoparticles allows two types of therapeutic approaches, photothermal and photodynamic therapies. Photothermal therapy (PTT) requires the use of GNPs which efficiently convert light into heat to induce localised temperature increase and, consequently, hyperthermia physiological responses which end into tumour cell death [44]. On the other hand, photodynamic therapy explores the generation of reactive oxygen species (ROS) through excitation of a photosensitiser to induce cell death by apoptosis, thus depending on the availability of tissue oxygen [44].

A great theranostic advantage of GNPs is the possibility of imaging at both macroscopic and microscopic levels. For example, GNP-loaded glioma xenografts in rats were shown to provide a higher spatial resolution of the tumour volume and shape through synchrotron-based heat CT when compared to PET and MRI [45]. However, a high radiation dose might be required which can be harmful for humans [45]. Thus, MRI continues as a method of choice for imaging, where the combination of gadolinium and GNPs allows an intense and lasting enhancement of brain tumour (more than 24 h), which correlate with the total tumour mass [45]. Apart from that, GNP-Gd allows intraoperative MRI with no need of further contrast injections, thus requiring only preoperative injection, allowing diagnostic accuracy and no Gd-induced toxicity [45]. At the microscopic level, GNPs can be combined with fluorescent markers for accurate intraoperative detection of residual tumour loci [45]. However, some problems might be associated to fluorescent probes such as false positives from biological structures, fast photochemical destruction and large spectral overlap with other imaging agents which do not allow multiple target detection [45]. Alternatively, GNPs allow the use of photoimaging which explores scattering by the nanoparticles, that is, surface-enhanced Raman scattering (SERS). This technique provides a stable, intense and persistent intraoperative detection and delineation of the tumour edges, loco-regional infiltration and satellite foci away from the main tumour mass, thus providing a precise identification of the tumour and healthy cells by the surgeons [44, 45].

10.2.2 Brain Theranostics with Plasmonic Nanoparticles

A target which has been commonly exploited as a strategy to enhance nanoparticle uptake is the transferrin receptor (TfR), which under normophysiological conditions is associated with the binding and endocytosis of iron-transferrin (Tf) complexes to subsequently transport iron into the brain parenchyma [46]. Recently, Johnsen et al. [46] showed that GNPs functionalised with low-affinity antibodies (anti-TfR^D) had an increased accumulation in the brain capillaries compared to the high-affinity antibodies (anti-TfR^A). Moreover, the use of a monovalent bispecific antibody (anti-TfR^A/BACE1) enhanced the uptake of GNPs by threefold compared to the low-affinity variant [46]. Alternatively, Dixit et al. [47] used a small transferrin peptide (HAIYPRH, Tf_{pep}) grafted on GNPs coated with tetraoctylammonium bromide (TOAB) and decadienealdehyde (DDA), which showed two- to threefold higher uptake of the photodynamic prodrug Pc4 compared to untargeted GNPs in human glioma cancer cell lines (LN229 and U87) overexpressing TfR. Moreover, targeted nanoparticles showed a 6 ± 2.2-fold increase in drug accumulation in glioma cells overexpressing TfR (U87 cells) 6 h after injection via the tail vein in mice, apart from the possibility of activating Pc4 delivery and cell death by the incidence of light at 670 nm [47]. Other functionalities include the angiopep-2, a shuttle peptide which can cross the BBB, which has been shown to enhance endocytosis in vitro and brain accumulation in vivo when functionalised onto polyethylene glycol (PEG)-coated gold nanorods (AuNRs) compared to nanorods solely coated with PEG [48]. Instead of incorporating drugs, GNPs can be explored in the development of multilayer complexes for gene delivery. For example, Bishop et al. [49] developed hybrid gold/polymer/DNA complexes comprising as the last layer a cationic polymer for DNA complex, containing tertiary amines to enhance proton sponge effect and endosomal escape, and either a disulphide bridge or ester functional group to trigger its degradation. The complexes contained either DNA for exogenous expression or small interfering RNA (siRNA) for mediated gene knockdown. The authors showed that polyethylenimine covered polyplexes were the most efficient to load nucleic acid polymers, while the polymer comprising the functional ester group exhibited better gene delivery (Fig. 10.6) [49]. Interestingly, the formulations showed superiority to the commercial Lipofectamine® 2000 at comparable dosages in human brain cancer cells [49].

Other approaches include the incorporation of GNPs in a matrix such as hydrogels or liposomes. For example, Ruan et al. [50] developed GNPs functionalised with doxorubicin (DOX) and Cy5.5 (a fluorescent dye) through a hydrazone bond which hydrolyses at low pH, and these GNPs were incorporated into a matrix of gelatine nanoparticles, which is a substrate for metalloproteinase-2 overexpressed in tumour cells, thus allowing a control on the size of the nanosystem. Moreover, the authors functionalised the GNPs with a tandem peptide, RRGD, which enhanced targeting effect and tumour penetration ability [50].

A potential and effective PTT was attained by Song et al. [51], who developed small vesicles (~60 nm) containing poly(lactic-*co*-glycolic acid) (PLGA) and AuNRs functionalised with PEG. The system can reach temperatures higher than 70°C after irradiation at 808 nm with a 0.8 W cm^{-2} laser for 5 min, which coupled to the high optical absorption coefficient and strong electromagnetic field upon laser irradiation provides an optimum system for photoacoustic diagnostic and thermal ablation of cancer cells [51]. Moreover, the nanosystem showed in PET a ~9.5% ID g^{-1} (injection dose per gram of tissue) at 24 h postinjection tumour uptake in a U87MG tumour mice model, where the tumour temperature increased 20°C after 5 min irradiation, thus surpassing the irreversible tissue damage threshold which resulted in the total ablation of the tumour without reoccurrence [51].

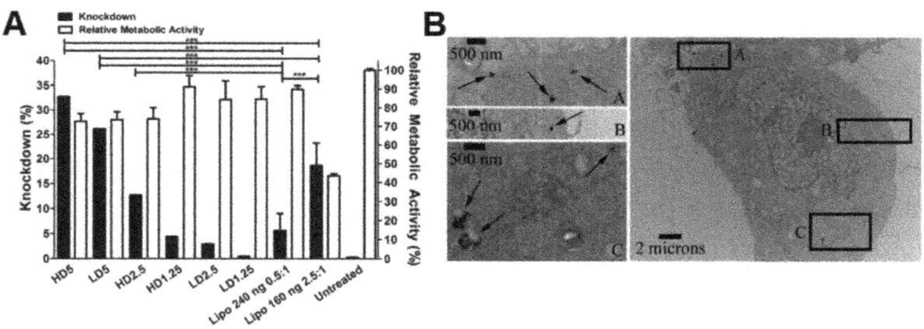

Figure 10.6 (A) The siRNA-mediated knockdown of eGFP-positive GBM319 cell line (human GBM cell line) by layer-by-layer particles containing either high-dose (HD) or low-dose (LD) nucleic acid content and 1.15, 2.5 or 5 mg/ml of a poly(bela-amino ester) compared to Lipofectamine® 2000 at a volume-to-siRNA mass ratio (μl:μg) of 0.5:1 and 2.5:1 on day 7 and relative metabolic activity at 24 h posttransfection. (B) Transmission electron microscopy (TEM) images showing cellular uptake of siRNA-containing HD5 nanoparticles in GBM319 cells, where nanoparticles of ~200 nm are observed (BA and BB), and putative endosomes with multiple gold nanoparticle aggregates are observed in BC. Reprinted from Ref. [49], Copyright (2015), with permission from Elsevier.

Recently, focused ultrasound (FUS) has been shown to be an alternative to the traditional active targeting, where the mechanical forces generated by FUS-activated microbubbles temporarily disrupt the BBB in the desired location, thus enhancing the penetration, retention and diffusion of negative, neutral and positive surface charged ^{64}Cu-integrated gold nanoclusters [52]. Hereby, it is expected that the combined use of ligand active targeting, FUS, PTT and a diagnostic imaging technique might confer GNPs as one of the most potent, biocompatible and flexible theranostic agents.

10.2.3 Magnetic Nanoparticles

Under a characteristic size limit, magnetic materials change from multidomain to single domain, their behaviour being similar to a single giant magnet. However, as the size is further reduced, these materials acquire superparamagnetism, where generation of heat occurs not through hysteresis losses but by means of different mechanisms when the material is subjected to an alternating field, without remnant magnetisation upon magnetic field removal [53–55]. Such mechanisms can be either Néel or Brownian relaxation, where the latter is dependent on the medium viscosity and the dominant relaxation process is dependent on size and on the particular magnetic material. Here, the heat generation is induced by the delayed relaxation of the magnetic moments under the application of an alternating magnetic field [53], thus making the Néel relaxation a preferable method, as it will avert free particle rotation associated with viscosity fluctuations of the medium. Thus, by exploring the dependency of the relaxation mechanisms on size and type of material, the concept of magnetic hyperthermia is made possible, where similarly to PTT, tissues are exposed to high temperatures (42°C–45°C), either to kill tumour cells by apoptosis or to prompt higher susceptibility to radiotherapy and chemotherapy [53, 56]. The produced thermal energy will promote denaturation of proteins required for replication and translation, thus leading to higher susceptibility of cancer cells to heat [53].

The recommendable temperature should be around 42°C, considering that higher temperatures (but lower than 46°C) lead to a decreased blood flux in tumour region, which hampers heat dissipation and enhances the sensitivity to hyperthermia therapies. Temperatures below 42°C might promote drug accumulation, assimilation and DNA damage, owing to increased blood flux and oxygenation in tumour tissues [53, 55, 57]. These properties and advantages have led hyperthermia as an adjuvant therapeutic technique suitable for combination with chemotherapy and radiotherapy, owing to the enhanced cytotoxic effect, perfusion facilitation and local oxygenation [56].

The most used magnetic nanoparticles have been the transition metal ferrites (Fe, Ni, Co, Mn, ...), a class of soft magnetic materials with great superparamagnetic behaviour, chemical stability and mechanical hardness [57–62]. The manganese ferrite has particularly gained increased attention due to the higher magnetic susceptibility than the other transition metal ferrites [63, 64]. Alternatively, ferrite nanoparticles containing other constituents, such as Ca^{2+} or Mg^{2+}, have also been showing promising results owing to the absence of toxic transition metals, promoting a higher biocompatibility than the other ferrites [65]. Nevertheless, an organic or inorganic shell may be used to reduce toxicity and control the bioaccumulation, bioelimination and tissue invasion [66], though it might hinder the magnetic properties of the core material.

Moreover, magnetic nanoparticles are particularly useful for MRI, owing to the higher and tuneable T_1 and T_2 relaxation values, reduced renal clearance, localisation through an externally applied magnetic field gradient, combination with other strategies (convection-enhanced delivery or high-intensity FUS) and materials such as liposomes (magnetoliposomes), hydrogels (magnetogels) and plasmonic nanoparticles [67].

10.2.4 Brain Theranostics with Magnetic Nanoparticles

Apart from the active targeting agents towards tumour cells previously described, other less explored ligands have been combined with magnetic nanoparticles, such as anti-Hsp70 specific antibody [68], which explores the Hsp70 large expression on high-grade glioma cell membranes owing to tumour-specific lipids which anchor this protein on the cell surface [67]. Other alternative ligand is the Cilengitide (a cyclic RGD peptide) which targets the integrins $\alpha_v\beta_3$ and $\alpha_v\beta_5$ overexpressed in glioblastoma cells, where the combination with ultrasound-targeted microbubble destruction has been shown to strongly increase the nanoparticle uptake [69]. Nevertheless, other recent strategies used in specific targeting with magnetic nanoparticles and their combination with MRI in glioma therapy are shown in Table 10.1.

Table 10.1 Recent strategies of active targeting combined with MRI using magnetite nanoparticles and respective hydrodynamic size

Coating	Ligand	Target	Model	Size (nm)	Reference
PMAO	Lf	LRP	C6 cell line	46–52	[70]
PEG	Lf	LRP	Sprague–Dawley rats	48.9	[71]
PVA/PAA	Lf	LRP	BALB/c nude mice	100–150	[72]
PEG	RGD	Integrin	U87-MG cell line	212.5	[73]
Caffeic acid	None	none	U87-MG cell line	17	[74]
PEG	Dimeric RGD	Integrin	U87-MG tumour-bearing nude mice	13.1	[75]
Dextran	EGF	EGFR	Wistar rats	47.6	[76]
DMSA	EGFRmAb	EGFR	Normal rats	161.5	[77]
Dextran	Interleukin-1 receptor antagonist	ILR	Wistar rats	43.1	[78]

PMAO, poly(maleic anhydride-alt-1-octadene); Lf, lactoferrin; LRP, low-density lipoprotein receptor-related protein; PVA, poly(vinyl alcohol); PAA, poly(acrylic acid); PEG, polyethylene glycol; RGD, arginylglycylaspartic acid; EGF, epidermal growth factor; EGFRmAb, epidermal growth factor receptor monoclonal antibody; DMSA, meso-2,3-dimercaptosuccinic acid.

Although iron oxide nanoparticles can generate ROS, Richard et al. [74] were able to reduce their impact by combining the nanoparticles with the antioxidant caffeic acid, showing a buffering effect within the cells which can be explored in future developments. Moreover, Luo et al. [73] pioneered on the development of RGD functionalised ultrasmall iron oxide nanoparticles with an r_1 relaxivity of 1.4 mM^{-1} s^{-1}, thus demonstrating that magnetic nanoparticles can be an interesting alternative to the nephrotoxicity associated with Gd(III)-based contrast agents on T_1-weighted MRI [75]. Indeed, the combination of magnetic hyperthermia or magnetic nanoparticles as contrast agents and common therapeutic methods has shown to be a safe and effective approach to increase the effectiveness of glioblastoma treatment. This has been verified in the past few years by the increasing number of available and approved products by the US Food and Drug Administration (FDA) and in Europe, such as Feridex®, Combidex®, Resovist®, Gastromark® and NanoTherm™, the latter being under clinical trials [79]. However, the four former products have ceased probably owing to the ambiguity of T_2-weighted images' dark contrast with some pathogenic conditions and generation of unclear images around disease regions, thus supporting the need for ultrasmall nanoparticles for the preferential r_1 relaxivity enhancement [75].

A great contribution for magnetic targeting was given by Chertok et al. [80–82], who demonstrated a simple setup to accurately evaluate and predict in vitro the effectiveness of magnetic nanoparticles selectivity towards the desired area through a simple flow system, where the carotid route has shown an increase compared to intravenous route [81, 82]. Hereby, it can be explored as a strategy to screen the designed nanoparticles in future developments without directly recurring to in vivo assays.

Besides the active ligand targeting, other strategies have appeared. For example, Stewart et al. [83] developed magnetoelectric nanoparticles of $CoFe_2O_4@BaTiO_3$. The nonzero magnetoelectric effect allows the control of the nanoparticle dipole moment and magnetic moment through a local magnetic field and electric field, respectively. Thus, drug delivery and release can be controlled by the application of direct current (DC) and alternating current (AC) magnetic field sequences, as the dipole moment influences the bond strength between the nanoparticle and the loaded drug [83]. The authors showed that the application of an AC magnetic field produced a 1.6-fold enhancement of the nanosystem uptake by U-87MG cells compared to 12 h DC only, and 11-fold to MIA690 alone treatment (a hypothalamic growth hormone-releasing hormone antagonist) [83]. Other possibilities recently developed consist on the combination of microRNA (miRNA) and hyperthermia to enhance apoptosis (Fig. 10.7), where the miRNA is explored to target and downregulate or inhibit the translation of proteins in heat shock proteins (HSP)-mediated pathways involved in the protection of cellular proteins from degradation [84]. The HSP pathways include the activation of DNA repair mechanisms (via the BRCA family) and the inhibition of apoptosis (via protein kinase B/phosphatidylinositol 3-kinase [Akt/PI3K] pathways) which will hinder hyperthermia-induced apoptosis [84]. The magnetic nanoparticles can also be combined with photothermal materials, such as carbon [85] or gold shells [86, 87]. For example, Sun et al. [88] developed micelles loaded with SPIONs and GNPs and coated with a PEG-polycaprolactone (PEG-PCL) polymer, where the GNPs might enhance the effective radiation dose by inducing free radicals which directly produce DNA damage and indirectly lead to cell apoptosis. The authors showed that nanoparticles doubled the density of double strand breaks compared to radiation treatment alone for both U251 and U373 cell lines, apart from providing MRI contrast enhancement with good delineation of tumour borders and the possibility of serving as blood pool contrast agents in computed tomography. A recent alternative to photothermia and magnetic hyperthermia is the magnetic-mechanical destruction of the plasma and lysosomal membranes through the elevated torque forces associated with cubic nanoparticle aggregates which can be attained under a low frequency rotating magnetic field, thus reducing the cost for instrumentation and side effects [89].

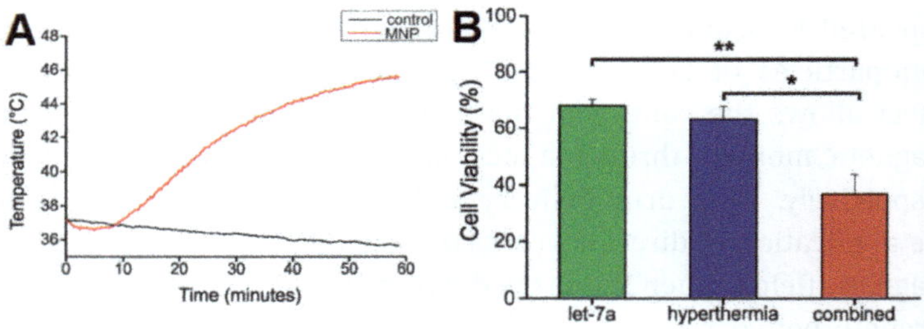

Figure 10.7 (A) Temperature increase in a solution of $ZnFe_2O_4$ nanoparticles through magnetic hyperthermia. (B) Cell viability of U87-EGFRvIII cells showing enhanced therapeutic effects of the combined lethal-7a miRNA delivery and magnetic hyperthermia treatment. Adapted with permission from Ref. [84]. Copyright (2014) John Wiley and Sons.

10.2.5 Advances in Brain Theranostics Using Magnetoliposomes

Magnetoliposomes combine liposomes and magnetic nanoparticles in a single nanosystem, which can be classified as aqueous magnetoliposomes (AMLs) or solid magnetoliposomes (SMLs), according to whether the nanoparticles are located in the inner aqueous phase of the liposomes or the inner phase consists on a cluster of magnetic nanoparticles (Fig. 10.8) [65]. Nevertheless, magnetoliposomes can also be nanoparticles embedded into or onto the surface of the lipid bilayer [65].

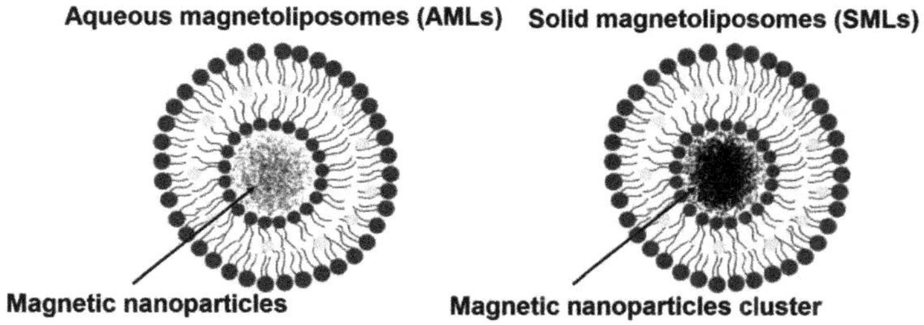

Figure 10.8 Schematic representation of aqueous magnetoliposomes (AMLs) and solid magnetoliposomes (SMLs).

Recently, magnetoliposomes have shown to be a promising nanosystem to cross the BBB. Skouras et al. [90] developed magnetoliposomes functionalised with apolipoprotein E-3 peptides and/or antitransferrin monoclonal antibody, containing ultrasmall SPIONs and loaded with DOX. This system was able to transport the drug across hCMEC/D3 monolayer cellular model of the BBB, showing the best results in the presence of both ligands and further enhancement in the presence of a permanent magnetic field. Moreover, the authors demonstrated that combined magnetic and ligand targeting significantly increased the cell death of melanoma B16 cells compared to ligand or magnetic targeting alone [90]. Another example is provided by Ding et al. [91], who showed a synergistic effect of the transferrin receptor-mediated transmigration and the externally applied magnetic field induced transendothelial extravasation of the magnetoliposomes through the BBB model comprising primary human brain microvascular endothelial cells (HBMECs) and human astrocytes. Indeed, magnetoliposomes provide several advantages, such as no requirement of covalently bound drugs, drug protection from enzymatic degradation, magnetic-helped remote guidance of the liposome content and the possibility of being used as contrast agents [92]. However, AMLs and SMLs have different MR contrast enhancement, where the AMLs can attain r_2/r_1 ratios between 6 and 18, while the SMLs (Fig. 10.9) have shown a ratio enhancement up to 80 [93, 94]. Furthermore, magnetoliposomes can be made of thermosensitive liposomes which change from the gel phase to the liquid-crystalline phase when the critical temperature is reached, thus providing the possibility of using hyperthermia as a trigger for drug release [93]. Another advantage of magnetoliposomes is the possibility of encapsulation and delivery of fatty acids with pharmaceutical properties, such as omega-3 fatty acids which exhibit anti-inflammatory effects [95]. Although the membrane is prone to Fe^{2+}- and Fe^{3+}-induced peroxidation, the nanosystem can be combined with an antioxidant such as quercetin, a natural-sourced bioflavonoid which will inhibit lipid peroxidation [96], thus favouring a higher stability of the magnetoliposomes for long-term therapies.

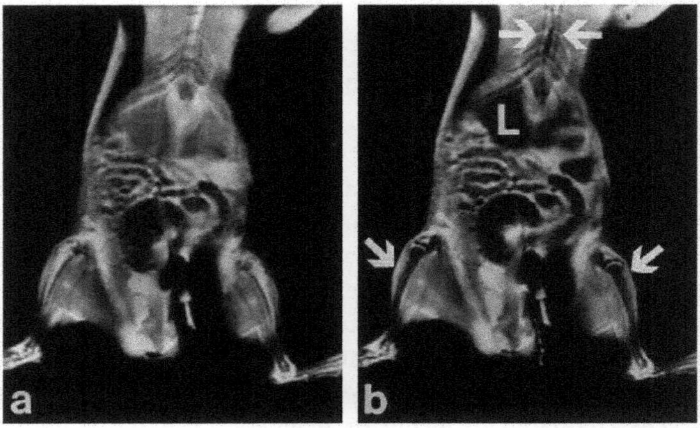

Figure 10.9 Fast spin echo magnetic resonance coronal images of Harlan Sprague–Dawley rats (a) pre- and (b) 1 h postintravenous (tail vein) administration of SMLs-PEG, where increased contrast is observed in bone marrow (arrows) and liver (L). Reprinted from Ref. [94], Copyright (1999), with permission from Elsevier.

A recent strategy on the use of magnetoliposomes as contrast agents was shown by Yan et al. [97] on breast cancer–bearing mice, which explores the strong avidin affinity towards biotin through a three-step pretargeting, where biotinylated anti-$\alpha_v\beta_3$ monoclonal antibodies are administered first, followed by avidin and streptavidin and, after, the biotinylated magnetoliposomes, affording a 7% enhancement compared with the 2% of the nontargeted magnetoliposomes.

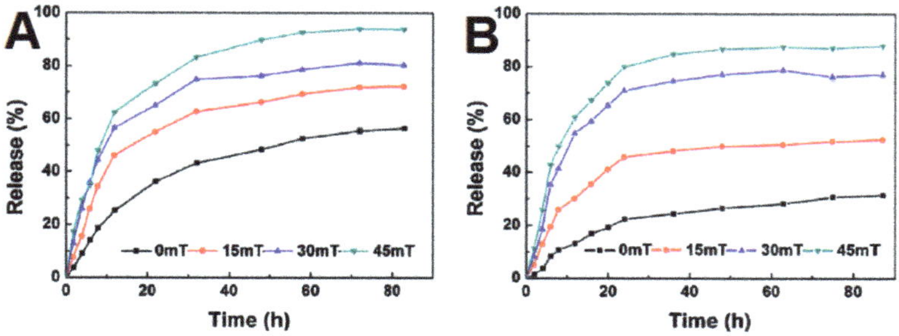

Figure 10.10 Release profiles of doxorubicin from carboxymethyl dextran–coated magnetoliposomes under (A) pH 5.0 and (B) pH 7.4 after exposure to a low-frequency alternating magnetic field at various intensities for 10 min. Reprinted from Ref. [99], Copyright (2015), with permission from Elsevier.

The combination of thermosensitive response with hyperthermia has shown promising results. Babincová et al. [98] reported that when magnetoliposomes were heated to the phase transition temperature, DOX was released in a controllable manner, where the synergy doubled the decrease on cell viability in 92.7%. In another example, Guo et al. [99] developed carboxymethyl dextran–coated magnetoliposomes, which showed an enhanced release of DOX under a low-frequency alternating magnetic field, without hyperthermia generation (Fig. 10.10). The latter might not be suitable for brain therapy, as the tissue is susceptible to changes in environmental temperature. Moreover, this nanosystem showed a 57 r_2/r_1 ratio which provides this system as an efficient T_2-weight contrast agent [99]. Besides the brain tumour therapy, magnetoliposomes can also be introduced in the brain-target human immunodeficiency virus (HIV) treatment, as demonstrated by Tomitaka et al. [100]. The authors developed magnetoliposomes containing core–shell iron oxide GNPs which showed higher T_2 relaxivity (424 mM^{-1} s^{-1}) than the T_2 contrast agent Feridex® (133 mM^{-1} s^{-1}), enhanced magnetic particle imaging (MPI) positive contrast, and higher X-ray CT contrast owing to the high X-ray attenuation coefficient of gold. Moreover, the presence of an external applied magnetic field induced a 1.8-fold increase on the transmigration efficiency through an in vitro BBB model and higher reduction of p24 (a HIV capsid protein) level than free tenofovir disoproxil fumarate in HIV-infected CHME-5 microglia cells [100].

10.3 Conclusion and Future Perspectives

Nanoparticles have shown remarkable results in in vitro and in vivo theranostics, though few got to clinical assays. This can be understood considering the wide parameters which still require optimisation, such as the size, functionalisation, biocompatibility, specificity and stability, but also the reproducibility and feasibility of the nanosystem. When the nanosystem is to be translated to clinical assays, it must be guaranteed that its effects, properties and in vivo behaviour will be reproducible to assure that the system can be safely applied in different patients, without unexpected side effects and that the desired objective will be accomplished. Hereby, although magnetite has shown potentiality in brain theranostics, its predisposition to peroxidation shall be prevented by combining with more biocompatible materials, such as gold. As previously observed, gold-based nanoparticles can be used as multimodal imaging contrast agents (e.g. MRI and X-ray CT) but also as multimodal therapeutic agents. The presence of a core magnetic material further enhances the therapeutic potentiality by combining different strategies (e.g. photothermia, photodynamic therapy, magnetic hyperthermia, magnetic-guided delivery) which have been shown to improve BBB transmigration. Nevertheless, some questions remain to be answered, as it must be understood if hyperthermia will locally affect brain tissue function and stability, whether it is required a continuous hyperthermia application or just a stimulus to trigger drug release, and if a magnetic-guided delivery combined with a magnetic-mechanical strategy can be a viable approach as an alternative to hyperthermia. Other aspect to be assessed is which active ligand delivery strategy, that is, the targeting ligand bond to the nanosystem or the described three-step pretargeting, has better cost/benefit ratio with the least side effects and unexpected outcomes. Moreover, magnetoliposomes appeared as a potential nanosystem for theranostics by improving T_2 contrast, BBB transmigration, better control onto nanoparticle properties and drugs passible of being incorporated, which extends their applicability not only on the glioma therapy, but also on diseases such as HIV. Therefore, it is expected that magnetoliposomes will lead the theranostic strategies in the upcoming years and potentially translate into clinical assays.

References

1. Khawaja, A. (2011). The legacy of nanotechnology: revolution and prospects in neurosurgery. *Int. J. Surg.*, **9**, 608–614.
2. Jaishree, V., Gupta, P. (2012). Nanotechnology: a revolution in cancer diagnosis. *Indian J. Clin. Biochem.*, **27**, 214–220.
3. Mohammadi, M., Nojoomi, A., Mozafari, M., Dubnika, A., Inayathullah, M., Rajadas, J. (2017). Nanomaterials engineering for drug delivery: a hybridization approach. *J. Mater. Chem. B*, **5**, 3995–4018.
4. Wei, M., Li, S., Le, W. (2017). Nanomaterials modulate stem cell differentiation: biological interaction and underlying mechanisms. *J. Nanobiotechnol.*, **15**, 1–13.
5. Smith, B., Gambhir, S. (2017). Nanomaterials for *in vivo* imaging. *Chem. Rev.*, **117**, 901–986.
6. Bae, K., Chung, H., Park, T. (2011). Nanomaterials for cancer therapy and imaging. *Mol. Cells*, **31**, 295–302.
7. Iavicoli, I., Leso, V., Ricciardi, W., Hodson, L., Hoover, M. (2014). Opportunities and challenges of nanotechnology in the green economy. *Environ. Health*, **13**, 1–11.
8. Kumari, P., Ghosh, B., Biswas, S. (2015). Nanocarriers for cancer-targeted drug delivery. *J. Drug Targeting*, **24**, 179–191.
9. Torre, L., Siegel, R., Ward, E., Jemal, A. (2015). Global cancer incidence and mortality rates and trends: an update. *Cancer Epidemiol. Biomark. Prev.*, **25**, 16–27.
10. Amy Lee, Y., Hashibe, M. (2014). Tobacco, alcohol, and cancer in low and high income countries. *Ann. Glob. Health*, **80**, 378–383.
11. Berger, N. (2014). Obesity and cancer pathogenesis. *Ann. N. Y. Acad. Sci.*, **1311**, 57–76.
12. Bhojani, M., Van Dort, M., Rehemtulla, A., Ross, B. (2010). Targeted imaging and therapy of brain cancer using theranostic nanoparticles. *Mol. Pharm.*, **7**, 1921–1929.

13. Mountz, J., Ahmed, R., Oborski, M., Lieberman, F., Hwang, M. (2014). Malignant gliomas: current perspectives in diagnosis, treatment, and early response assessment using advanced quantitative imaging methods. *Cancer Manag. Res.*, **6**, 149–170.

14. Blystad, I., Warntjes, J., Smedby, Ö., Lundberg, P., Larsson, E., Tisell, A. (2017). Quantitative MRI for analysis of peritumoral edema in malignant gliomas. *PLoS One*, **12**, 1–12.

15. Gao, H. (2016). Progress and perspectives on targeting nanoparticles for brain drug delivery. *Acta Pharm. Sin. B*, **6**, 268–286.

16. Krol, S. (2012). Challenges in drug delivery to the brain: nature is against us. *J. Control. Release*, **164**, 145–155.

17. Tabansky, I., Messina, M., Bangeranye, C., Goldstein, J., Blitz-Shabbir, K., Machado, S., Jeganathan, V., Wright, P., Najjar, S., Cao, Y., Sands, W., Keskin, D., Stern, J. (2015). Advancing drug delivery systems for the treatment of multiple sclerosis. *Immunol. Res.*, **63**, 58–69.

18. Chaichana, K., Pinheiro, L., Brem, H. (2015). Delivery of local therapeutics to the brain: working toward advancing treatment for malignant gliomas. *Ther. Deliv.*, **6**, 353–369.

19. Ozdemir-Kaynak, E., Qutub, A., Yesil-Celiktas, O. (2018). Advances in glioblastoma multiforme treatment: new models for nanoparticle therapy. *Front. Phys.*, **9**, 1–14.

20. Nam, L., Coll, C., Erthal, L., de la Torre, C., Serrano, D., Martínez-Máñez, R., Santos-Martínez, M., Ruiz-Hernández, E. (2018). Drug delivery nanosystems for the localized treatment of glioblastoma multiforme. *Materials*, **11**, 779.

21. Ghalamfarsa, G., Hojjat-Farsangi, M., Mohammadnia-Afrouzi, M., Anvari, E., Farhadi, S., Yousefi, M., Jadidi-Niaragh, F. (2016). Application of nanomedicine for crossing the blood–brain barrier: theranostic opportunities in multiple sclerosis. *J. Immunotoxicol.*, **13**, 603–619.

22. Dong, X. (2018). Current strategies for brain drug delivery. *Theranostics*, **8**, 1481–1493.

23. De Souza, R., Zahedi, P., Allen, C., Piquette-Miller, M. (2010). Polymeric drug delivery systems for localized cancer chemotherapy. *Drug Deliv.*, **17**, 365–375.

24. Xie, J., Lee, S., Chen, X. (2010). Nanoparticle-based theranostic agents. *Adv. Drug Deliv. Rev.*, **62**, 1064–1079.

25. Fan, Z., Fu, P., Yu, H., Ray, P. (2014). Theranostic nanomedicine for cancer detection and treatment. *J. Food Drug Anal.*, **22**, 3–17.

26. Muthu, M., Leong, D., Mei, L., Feng, S. (2014). Nanotheranostics: application and further development of nanomedicine strategies for advanced theranostics. *Theranostics*, **4**, 660–677.

27. Chan, M., Lux, J., Nishimura, T., Akiyoshi, K., Almutairi, A. (2015). Long-lasting and efficient tumor imaging using a high relaxivity polysaccharide nanogel magnetic resonance imaging contrast agent. *Biomacromolecules*, **16**, 2964–2971.

28. Mikhail, A., Partanen, A., Yarmolenko, P., Venkatesan, A., Wood, B. (2015). Magnetic resonance-guided drug delivery. *Magn. Reson. Imaging Clin. N. Am.*, **23**, 643–655.

29. Pankhurst, Q., Thanh, N., Jones, S., Dobson, J. (2009). Progress in applications of magnetic nanoparticles in biomedicine. *J. Phys. D: Appl. Phys.*, **42**, 224001.

30. de Haan, H. (2011). Mechanisms of proton spin dephasing in a system of magnetic particles. *Magn. Reson. Med.*, **66**, 1748–1758.

31. de Haan, H., Paquet, C. (2011). Enhancement and degradation of the R_2* relaxation rate resulting from the encapsulation of magnetic particles with hydrophilic coatings. *Magn. Reson. Med.*, **66**, 1759–1766.

32. Sonali, Viswanadh, M., Singh, R., Agrawal, P., Mehata, A., Pawde, D. (2018). Nanotheranostics: emerging strategies for early diagnosis and therapy of brain cancer. *Nanotheranostics*, **2**, 70–86.

33. Zwicke, G., Ali Mansoori, G., Jeffery, C. (2012). Utilizing the folate receptor for active targeting of cancer nanotherapeutics. *Nano Rev.*, **3**, 18496.

34. Daniels, T., Bernabeu, E., Rodríguez, J., Patel, S., Kozman, M., Chiappetta, D. (2012). The transferrin receptor and the targeted delivery of therapeutic agents against cancer. *Biochim. Biophys. Acta Gen. Subj.*, **1820**, 291–317.

35. Das, M., Shim, K., An, S., Yi, D. (2011). Review on gold nanoparticles and their applications. *Toxicol. Environ. Health Sci.*, **3**, 193–205.

36. Hornos Carneiro, M., Barbosa, F. (2016). Gold nanoparticles: a critical review of therapeutic applications and toxicological aspects. *J. Toxicol. Environ. Health, Part B*, **19**, 129–148.

37. Yeh, Y., Creran, B., Rotello, V. (2012). Gold nanoparticles: preparation, properties, and applications in bionanotechnology. *Nanoscale*, **4**, 1871–1880.

38. Nealon, G., Donnio, B., Greget, R., Kappler, J., Terazzi, E., Gallani, J. (2012). Magnetism in gold nanoparticles. *Nanoscale*, **4**, 5244–5258.

39. Amendola, V., Pilot, R., Frasconi, M., Maragò, O., Iatì, M. (2017). Surface plasmon resonance in gold nanoparticles: a review. *J. Phys. Condens. Matter*, **29**, 203002.
40. Huang, X., El-Sayed, M. (2010). Gold nanoparticles: optical properties and implementations in cancer diagnosis and photothermal therapy. *J. Adv. Res.*, **1**, 13–28.
41. Stockman, M. (2011). Nanoplasmonics: the physics behind the applications. *Phys. Today*, **64**, 39–44.
42. Elsherbini, E. (2011). Laser and radiofrequency-induced hyperthermia treatment via gold-coated magnetic nanocomposites. *Int. J. Nanomed.*, **6**, 2155–2165.
43. Hashimoto, S., Werner, D., Uwada, T. (2012). Studies on the interaction of pulsed lasers with plasmonic gold nanoparticles toward light manipulation, heat management, and nanofabrication. *J. Photochem. Photobiol. C*, **13**, 28–54.
44. Singh, P., Pandit, S., Mokkapati, V., Garg, A., Ravikumar, V., Mijakovic, I. (2018). Gold nanoparticles in diagnostics and therapeutics for human cancer. *Int. J. Mol. Sci.*, **19**, 1979.
45. Meola, A., Rao, J., Chaudhary, N., Sharma, M., Chang, S. (2018). Gold nanoparticles for brain tumor imaging: a systematic review. *Front. Neurol.*, **9**, 328.
46. Johnsen, K. B., Bak, M., Kempen, P. J., Melander, F., Burkhart, A., Thomsen, M. S., Nielsen, M. S., Moos, T., Andresen, T. L. (2018). Antibody affinity and valency impact brain uptake of transferrin receptor-targeted gold nanoparticles. *Theranostics*, **8**, 3416–3436.
47. Dixit, S., Novak, T., Miller, K., Zhu, Y., Kenney, M., Broome, A. (2015). Transferrin receptor-targeted theranostic gold nanoparticles for photosensitizer delivery in brain tumors. *Nanoscale*, **7**, 1782–1790.
48. Velasco-Aguirre, C., Morales-Zavala, F., Salas-Huenuleo, E., Gallardo-Toledo, E., Andonie, O., Muñoz, L., Rojas, X., Acosta, G., Sánchez-Navarro, M., Giralt, E., Araya, E., Albericio, F., Kogan, M. J. (2017). Improving gold nanorod delivery to the central nervous system by conjugation to the shuttle Angiopep-2. *Nanomedicine*, **12**, 2503–2517.
49. Bishop, C., Tzeng, S., Green, J. (2015). Degradable polymer-coated gold nanoparticles for co-delivery of DNA and siRNA. *Acta Biomater.*, **11**, 393–403.
50. Ruan, S., He, Q., Gao, H. (2015). Matrix metalloproteinase triggered size-shrinkable gelatin-gold fabricated nanoparticles for tumor microenvironment sensitive penetration and diagnosis of glioma. *Nanoscale*, **7**, 9487–9496.

51. Song, J., Yang, X., Jacobson, O., Huang, P., Sun, X., Lin, L., Yan, X., Niu, G., Ma, Q., Chen, X. (2015). Ultrasmall gold nanorod vesicles with enhanced tumor accumulation and fast excretion from the body for cancer therapy. *Adv. Mater.*, **27**, 4910–4917.

52. Sultan, D., Ye, D., Heo, G., Zhang, X., Luehmann, H., Yue, Y., Detering, L., Komarov, S., Taylor, S., Tai, Y. C., Rubin, J. B., Chen, H., Liu, Y. (2018). Focused ultrasound enabled trans-blood brain barrier delivery of gold nanoclusters: effect of surface charges and quantification using positron emission tomography. *Small*, **14**, 1703115.

53. Hervault, A., Thanh, N. (2014). Magnetic nanoparticle-based therapeutic agents for thermo-chemotherapy treatment of cancer. *Nanoscale*, **6**, 11553–11573.

54. Akbarzadeh, A., Samiei, M., Davaran, S. (2012). Magnetic nanoparticles: preparation, physical properties, and applications in biomedicine. *Nanoscale Res. Lett.*, **7**, 144.

55. Veloso, S. R. S., Ferreira, P. M. T., Martins, J. A., Coutinho, P. J. G., Castanheira, E. M. S. (2018). Magnetogels: prospects and main challenges in biomedical applications. *Pharmaceutics*, **10**, 145.

56. Zhang, Z. Q., Song, S. C. (2016). Thermosensitive/superparamagnetic iron oxide nanoparticle-loaded nanocapsule hydrogels for multiple cancer hyperthermia. *Biomaterials*, **106**, 13–23.

57. Issa, B., Obaidat, I. M., Albiss, B. A., Haik, Y. (2013). Magnetic nanoparticles: surface effects and properties related to biomedicine applications. *Int. J. Mol. Sci.*, **14**, 21266–21305.

58. Indira, T. K., Lakshmi, P. K. (2010). Magnetic nanoparticles: a review. *Int. J. Pharm. Sci. Nanotechol.*, **3**, 1035–1042.

59. Rodrigues, A. R. O., Ramos, J. M. F., Gomes, I. T., Almeida, B. G., Araújo, J. P., Queiroz, M. J. R. P., Coutinho, P. J. G., Castanheira, E. M. S. (2016). Magnetoliposomes based on manganese ferrite nanoparticles as nanocarriers for antitumor drugs. *RSC Adv.*, **6**, 17302–17313.

60. Datta, N. R., Krishnan, S., Speiser, D. E., Neufeld, E., Kuster, N., Bodis, S., Hofmann, H. (2016). Magnetic nanoparticle-induced hyperthermia with appropriate payloads: Paul Ehrlich's "magic (nano)bullet" for cancer theranostics? *Cancer Treat. Rev.*, **50**, 217–227.

61. Pereira, C., Pereira, A. M., Fernandes, C., Rocha, M., Mendes, R., Garcia, M. P. F., Guedes, A.,Tavares, P. B., Grenèche, J. M., Araújo, J. P., Freire., C. (2012). Superparamagnetic MFe_2O_4 (M = Fe, Co, Mn) nanoparticles: tuning the particle size and magnetic properties through a novel one-step coprecipitation route. *Chem. Mater.*, **24**, 1496–1504.

62. Carta, D., Casula, M. F., Floris, P., Falqui, A., Mountjoy, G., Boni, A., Sangregorio, C., Corrias, A. (2010). Synthesis and microstructure of manganese ferrite colloidal nanocrystals. *Phys. Chem. Chem. Phys.*, **12**, 5074–5083.

63. Cabrera, L. I., Somoza, A., Marco, J. F., Serna, C. J., Morales, M. P. (2012). Synthesis and surface modification of uniform MFe_2O_4 (M = Fe, Mn, and Co) nanoparticles with tunable sizes and functionalities. *J. Nanopart. Res.*, **14**, 873.

64. Colombo, M., Carregal-Romero, S., Casula, M. F., Gutiérrez, L., Morales, M. P., Böhm, I. B., Heverhagen, J. T., Prosperi, D., Parak, W. J. (2012). Biological applications of magnetic nanoparticles. *Chem. Soc. Rev.*, **41**, 4306–4334.

65. Rodrigues, A. R. O., Almeida, B. G., Araújo J. P., Queiroz, M. J. R. P., Coutinho, P. J. G., Castanheira, E. M. S. (2018). Magnetoliposomes for dual cancer therapy, in *Inorganic Frameworks as Smart Nanomedicines*, Grumezescu, A. M., ed., William Andrew, Oxford, UK, pp. 489–527.

66. Kafrouni, L., Savadogo, O. (2016). Recent progress on magnetic nanoparticles for magnetic hyperthermia. *Prog. Biomater.*, **5**, 147–160.

67. Shevtsov, M., Multhoff, G. (2016). Recent developments of magnetic nanoparticles for theranostics of brain tumor. *Curr. Drug Metab.*, **17**, 737–744.

68. Shevtsov, M., Nikolaev, B., Ryzhov, V., Yakovleva, L., Marchenko, Y., Parr, M., Rolich, V. I., Mikhrina, A. L., Dobrodumov, A. V., Pitkin, E., Multhoff, G. (2015). Ionizing radiation improves glioma-specific targeting of superparamagnetic iron oxide nanoparticles conjugated with cmHsp70.1 monoclonal antibodies (SPION–cmHsp70.1). *Nanoscale*, **7**, 20652–20664.

69. Zhao, Y. Z., Lin, Q., Wong, H. L., Shen, X. T., Yang, W., Xu, H. L., Mao, K. L., Tian, F. R., Yang, J. J., Xu, J., Xiao, J., Lu, C. T. (2016). Glioma-targeted therapy using Cilengitide nanoparticles combined with UTMD enhanced delivery. *J. Control. Release*, **224**, 112–125.

70. Tomitaka, A., Arami, H., Gandhi, S., Krishnan, K. (2015). Lactoferrin conjugated iron oxide nanoparticles for targeting brain glioma cells in magnetic particle imaging. *Nanoscale*, **7**, 16890–16898.

71. Qiao, R., Jia, Q., Hüwel, S., Xia, R., Liu, T., Gao, F., Galla, H. J., Gao, M. (2012). Receptor-mediated delivery of magnetic nanoparticles across the blood-brain barrier. *ACS Nano*, **6**, 3304–3310.

72. Fang, J., Lai, Y., Chiu, T., Chen, Y., Hu, S., Chen, S. (2014). Magnetic core-shell nanocapsules with dual-targeting capabilities and co-delivery of multiple drugs to treat brain gliomas. *Adv. Healthcare Mater.*, **3**, 1250–1260.

73. Luo, Y., Yang, J., Yan, Y., Li, J., Shen, M., Zhang, G., Mignani, S., Shi, X. (2015). RGD-functionalized ultrasmall iron oxide nanoparticles for targeted T1-weighted MR imaging of gliomas. *Nanoscale*, **7**, 14538–14546.

74. Richard, S., Saric, A., Boucher, M., Slomianny, C., Geffroy, F., Mériaux, S., Lalatonne, Y., Petit, P. X., Motte, L. (2016). Antioxidative theranostic iron oxide nanoparticles toward brain tumors imaging and ROS production. *ACS Chem. Biol.*, **11**, 2812–2819.

75. Shen, Z., Chen, T., Ma, X., Ren, W., Zhou, Z., Zhu, G., Zhang, A., Liu, Y., Song, J., Li, Z., Ruan, H., Fan, W., Lin, L., Munasinghe, J., Chen, X., Wu, A. (2017). Multifunctional theranostic nanoparticles based on exceedingly small magnetic iron oxide nanoparticles for t1-weighted magnetic resonance imaging and chemotherapy. *ACS Nano*, **11**, 10992–11004.

76. Shevtsov, M. A., Nikolaev, B. P., Yakovleva, L. Y., Marchenko, Y. Y., Mikhrina, A. L., Martynova, M. G., Bystrova, O. A., Yakovenko, I. V., Ischenko, A. M. (2014). Superparamagnetic iron oxide nanoparticles conjugated with epidermal growth factor (SPION-EGF) for targeting brain tumors. *Int. J. Nanomed.*, **9**, 273–287.

77. Mu, K., Zhang, S., Ai, T., Jiang, J., Yao, Y., Jiang, L., Zhou, Q., Xiang, H., Zhu, Y., Yang, X., Zhu, W. (2015). Monoclonal antibody–conjugated superparamagnetic iron oxide nanoparticles for imaging of epidermal growth factor receptor–targeted cells and gliomas. *Mol. Imaging*, **14**, 1–12.

78. Shevtsov, M., Nikolaev, B., Yakovleva, L., Dobrodumov, A., Zhakhov, A., Mikhrina, A., Pitkin, E., Parr, M. A., Rolich, V. I., Simbircev, A. S., Ischenko, A. M. (2015). Recombinant interleukin-1 receptor antagonist conjugated to superparamagnetic iron oxide nanoparticles for theranostic targeting of experimental glioblastoma. *Neoplasia*, **17**, 32–42.

79. Zhu, L., Zhou, Z., Mao, H., Yang, L. (2017). Magnetic nanoparticles for precision oncology: theranostic magnetic iron oxide nanoparticles for image-guided and targeted cancer therapy. *Nanomedicine*, **12**, 73–87.

80. Chertok, B., David, A., Huang, Y., Yang, V. (2007). Glioma selectivity of magnetically targeted nanoparticles: a role of abnormal tumor hydrodynamics. *J. Control. Release*, **122**, 315–323.

81. Chertok, B., David, A., Yang, V. (2010). Polyethyleneimine-modified iron oxide nanoparticles for brain tumor drug delivery using magnetic targeting and intra-carotid administration. *Biomaterials*, **31**, 6317–6324.

82. Chertok, B., David, A., Yang, V. (2011). Brain tumor targeting of magnetic nanoparticles for potential drug delivery: effect of administration route and magnetic field topography. *J. Control. Release*, **155**, 393–399.

83. Stewart, T. S., Nagesetti, A., Guduru, R., Liang, P., Stimphil, E., Hadjikhani, A., Salgueiro, L., Horstmyer, J., Cai, R., Schally, A., Khizroev, S. (2018). Magnetoelectric nanoparticles for delivery of antitumor peptides into glioblastoma cells by magnetic fields. *Nanomedicine*, **13**, 423–438.

84. Yin, P., Shah, B., Lee, K. (2014). Combined magnetic nanoparticle-based microRNA and hyperthermia therapy to enhance apoptosis in brain cancer cells. *Small*, **10**, 4106–4112.

85. Wang, H., Mu, Q., Revia, R., Wang, K., Tian, B., Lin, G., Lee, W., Hong, Y. K., Zhang, M. (2018). Iron oxide-carbon core-shell nanoparticles for dual-modal imaging-guided photothermal therapy. *J. Control. Release*, **289**, 70–78.

86. Menichetti, L., Manzoni, L., Paduano, L., Flori, A., Kusmic, C., De Marchi, D., Casciaro, S., Conversano, F., Lombardi, M., Positano, V., Arosio, D. (2013). Iron oxide-gold core-shell nanoparticles as multimodal imaging contrast agent. *IEEE Sens. J.*, **13**, 2341–2347.

87. Sood, A., Arora, V., Shah, J., Kotnala, R., Jain, T. (2017). Multifunctional gold coated iron oxide core-shell nanoparticles stabilized using thiolated sodium alginate for biomedical applications. *Mater. Sci. Eng. C*, **80**, 274–281.

88. Sun, L., Joh, D. Y., Al-Zaki, A., Stangl, M., Murty, S., Davis, J. J., Baumann, B. C., Alonso-Basanta, M., Kaol, G. D., Tsourkas, A., Dorsey, J. F. (2016). Theranostic application of mixed gold and superparamagnetic iron oxide nanoparticle micelles in glioblastoma multiforme. *J. Biomed. Nanotechnol.*, **12**, 347–356.

89. Shen, Y., Wu, C., Uyeda, T. Q. P., Plaza, G. R., Liu, B., Han, Y., Lesniak, M. S., Cheng, Y. (2017). Elongated nanoparticle aggregates in cancer cells for mechanical destruction with low frequency rotating magnetic field. *Theranostics*, **7**, 1735–1748.

90. Skouras, A., Papadia, K., Mourtas, S., Klepetsanis, P., Antimisiaris, S. (2018). Multifunctional doxorubicin-loaded magnetoliposomes with active and magnetic targeting properties. *Eur. J. Pharm. Sci.*, **123**, 162–172.

91. Ding, H., Sagar, V., Agudelo, M., Pilakka-Kanthikeel, S., Atluri, V., Raymond, A., Samikkannu, T., Nair, M. P. (2014). Enhanced blood–brain barrier transmigration using a novel transferrin embedded fluorescent magneto-liposome nanoformulation. *Nanotechnology*, **25**, 055101.

92. Thomsen, L., Thomsen, M., Moos, T. (2015). Targeted drug delivery to the brain using magnetic nanoparticles. *Ther. Deliv.*, **6**, 1145–1155.

93. Soenen, S., Velde, G., Ketkar-Atre, A., Himmelreich, U., De Cuyper, M. (2011). Magnetoliposomes as magnetic resonance imaging contrast agents. *Wiley Interdiscip. Rev. Nanomed. Nanobiotechnol.*, **3**, 197–211.

94. Bulte, J., Cuyper, M., Despres, D., Frank, J. (1999). Preparation, relaxometry, and biokinetics of PEGylated magnetoliposomes as MR contrast agent. *J. Magn. Magn. Mater.*, **194**, 204–209.

95. Calle, D., Negri, V., Ballesteros, P., Cerdán, S. (2015). Magnetoliposomes loaded with poly-unsaturated fatty acids as novel theranostic anti-inflammatory formulations. *Theranostics*, **5**, 489–503.

96. Santos, S. C., Silva, N. O., Espinelli, J. B. J. S., Marinho, M. A. G., Borges, Z. V., Branco, N. B. C., Faita, F. L., Soares, B. M., Horn, A. P., Parize, A. L., Lima, V. R. (2018). Molecular interactions and physico-chemical characterization of quercetin-loaded magnetoliposomes. *Chem. Phys. Lipids*, **218**, 22–33.

97. Yan, C., Wu, Y., Feng, J., Chen, W., Liu, X., Hao, P., Yang, R., Zhang, J., Lin, B., Xu, Y., Liu, R. (2013). Anti-$\alpha_v\beta_3$ antibody guided three-step pretargeting approach using magnetoliposomes for molecular magnetic resonance imaging of breast cancer angiogenesis. *Int. J. Nanomed.*, **8**, 245–255.

98. Babincová, N., Sourivong, P., Babinec, P., Bergemann, C., Babincová, M., Durdík, Š. (2018). Applications of magnetoliposomes with encapsulated doxorubicin for integrated chemotherapy and hyperthermia of rat C6 glioma. *Z. Naturforsch. C*, **73**, 265–271.

99. Guo, H., Chen, W., Sun, X., Liu, Y., Li, J., Wang, J. (2015). Theranostic magnetoliposomes coated by carboxymethyl dextran with controlled release by low-frequency alternating magnetic field. *Carbohydr. Polym.*, **118**, 209–217.

100. Tomitaka, A., Arami, H., Huang, Z., Raymond, A., Rodriguez, E., Cai, Y., Febo, M., Takemura, Y., Nair, M. (2018). Hybrid magneto-plasmonic liposomes for multimodal image-guided and brain-targeted HIV treatment. *Nanoscale*, **10**, 184–194.

Part III

Development and Translation

Chapter 11

Quality by Design for Nanocarriers

Branca M. A. Silva[a] **and Cláudia Silva**[a,b]
[a]*Bluepharma, Indústria Farmacêutica, S.A.,*
3045-016 Coimbra, Portugal
[b]*Colep, Rua Manuel Pinto de Azevedo, 272 – 5°, 4100-320 Porto, Portugal*
branca.silva@bluepharmagroup.com

The chapter aims to introduce the quality-by-design (QbD) principles to those who want to acquire a better understanding or to find out more about this subject. It is applicable to scientists in early development stages but also for formulation, analytical and quality scientists. An introduction to the pharmaceutical development is provided in order to highlight the importance of following a systematic approach when working with nanocarriers. The QbD approach is then presented in sections for ease of understanding, but it should be considered as a whole.

11.1 Introduction

There are different types of neurological disorders which can affect the central nervous system (CNS), such as epilepsy, schizophrenia, Alzheimer's disease, Parkinson's disease, lysosomal storage diseases,

Nanoparticles for Brain Drug Delivery
Edited by Carla Vitorino, Andreia Jorge and Alberto Pais

ISBN 978-981-4877-31-2 (Hardcover), 978-1-003-11932-6 (eBook)
www.jennystanford.com

brain tumours, brain stroke and so on [1–3]. For many of them there are no effective treatment because, as already mentioned in previous chapters, the drug delivery to the CNS is quite challenging. The blood–brain barrier (BBB) is almost impenetrable to most of the available drugs due to the presence of thigh junctions which prevent the passage of molecules as well as the presence of efflux pumps which remove the molecules which were able to cross the BBB. Therefore, to passively cross the BBB, the drug molecules should have less than 150 Da and be hydrophilic or, be lipophilic and have less than 500 Da. The use of nanocarriers for brain delivery has been widely explored because it does not require drug modifications and the nanocarriers surface can be modulated in several ways to facilitate its entry in the CNS [1–3].

The traditional approach for pharmaceutical process and product development has been based on empirical experimentation rather than science and risk-based analysis. Also, the product quality was ensured by following batch operations and end product testing. The poor understanding of how process and material variables influence the target product profile led to endless tests of trial and error, product variability and, in the end, supplement submissions to the authorities for revision and approval. The quality-by-design (QbD) approach applied to the pharmaceutical development emerged as part of the regulatory authorities initiatives to improve the quality of the product as well as the efficiency of the manufacturing processes [4, 5].

The development of nanocarriers as drug delivery systems is challenging, involving complex and nonstandard manufacturing process, which encompasses greater difficulties in the assessment of potential risks and impact of raw materials' attributes and process parameters (PPs). In addition, the physical, biological and chemical properties of the raw materials used in the manufacturing of nanotechnology products are different from the raw materials used in the conventional dosage forms. These facts have raised many questions regarding the quality and safety of nanotechnology products, which prompted the regulatory authorities to the creation of working groups dedicated to the nanopharmaceuticals and/or nanotechnology products [6, 7]. Altogether, these complex drug products would benefit from a systematic and integrative approach starting at early development stages up to the end of the product life cycle.

11.2 The QbD Approach

Juran first introduced the QbD concept in the 1970s as part of his work in the field of the quality and quality management. The well-known Juran Trilogy (quality planning, quality control and quality improvement) are still up-to-date and it can be considered the foundation of the modern process and quality improvement not only in the pharmaceutical industry but also in other industries. The QbD methodology is a multistep approach aiming to build quality into products by design [5, 8]. The International Conference of Harmonization (ICH) Q8 defines the QbD as 'a systematic approach to development that begins with predefined objectives and emphasizes product and process understanding and process control, based on sound science and quality risk management' [9]. In other words, the pharmaceutical development following the QbD methodology provides a thorough knowledge of how PPs and material attributes (MAs) influence product performance. This understanding is then used to establish a design space, product and process specifications and suitable manufacturing controls in order to ensure that the quality targets and product requirements are consistently achieved [9, 10].

The roadmap for QbD implementation is illustrated in Fig. 11.1. It starts with the definition of the quality target product profile (QTPP) and the identification of potential critical quality attributes (CQAs), critical material attributes (CMAs) and critical process parameters (CPPs). As part of the QbD and integrated with the quality risk management principles, a control strategy should be defined and a continuous monitoring implemented [9–12].

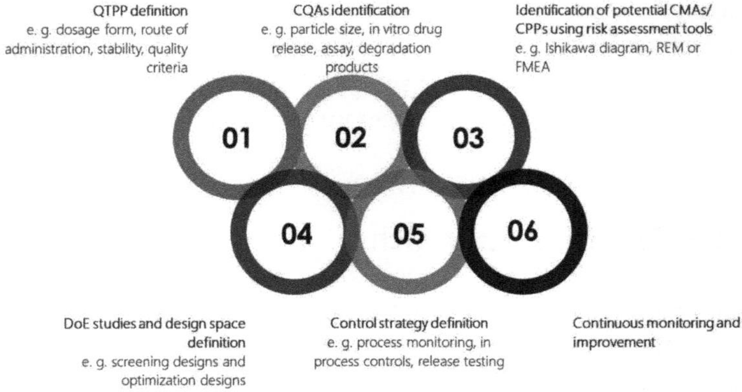

Figure 11.1 Quality-by-design approach, as defined in the ICH Q8, Q9 and Q10.

11.2.1 QTPP

The QTPP is a summary of the product quality characteristics which is defined according to the product objectives, the relevant physicochemical characteristics and the intended product performance. It usually includes quality characteristics related to the intended use, route of administration, dosage form, dosage strength, container closure system, drug product quality criteria (e.g. assay, impurities profile, sterility), characteristics affecting the pharmacokinetic (PK) parameters (e.g. drug release, particle size) and so on [8, 9, 13]. The QTPP works as the bridge between drug products attributes and the patient needs. In Table 11.1 is represented a general QTPP for nanocarriers aimed at the drug delivery to the brain. It contains the attribute, the target and the rationale behind it. This QTPP was built based on the authors experience in the development of nanocarriers in the pharmaceutical industry context and literature examples. Not all the attributes have a general target profile, since in most of the cases the target is dependent on the specificities of the drug substance and/or drug product. A typical QTPP for nanocarriers should include particle size, particle size distribution, morphology, zeta potential, vitro drug release [13–15] in addition to applicable requirements considering the route of drug administration (e.g. parenteral or nasal). Depending on the dosage form, some other attributes should be present as well. For injectable liquid products pH, subvisible particles, clarity, sterility, etc., should be identified. Moisture content, cake appearance and reconstitution time should be considered for lyophilised products.

11.2.2 CQAs

The CQAs are chemical, physical or microbiological properties of the drug product which must be within an appropriate limit or range to ensure the desired product quality [9]. The CQAs identification is based on the QTPP; which CQAs impact safety and efficacy (impurities profile, mean particle size), drug product performance (morphology, in vitro drug release, leakage) and drug product manufacturability (uniformity of dosage units, viscosity) should be determined. For conventional dosage forms there is a strong understanding of how product attributes correlate with the safety, efficacy, performance and manufacturing. Yet, for new technologies such as the ones available to obtain nanocarriers, there is a need to establish these correlations, especially the in vivo performance. This knowledge should be established in a systematic way, at an early stage of development, and should include less obvious attributes (e.g. residual solvents, extractables, leachables, container closure system, impurities profile). In Table 11.2 are listed commonly identified CQAs as well as others which are product specific and often omitted. The consultation of the general chapters/monographs on specific drug products of the European Pharmacopeia (EP) and the United States Pharmacopeia (USP) are recommended. For example, the general Chapter 5 of the USP provides information about the quality tests which should be performed for inhalation and nasal drug products, while the general Chapter 1 refers to injections and implanted drug products.

11.2.3 Risk Assessment

Risk assessment is essential to identify the unit operations of drug product manufacturing process with the potential to impact on product CQAs. The ICH Q8(R2) recommends the use of risk assessment tools during product development in order to select

Table 11.1 Quality target product profile (QTPP) for nanocarriers aimed for drug delivery to the brain

Attribute	Target product profile	Rationale
Dosage form	Polymeric nanoparticle, carbon-based vehicle, polymeric micelles, liposomes, solid lipid nanoparticles, niosomes, transferosomes, nanogel, nanoemulsion	The nanocarriers were identified as potential drug delivery systems for the brain, due to the different strategies to surpass the BBB [2, 3].
Dosage form design	Injectables: lyophilised, concentrate for dilution Nasal sprays: liquid, powder and semisolid	Some products may require lyophilisation to increase the stability of the finished product [16]. However, it is desirable to avoid this complex process which increases the development time and cost of the drug product.
Route of administration	Intravenous, nasal	Intravenous administration is known to provide the highest drug bioavailability. However, it is invasive and the manufacturing process is costly. Other routes of administration should be explored. For example, the nasal route could provide a fast delivery from the nasal cavity to the brain, and it is less invasive [14, 17, 18].

Attribute		Target product profile	Rationale
Dosage strength		Product specific	The selected strength should guarantee the pharmacological effect. It depends on the drug, the route of administration and the ability of the formulation to deliver the drug to the site of action.
Pharmacokinetics		Product specific	The determination of the PK is essential to define the drug bioavailability, the safety and the toxicity of the medicinal product.
Stability		Long-term physicochemical stability Protection from light and freezing (when applicable) Shelf-life of at least 24 months	The quality of the product should be maintained during storage in order to define the product shelf-life and to ensure the commercial viability of the product. Some products may require special storage conditions to avoid degradation and maintain the quality of the product [19].
Drug product quality attributes	Appearance	According to the dosage form and intended application site, there are acceptance limits defined in the pharmacopoeias and in the regulatory authorities' guidance documents (e.g. FDA, EMA, ICH). Detailed target limits are depicted in the CQAs (Table 11.2).	The appearance of the drug product depends on the raw materials' characteristics as well as on the dosage form design. Nevertheless, the colour, clarity (liquid dosage forms) and cake appearance (lyophilised products) should be defined [20].

(Continued)

Table 11.1 (*Continued*)

Attribute		Target product profile	Rationale
	Mean particle size		The nanocarriers' small dimensions are comparable to endogenous molecules and, therefore, offer the potential to overcome the BBB [21].
	Particle size distribution		High variability in the nanocarriers' size is not desirable because of the possibility of having different drug release behaviour and intra- and intersubject drug biodistribution [13, 22].
	Morphology		The nanocarriers' morphology may influence the drug loading, retention and release [23]. For each nanocarrier the best morphology should be defined.
	Surface charge		A balance should be established between neutral, positive and negative surface charge: a neutral surface charge allows the nanocarriers to escape the reticuloendothelial system; a positive surface charge facilitates the interaction with the lipid membranes which are negatively charged; a negative surface promotes the colloidal stability of the drug product [13, 24, 25].

Attribute		Target product profile	Rationale
	DS and raw materials Identification		From a quality standpoint, it is crucial to ensure the correct identification of the selected materials [26, 27].
	DS polymorphism		In the majority of nanocarriers, the drug substance is solubilised before the encapsulation. In these cases, the polymorphism does not represent an issue in terms of drug bioavailability but may influence the formulation composition (e.g. solvent selection) as well as the manufacturing process (e.g. solubilisation time and/or order of addition).
	Uniformity of dosage units		The uniformity in the amount of the drug substance is mandatory to ensure the consistency of the dosage administered to the patients.
	DS and functional excipients assay		The DS must be present in the amount stated in the label claim, which means present in the amount which provides the desired efficacy [28, 29]. In addition, the ratio between the raw materials could influence the product performance.

(*Continued*)

Table 11.1 (*Continued*)

Attribute		Target product profile	Rationale
	Encapsulated and free drug substance (DS)		High encapsulation efficiency is indicative of an efficient and cost-effective process. Also, the high drug concentration can establish a suitable gradient for drug delivery [2].
	DS and functional excipients degradation products		There are limits for degradation products in order to guarantee the quality and stability of the drug product, as well as to limit the exposure to potentially toxic impurities [30].
	Residual solvents		The use of organic solvents is very common in the development and manufacturing of nanocarriers. There are recommendations regarding the admitted solvents and their limits [31].
	In vitro release of the DS		An in vitro drug release method, capable of providing a good IVIV correlation, is useful to demonstrate consistent quality and performance of the drug product [32]. Keep in mind that it may be possible to develop a method for quality control purposes only and a method with the ability to provide a better insight on the product performance in vivo.

Attribute		Target product profile	Rationale
	Osmolality		An isotonic product is desirable, both for the intravenous and nasal route, in order to avoid tissue irritation and cells damage.
	pH		pH values different from the pH of the intended administration site may cause irritation. Nevertheless, a balance should be established between the drug permeability, stability and patient safety.
	Viscosity		No special equipment or devices are required for manufacturing, storage and delivery when the product has a low viscosity.
	Moisture content		The moisture content is applicable for lyophilised products in order to ensure a suitable shelf-life.
	Microbial limits		For nonsterile products, the microbiological quality should limit/prevent the occurrence of adverse reactions due to the presence of a high level of microorganisms. The microbiological quality must be maintained throughout the product shelf-life.

(*Continued*)

Table 11.1 (*Continued*)

Attribute		**Target product profile**	**Rationale**
	Sterility		Injectable drug products are meant to enter directly to the blood circulation. Therefore, it is mandatory to have a product free from microorganisms, pyrogen content and bacterial endotoxins.
	Pyrogen test		
	Bacterial endotoxins		
Drug product composition		Biocompatible, biodegradable, nontoxic, compliant with GMP and other compendial requirements	All the raw materials used in the manufacturing of drug products should have certain properties which ensure its quality and safety. Also, for the US market it is desirable to choose raw materials present in the Inactive Ingredients Database, to avoid additional toxicological tests prior to the approval of the drug product.
Dilution/ reconstitution buffer		To be determined	The product properties and performance must be maintained after dilution and/or reconstitution.
Dilution/ reconstitution process		To be determined	The process for dilution/reconstitution must guarantee the product properties and performance. The stability of the diluted product must be determined as well.

Attribute		Target product profile	Rationale
Container closure system		Injectables: clear type I glass vial with an elastomeric stopper	Needed to achieve the target shelf-life and to ensure the container integrity during shipment. In the case of sprays, the performance and usability should also be evaluated.
		Nasal sprays: type I glass bottles or plastic bottles (e.g. polyethylene, polypropylene, PET)	
Fill volume		A volume which enables the extraction of the labelled volume which is to be withdrawn.	The volume present must ensure correct dosing.

Table 11.2 Critical quality attributes (CQAs) of nanocarriers aimed for drug delivery to the brain

Quality attributes		Target	Is this a CQA?	Justification
Physical attributes	Appearance	Depends on formulation (to be determined)	Yes	The colour and clarity of the drug product may be quality- and stability-indicating, which can be linked to safety and efficacy. Therefore, they should be evaluated during development.
	Mean particle size	Below 200 nm	Yes	The particle size and particle size distribution will affect drug PK. Process variables may affect the nanocarrier size. Thus, mean particle size and size distribution should be evaluated throughout product and process development.
	Particle size distribution	Narrow	Yes	
	Morphology/ lamellarity	Depends on formulation (to be determined)	Yes	Nanocarrier morphology and lamellarity (in the case of liposomes) influence drug loading, drug retention, and the rate of drug release. These CQAs may be affected by process variables. Therefore, morphology and lamellarity should be investigated throughout product and process development.
	Surface charge	–30 mV to 30 mV	Yes	Surface charge on nanocarriers can affect the clearance, tissue distribution and cellular uptake. The surface charge may be influenced by formulation and process parameters, so the zeta potential will be investigated throughout formulation and process development.

Quality attributes	Target	Is this a CQA?	Justification
Identification	Positive for the materials in use	Yes	Identification is critical for safety and efficacy. However, it can be effectively controlled by the quality management system and should be monitored at drug product quality control release.
Assay DS	USP: 90%–110% of label claim EP: 95%–105% of label claim	Yes	Assay variability will affect safety and efficacy. Process variables may affect the assay of the drug product. Thus, assay should be evaluated throughout product and process development.
Assay of functional excipients	Molar ratio drug substance:total lipids Molar ratio drug substance:polymer Molar ratio lipid:lipid	Yes	The molar ratio between the formulation components demonstrates consistency with the intended formulation and influence the drug loading. Changes in the molar ratio can influence the bioavailability and efficacy of the product. Process variables may affect the assay of the drug product, so this CQA should be evaluated throughout product and process development.
Uniformity of dosage units	Conforms to USP <905>	Yes	The consistency of dosage units is linked to the safety and efficacy of the drug products. Formulation, process parameters and container closure influence this CQA.

(*Continued*)

Table 11.2 (*Continued*)

Quality attributes	Target	Is this a CQA?	Justification
Fill volume	Injectables: Fill volume per vial according to the compendial recommendation (USP <697>) Nasal sprays: Minimum fill according to the compendial recommendation (USP <755>)	Yes	Inadequate volume in the container may lead to insufficient dosing. Process parameters and the container closure affect this CQA. Fill volume per vial should be investigated during product and process development.
DS and functional excipients degradation products	Meet ICH Q3B(R2) requirements	Yes	Degradation products can impact safety and must be controlled based on compendial/ICH requirements to limit patient exposure. Formulation and process variables can impact degradation products. Therefore, degradation products should be assessed during product and process development.
In vitro drug release	Depends on formulation (to be determined)	Yes	Failure to meet the in vitro drug release specification can impact safety and efficacy. Both physical and chemical formulation stability as well as process variables affect the in vitro drug release. This CQA should be investigated throughout formulation and process development.

Quality attributes	Target	Is this a CQA?	Justification
Leakage	As low as possible	Yes	Leakage during storage could have an impact on drug PK. Formulation and manufacturing variables may affect this CQA. This CQA should be investigated throughout formulation and process development.
Percentage of encapsulated DS	As high as possible	Yes	Free DS content could have an impact on drug PK. Formulation and manufacturing parameters may affect this CQA.
State of encapsulated DS	To be determined	Yes	The salt form/precipitated form of the DS could influence its release from the nanocarrier and, consequently, the PK. This CQA should be evaluated during process and formulation development.
Osmolality	Conforms to USP <785>	Yes	The osmolality should be compatible with the application site and the formulation stability. Osmolality values different from plasma osmolality may cause tissue irritation and damage to blood cells. The integrity of the nanocarriers may also be influenced by osmolality which can cause leakage of the drug substance. The osmolality may be affected by process and formulation variables, so this CQA should be evaluated during product and process development.

(*Continued*)

Table 11.2 (*Continued*)

Quality attributes	Target	Is this a CQA?	Justification
pH	Close to the pH of the intended administration site	Yes	The pH is critical for drug permeability, stability and patient safety. Both formulation and process variables affect the pH. Thus, pH should be assessed during product and process development.
Viscosity	As low as possible	Yes	No special equipment or devices are required for manufacturing, storage and delivery when the product has a low viscosity. Formulation and process variables impact on viscosity. Thus, this CQA should be evaluated throughout the development.
Residual solvents	Meet ICH Q3C(R6) requirements	Yes	Residual solvents can impact patient safety. Considering that solvents may not be completely removed during manufacturing, they should be quantified during product and process development.
Leachables and extractables	Conforms to USP <1663> and <1664>	Yes	Nanocarrier formulations have the potential to present leachables and extractables from plastic and rubber components. This may influence patient safety, so these should be evaluated throughout product and process development.

Quality attributes	Target	Is this a CQA?	Justification
Microbial limits	Conforms to USP <1111>	Yes	Noncompliance with microbial limits will impact patient safety. The sterility, pyrogen content and bacterial endotoxins may be influenced by process and formulation parameters. Therefore, these CQAs should be investigated during product and process development.
Sterility	Conforms to USP <71>	Yes	
Pyrogen test	Conforms to USP <151>	Yes	
Bacterial endotoxins	Conforms to USP <85>	Yes	
Particulate matter in injections	Conforms to USP <788> and USP <790>	Yes	The presence of particulate matter in intravenous injections represents a potentially life-threatening health hazard. Both formulation and process variables may influence this CQA, so it should be evaluated throughout product and process development.
Lipid bilayer phase transition temperature	Depends on formulation (to be determined)	Yes	Equivalence in lipid bilayer phase transitions will contribute to demonstrating equivalence in bilayer fluidity and uniformity (FDA, 2018a). This affects drug release from the nanocarrier and drug PK. Formulation and manufacturing parameters may impact phase transition temperature. Thus, phase transition temperature should be assessed during product and process development.

(Continued)

Table 11.2 (*Continued*)

Quality attributes	Target	Is this a CQA?	Justification
Moisture content	Depends on formulation (to be determined)	Yes	The residual water present in the lyophilised products may lead to the formation of degradation products, which could compromise the patient's safety. The moisture content is determined by formulation and process parameters, and for that it should be evaluated during development.

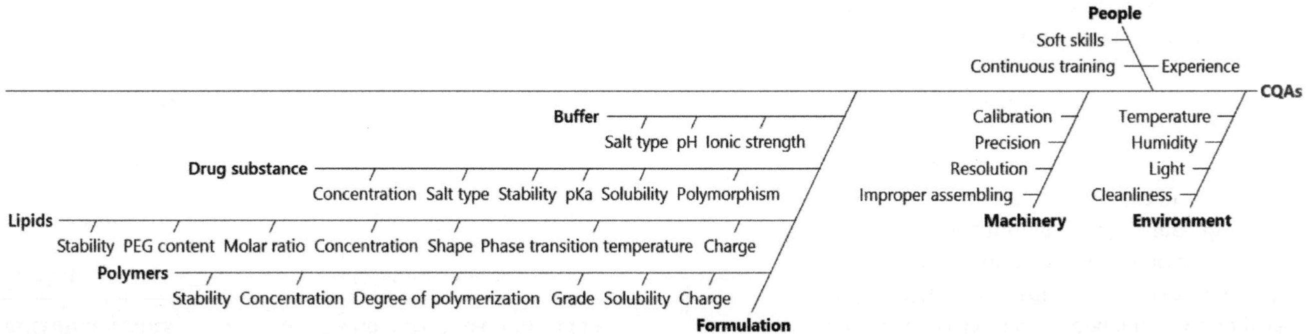

Figure 11.2 Identification of environmental, man, equipment and raw materials with the potential to influence nanocarriers' CQAs based on the cause-and-effect diagram.

and prioritise which material attributes and PPs should be studied (the factors or variables) [9]. Cause-and-effect diagram/fishbone/Ishikawa diagram, risk estimation matrix (REM) and the failure mode and effects analysis (FMEA) are widely used tools for this purpose [4, 9, 10, 12]. The cause-and-effect diagram is a qualitative tool, where environmental, man, equipment, raw materials and process variables are categorised according to their a priori importance aiming to explain the CQAs variation. Common variables can be defined for all types of nanocarriers (Fig. 11.2) and other variables are only applicable to specific manufacturing process of nanocarriers where the potential critical unit operations are linked to the CQAs. In the case of liposomes (Fig. 11.3) the manufacturing process might include the following major process steps: formation of multilamellar vesicles (MLVs) through ethanol injection, extrusion for size reduction and manufacturing of small unilamellar vesicles, tangential flow filtration for buffer exchange, active drug loading and finally a new tangential flow filtration for the removal of unencapsulated drug. The manufacturing of solid lipid nanoparticles (Fig. 11.4) starts with the formation of a coarse dispersion by high-speed homogenisation of the organic and aqueous phase, during the ultrasonication a pre-emulsion is formed and the final emulsion is obtained by high-speed homogenisation, and in the last step occurs the recrystallisation of the lipid nanoparticles. For each of these unit operations it is possible do identify PPs which have the potential to influence the product CQAs and construct cause-and-effect diagrams, as depicted in Figs. 11.3 and 11.4.

The FMEA and REM are quantitative tools which can be used alone or in combination with the cause-and-effect diagram [10, 12]. Design of experiment (DoE) studies for formulation/process understanding and design space definition are recommend during development. Because it is not feasible to study all possible formulation and process variables during product development using DoE, the REM is often used to prioritise which ones are more likely to be critical and should be investigated – CMA and CPP identification [33]. The

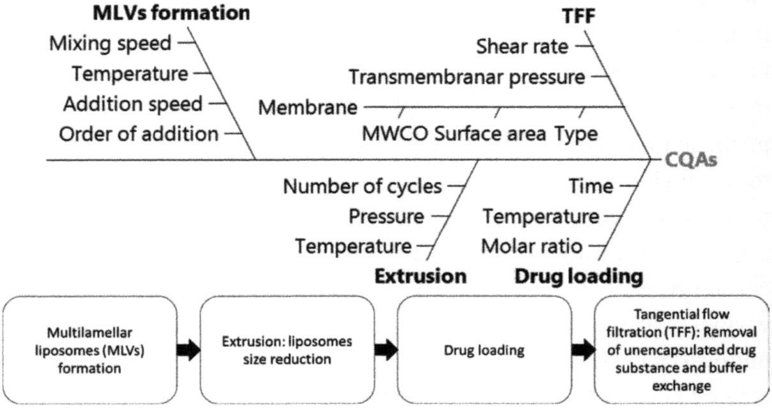

Figure 11.3 Cause-and-effect diagram representing the link between process parameters in the manufacturing of liposomes which can interfere with the CQAs.

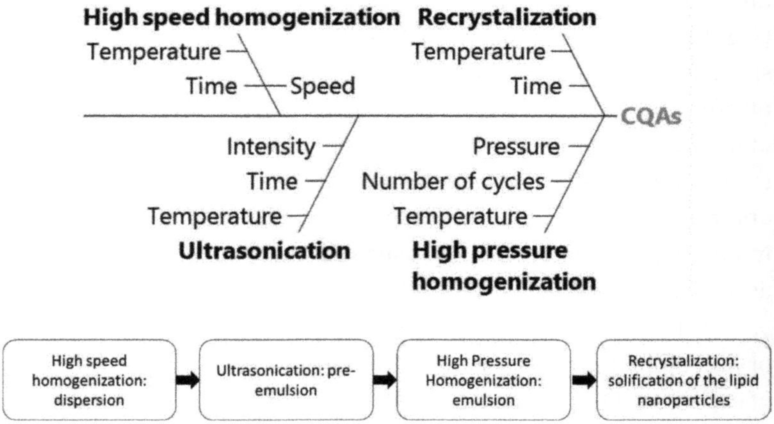

Figure 11.4 Cause-and-effect diagram representing the link between process parameters in the manufacturing of solid lipid nanoparticles which can interfere with the CQAs.

REM ranks the variables considering the potential critically in terms of risk (high, medium or low risk level). REM considers the severity and the probability of occurrence of each variable but does not take into consideration the detection, which is present in the FMEA risk assessment tool. The goal of the DoE studies is to increase the knowledge about the product and the process; therefore, it is important to study as much variables as possible, including the ones which are easily detected. When the probability of detection is included in the risk assessment, as in the case of FMEA tool, it is possible to document the actions related to the risk of failure, and in this sense, it is used for prevention and control during development and throughout product life cycle management. A REM (Table 11.3) was constructed to highlight the relation between five CQAs of liposomes (particle size, particle size distribution, in vitro release, assay and degradation products) and the PPs of the manufacturing of liposomes previously identified in the cause-and-effect diagram depicted on Fig. 11.2. The parameters with a high risk of influencing the CQAs are shaded in red, the medium risk in yellow and the low risk in green. For example, in the MLVs formation the temperature, addition and mixing speed were considered as high-risk factors for the particle size and particle distribution. The lipids present in the liposomes composition have a phase transition temperature which should be reached in order to promote the alignment of the polar heads and the vesicles' formation [34, 35]. Therefore, there is a high probability that changes in the temperature impact on the CQAs mentioned, and when it occurs, the severity is very high because different particle sizes results in changes in the PK of the product. When different addition speed and mixing speed are applied, different mechanical stress is generated which will impact on the particle size and particle size distribution [34, 35]. In these cases, the probability of occurrence is high and the severity very high.

11.3 Design of Experiments, Design Space and Control Strategy

The DoE is a useful and effective tool which allows the determination of how the variables being studied (CMAs and CPPs) interact and how their interaction influences the responses (CQAs). Therefore, the DoE is the preferred approach to define the design space

Table 11.3 Examples of initial risk assessment of the manufacturing of liposomes based on the risk estimation matrix (REM)

Process steps	MLVs				Extrusion						Drug loading			Tangential flow filtration				
Process parameters/ CQ As	Order of addition	Temperature	Addition speed	Mixing speed	Temperature	Pressure	Number of cycles	Membrane type	Membrane pore size	Membrane stacking	Temperature	Molar ratio	Time	Membrane type	Membrane surface area	Membrane MWCO	Transmembrane pressure	Shear rate
Particle size	Med	High	High	High	High	Med	High	Low	High	High	Low	Low	Low	Low	Med	Med	Low	Med
Particle size distribution	Med	High	High	High	High	Med	High	Low	High	High	Low	Low	Low	Low	Med	Med	Low	Med
In vitro drug release	Med	High	High	High	High	Low	High	Low	Low	Low	Low	Low	Low	Low	Low	Med	Low	Med
Assay DS	Low	Low	Low	Low	Low	Low	Low	Low	Low	Low	High	High	High	Med	Med	Low	Med	Low
Degradation products DS	Low	Low	Low	Low	Low	Low	Low	Low	Low	Low	High	Low	Low	Low	Low	Low	Low	Low

during product development. Several advantages are offered over the traditional approach of changing one factor at a time such as: maximising knowledge with less resources, definition of the relative significance of each factor, construction of prediction models and optimisation of multiple CQAs [5, 36, 37].

The choice of a suitable experimental design is critical for the success of the DoE approach and it depends on the study goals (screening, optimisation and/or robustness testing), the investigator's experience, previous knowledge, the available resources and number and level of variables [5, 36, 37]. Screening designs such as response surface design, factorial designs, Placket-Burman and Taguchi are useful to determine the most influential factors and require few experiments in relation to the number of factors being studied. Optimisation designs (e.g. Box-Behnken, central composite design, optimal designs) can be employed following the application of screening designs and aim to find optimal operating conditions and to predict the response values. The robustness testing allows to determine the sensitivity of CQAs to small changes in the factors levels. It is important to note, that in most of the studies related to the development of nanocarriers for brain delivery the only QbD element used is DoE [16–18, 24, 38–42]. This finding is transversal to many other research papers and should be emphasised that this is not the most appropriate approach. A successful DoE study must be preceded by the definition of solid objectives through QTPP and CQAs definition and the identification and selection of factors (CPPs and CMAs) based on risk assessment tools [4, 5, 9, 43].

The ICH Q8 defines the design space as 'the multidimensional combination and interaction of input variables (e. g. material attributes) and process parameters that have been demonstrated to provide assurance of quality' [9]. The data obtained in the DoE is used to estimate each CQA (dimension) through statistical modelling. The prediction profiles obtained for each CQA (dimension) can be combined to find the region where the product meets the QTPP. The ranges/levels studied (characterisation range) in the DoE experiments represent the knowledge space while with the design space is possible to find the acceptable working range and the operating range (Fig. 11.5) [4, 5, 9, 43].

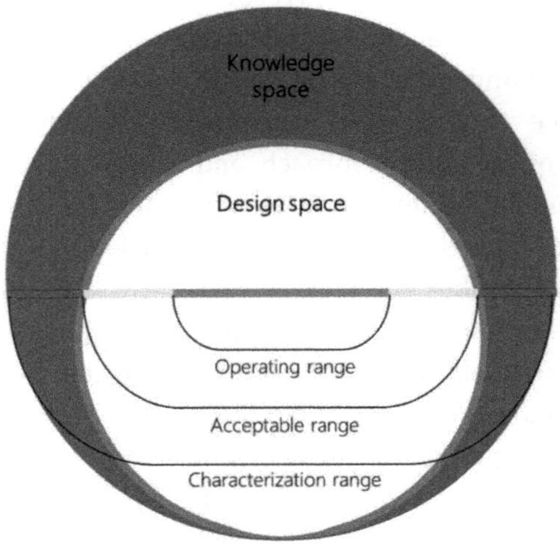

Figure 11.5 Schematic representation of different regions which can be defined during QbD implementation. The characterisation range is studied during design of experiments (DoE) and constitutes the knowledge space. Within the design space it is possible to find the acceptable range, which is the output of the DoE, and the operating range, which constitutes the ranges defined for the manufacturing procedures. Adapted from Refs. [4, 43].

Mendes et al. [13] and Xu et al. [35] could be a good starting point for those interested in following the QbD approach for their product development. Although not exhaustively, the QTPP was defined, the CQAs were selected, the risks were identified and analysed and DoE studies were conducted for formulation/process understanding and design space definition. In Xu et al. [35] a Placket-Burman design was used for the initial screening of eight formulation and process variables (lipid concentration, drug concentration, cholesterol concentration, buffer concentration, hydration time, sonication time, freeze–thaw cycles and extrusion pressure) which could impact on the encapsulation efficiency of liposomes. A composite design was selected for product optimisation and design space definition using the two statistically significant variables (lipid concentration and drug concentration) identified in the screening DoE. In the end, it was demonstrated that the higher the lipid concentration the higher the encapsulation efficiency, probably due to the increase in the number of vesicles and, consequently, in the internal volume available for encapsulation. On the other hand, the increase in drug concentration resulted in a decrease of the encapsulation efficiency, which may be related with a decrease in the bound between the drug and lipid.

The control strategy is established based on the knowledge and understanding gained during the development and the DoE application. It can include the control of input MAs, the control of the unit operations (CPPs) and in-process and real-time testing of the CQAs [9, 12, 44]. In-process controls of nanocarriers and liposomes, in particular, may include visual inspection, particle size and particle size distribution, residual solvents, extrusion membrane integrity, lipid content, percentage of free drug, pH, filter integrity and so on [44, 45]. The end-product testing is the bottom line of the control strategy and can be reduced to a minimum provided that the sources of variability were well characterised and are broadly understood.

11.3.1 Continuous Monitoring and Improvement

The continuous monitoring throughout the product life cycle allows to obtain additional understanding of the product and process performance and to manage the impact of any changes [9, 11, 12]. This new information can trigger the need to perform adjustments and, in this way, continuously improve the product and the process. When a design space is defined, the adjustments performed within the design space are not considered a change to the approved dossier. Therefore, no new review or approval by the regulatory authorities are required. The expansion, reduction or redefinition of the design space is subjected to post-approval submission. Control charts and product quality review reports are tools which can be used for the continuous monitoring of the product quality and the process performance.

11.4 Conclusion

The ultimate goal of the QbD implementation is to develop products and processes which have a higher quality and robustness through a deeper understanding about the science behind it. In this way go/no-go decisions are more based on sound scientific knowledge. The application of this approach from early stages will facilitate the scale-up stages, which is even more critical when working with complex products such as nanocarriers. Altogether, the project costs can be reduced because there is less waste and fewer failures; the manufacturing efficiency can be increased, and the product quality is increased when the QbD approach is followed. Additionally, in nanotechnology products where there is still uncertainty and lack of knowledge regarding their quality and safety, an integrative approach, such as the QbD, could facilitate their acceptance by the regulatory authorities. Despite that, many challenges and questions still remain to be answered regarding these complex drug products and manufacturing processes. Therefore, multidisciplinary working groups (academia, industry and regulators) must continue to work together to ensure a smooth introduction of the nanocarriers into the market.

References

1. Tam, V. H., Sosa, C., Liu, R., Yao, N., Priestley, R. D. (2016). Nanomedicine as a non-invasive strategy for drug delivery across the blood brain barrier. *Int. J. Pharm.*, **515**(1–2), 331–342.
2. Masserini, M. (2013). Nanoparticles for brain drug delivery. *ISRN Biochem.*,**2013**, 1–18.
3. Khan, A. R., Yang, X., Fu, M., Zhai, G. (2018). Recent progress of drug nanoformulations targeting to brain. *J. Control. Release*, **291**, 37–64.
4. Rathore, A. S., Winkle, H. (2009). Quality by design for biopharmaceuticals. *Nat.Biotechnol.*, **27**(1), 26–34.
5. Schlindwein, W. S., Gibson, M. (eds.) (2018). *Pharmaceutical Quality by Design*, John Wiley & Sons, Chichester, UK.
6. Food and Drug Administration (2018b). Nanotechnology fact sheet. Retrieved January 31, 2019, from https://www.fda.gov/ScienceResearch/SpecialTopics/Nanotechnology/ucm402230.htm.
7. Pepic, I., Hafner, A., Lovric, J., PerinaLakos, G. (2014). Nanotherapeutics in the EU: an overview on current state and future directions. *Int. J.Nanomed.*, **9**, 1005–1023.
8. Bastogne, T. (2017). Quality-by-design of nanopharmaceuticals: a state of the art. *Nanomed.Nanotechnol. Biol. Med.*, **13**(7), 2151–2157.

9. International Conference of Harmonization (2009). *ICH Harmonized Tripartite Guideline: Q8 (R2) Pharmaceutical Development*. Retrieved from http://www.ich.org/fileadmin/Public_Web_Site/ICH_Products/Guidelines/Quality/Q8_R1/Step4/Q8_R2_Guideline.pdf.

10. Yu, L. X., Amidon, G., Khan, M. A., Hoag, S. W., Polli, J., Raju, G. K., Woodcock, J. (2014). Understanding pharmaceutical quality by design. *AAPS J.*, **16**(4), 771–783.

11. International Conference of Harmonization (2008). *ICH Harmonized Tripartite Guideline: Q10 Pharmaceutical Quality System*. Retrieved from http://www.ich.org/fileadmin/Public_Web_Site/ICH_Products/Guidelines/Quality/Q10/Step4/Q10_Guideline.pdf.

12. International Conference of Harmonization (2005). *ICH Harmonized Tripartite Guideline: Q9 Quality Risk Management*. Retrieved from http://www.ich.org/fileadmin/Public_Web_Site/ICH_Products/Guidelines/Quality/Q9/Step4/Q9_Guideline.pdf.

13. Mendes, M., Miranda, A., Cova, T., Gonçalves, L., Almeida, A. J., Sousa, J. J., do Vale, M. L. C., Marques, E. F., Pais, A.,Vitorino, C. (2018). Modeling of ultra-small lipid nanoparticle surface charge for targeting glioblastoma. *Eur. J. Pharm. Sci.*, **117**(2), 255–269.

14. Shah, B., Khunt, D., Bhatt, H., Misra, M., Padh, H. (2015). Application of quality by design approach for intranasal delivery of rivastigmine loaded solid lipid nanoparticles: effect on formulation and characterization parameters. *Eur. J. Pharm. Sci.*, **78**, 54–66.

15. Sánchez-López, E., Ettcheto, M., Egea, M. A., Espina, M., Cano, A., Calpena, A. C., Camins, A., Carmona, N., Silva, A. M., Souto, E. B.,García, M. L. (2018). Memantine loaded PLGA PEGylated nanoparticles for Alzheimer's disease: in vitro and in vivo characterization. *J.Nanobiotechnol.*, **16**(1), 32.

16. Ćurić, A., Keller, B. L., Reul, R., Möschwitzer, J., Fricker, G. (2015). Development and lyophilization of itraconazole loaded poly(butyl cyanoacrylate) nanospheres as a drug delivery system. *Eur. J. Pharm. Sci.*, **78**, 121–131.

17. Kumar, S., Ali, J., Baboota, S. (2016). Design Expert® supported optimization and predictive analysis of selegilinenanoemulsion via the olfactory region with enhanced behavioural performance in Parkinson's disease. *Nanotechnology*, **27**(43), 1–24.

18. Wang, Q., Wong, C. H., Chan, H. Y. E., Lee, W. Y., Zuo, Z. (2018). Statistical design of experiment (DoE) based development and optimization of DB213 in situ thermosensitive gel for intranasal delivery. *Int. J. Pharm.*, **539**(1–2), 50–57.

19. International Conference of Harmonization (2003). *ICH Harmonized Tripartite Guideline: Q1A(R2) Stability Testing of New Drug Substances and Products.*
20. Smith, M. K., French, J. L., Kowalski, K. G., Hutmacher, M. M., Ewy, W. (2015). *Quality by Design for Biopharmaceutical Drug Product Development*, Vol. 18, Jameel, F., Hershenson, S., Khan, M. A., Martin-Moe, S., eds., Springer New York, New York.
21. Poovaiah, N., Davoudi, Z., Peng, H., Schlichtmann, B., Mallapragada, S., Narasimhan, B., Wang, Q. (2018). Treatment of neurodegenerative disorders through the blood–brain barrier using nanocarriers. *Nanoscale*, **10**(36), 16962–16983.
22. Lundy, D. J., Chen, K.-H., Toh, E. K.-W., Hsieh, P. C.-H. (2016). Distribution of systemically administered nanoparticles reveals a size-dependent effect immediately following cardiac ischaemia-reperfusion injury. *Sci. Rep.*, **6**(1), 25613.
23. Smith, B. R., Kempen, P., Bouley, D., Xu, A., Liu, Z., Melosh, N., Dai, H., Sinclair, R., Gambhir, S. S. (2012). Shape matters: intravital microscopy reveals surprising geometrical dependence for nanoparticles in tumor models of extravasation. *Nano Lett.*, **12**(7), 3369–3377.
24. Joseph, E., Reddi, S., Rinwa, V., Balwani, G., Saha, R. (2018). DoE based Olanzapine loaded poly-caprolactone nanoparticles decreases extrapyramidal effects in rodent model. *Int. J. Pharm.*, **541**(1–2), 198–205.
25. Đorđević, S. M., Cekić, N. D., Savić, M. M., Isailović, T. M., Ranđelović, D. V., Marković, B. D., Savić, S. R., Stamenić, T. T., Daniels, R., Savić, S. D. (2015). Parenteral nanoemulsions as promising carriers for brain delivery of risperidone: design, characterization and in vivo pharmacokinetic evaluation. *Int. J. Pharm.*, **493**(1–2), 40–54.
26. European Commission (2015). Production, in *EudraLex- Volume 4- Good Manufacturing Practice Guidelines.*
27. European Commission (2013). Pharmaceutical quality system, in *EudraLex- Volume 4- Good Manufacturing Practice Guidelines.* Retrieved from https://ec.europa.eu/health/sites/health/files/files/eudralex/vol-4/vol4-chap1_2013-01_en.pdf.
28. International Conference of Harmonization (1999b). *ICH Harmonized Tripartite Guideline: Q6B Specifications: Test Procedures and Acceptance Criteria for Biotechnological/Biological Products.*
29. International Conference of Harmonization (1999a). *ICH Harmonized Tripartite Guideline: Q6A Specifications: Test Procedures and Acceptance Criteria for New Drug Substances and New Drug Products: Chemical Substances.*

30. International Conference of Harmonization (2006). *ICH Harmonized Tripartite Guideline: Q3B(R2) Impurities in New Drug Products.*

31. International Conference of Harmonization (2018). *ICH Harmonized Tripartite Guideline: Q3C(R8) Impurities: Guideline for Residual Solvents.*

32. Food and Drug Administration (2018a). *Liposome Drug Products.*

33. Food and Drug Administration (2012). *Quality by Design for ANDAs: An Example for Immediate-Release Dosage Forms.*

34. Lohan, S., Raza, K., Mehta, S. K., Bhatti, G. K., Saini, S., Singh, B. (2017). Anti-Alzheimer's potential of berberine using surface decorated multi-walled carbon nanotubes: a preclinical evidence. *Int. J. Pharm.*, **530**(1–2), 263–278.

35. Xu, X., Khan, M. A., Burgess, D. J. (2011). A quality by design (QbD) case study on liposomes containing hydrophilic API: I. Formulation, processing design and risk assessment. *Int. J. Pharm.*, **419**(1–2), 52–59.

36. Eriksson, L. (2000). *Design of Experiments: Principles and Applications*, 3rd ed., Umetrics Academy.

37. Politis, S.N., Colombo, P., Colombo, G., Rekkas, D. M. (2017). Design of experiments (DoE) in pharmaceutical development. *Drug Dev. Ind. Pharm.*, **43**(6), 889–901.

38. Bragagni, M., Mura, P., Mennini, N., Ghelardini, C., Orlandini, S., Furlanetto, S. (2014). Development and characterization of functionalized niosomes for brain targeting of dynorphin-B. *Eur. J. Pharm.Biopharm.*, **87**(1), 73–79.

39. Shah, V., Sharma, M., Pandya, R., Parikh, R. K., Bharatiya, B., Shukla, A., Tsai, H. C. (2017). Quality by design approach for an in situ gelling microemulsion of Lorazepam via intranasal route. *Mater. Sci. Eng. C*, **75**, 1231–1241.

40. Toyota, H., Asai, T., Oku, N. (2017). Process optimization by use of design of experiments: application for liposomalization of FK506. *Eur. J. Pharm. Sci.*, **102**, 196–202.

41. Đorđević, S. M., Radulović, T. S., Cekić, N. D., Randelović, D. V., Savić, M. M., Krajišnik, D. R., Milić, J. R.,Savić, S. D. (2013). Experimental design in formulation of diazepam nanoemulsions: physicochemical and pharmacokinetic performances. *J. Pharm. Sci.*, **102**(11), 4159–4172.

42. Kamal, N., Cutie, A. J., Habib, M. J., Zidan, A. S. (2015). QbD approach to investigate product and process variabilities for brain targeting liposomes. *J. Liposome Res.*, **25**(3), 175–190.

43. Boukouvala, F., Muzzio, F. J., Ierapetritou, M. G. (2010). Design space of pharmaceutical processes using data-driven-based methods. *J. Pharm. Innovation*, **5**(3), 119–137.

44. American Pharmaceutical Review (2018). Process control and monitoring for continuous production of biopharmaceuticals. Retrieved March 16, 2019, from https://www.americanpharmaceuticalreview.com/Featured-Articles/348877-Process-Control-and-Monitoring-for-Continuous-Production-of-Biopharmaceuticals/.

45. Kapoor, M., Lee, S. L., Tyner, K. M. (2017). Liposomal drug product development and quality: current US experience and perspective. *AAPS J.*, **19**(3), 632–641.

Chapter 12

Recent in vitro Models for the Blood–Brain Barrier

João Basso,[a,b,*] Maria Mendes,[a,c,*] Maria Ferreira,[a] João Sousa,[a,b] Alberto Pais[b] and Carla Vitorino[a,b,c]
[a]*Faculty of Pharmacy, University of Coimbra, Pólo das Ciências da Saúde, Azinhaga de Santa Comba, 3000-548 Coimbra, Portugal*
[b]*Coimbra Chemistry Centre, Department of Chemistry, University of Coimbra, Rua Larga, 3004-535 Coimbra, Portugal*
[c]*Centre for Neurosciences and Cell Biology (CNC), University of Coimbra, Faculty of Medicine, Rua Larga, Pólo I, 1st floor, 3004-504 Coimbra, Portugal*
csvitorino@ff.uc.pt

The blood–brain barrier (BBB) is essential for the regulation and maintenance of the neurological function and homeostasis of the brain, being a complex cellular system which strictly controls the transport of substances between the blood circulation and brain tissue. Several central nervous system (CNS) disorders may, however, lead to impairment in the BBB integrity. As such, further insights on the brain pathophysiology are required. An understanding of the brain microenvironment and underlying response mechanisms is

*These authors contributed equally to this chapter.

Nanoparticles for Brain Drug Delivery
Edited by Carla Vitorino, Andreia Jorge and Alberto Pais

ISBN 978-981-4877-31-2 (Hardcover), 978-1-003-11932-6 (eBook)
www.jennystanford.com

crucial for the development of several in vitro models which mimic in vivo conditions, designed for diverse purposes and studies. Through the correlation between BBB function and the pathogenicity of the target disease, in vitro models enable both the analysis of the BBB influence in the CNS disorders and the exploration of the BBB as a promising target for pharmacological modulation.

This chapter provides a comprehensive and detailed description of the currently existing in vitro models of the BBB, addressing the advantages and drawbacks of each mentioned model (monolayer cultures, Transwell cultures and microfluidic systems), on a comparative perspective.

12.1 Introduction to Blood–Brain Barrier Models

The concept of the blood-brain barrier (BBB) is not new. In fact, it arose between the late ends of the 19th and the beginning of the 20th century, after the intravenous or intrathecal administration of dyes resulted in selective compartmental organ staining [1]. The BBB is a physical and chemical barrier which plays a vital role in maintaining the homeostasis of the central nervous system (CNS) by controlling the transport of substances and drugs between the systemic blood circulation and the brain tissue. Therefore, not only the BBB mediates the transport of nutrients and metabolites to the brain, it also prevents the crossover of toxic substances and pathogens and their action within the CNS [2]. The dysfunction or disruption of this barrier is associated to several neurological conditions, including Alzheimer's disease, brain infections, brain tumours, epilepsy, ischaemic stroke, multiple and amyotrophic lateral sclerosis and traumatic brain injuries [3, 4].

The anatomical and physiological structure of the BBB includes the relationship between endothelial cells, pericytes, neurons, astrocytes and the extracellular matrix (ECM), thus establishing a neurovascular unit [2]. Cerebral capillaries are composed of series of endothelial cells which completely surround the lumen and are connected by junctional complexes which include tight, adherens and gap junctions [5].

Studies on the structure and function of the BBB are extremely importance, as neurological disorders are considered the second leading cause of death worldwide [6].

Clarifying the details of the BBB transport mechanism is a very important step towards a successful drug delivery to the brain and understanding what occurs within this organ. As a result, various strategies are being developed to accurately reproduce the microenvironmental complex and predominant extracellular conditions of the brain. These models also aim at easing the measurement of biological phenomena with high resolution and high throughput.

Hence, BBB models are a powerful tool for the pharmaceutical industry and academia to identify novel and commercialised drugs and compounds which easily pass the BBB and are effective at treating CNS disorders. Ideally, and to approximate in vitro assays to in vivo conditions, a BBB-on-chip model should be able to simulate the organisation and unique characteristics of the BBB, thus reflecting its physiological complexity and endothelium with barrier function. These models should not only possess the same cell types, distribution (3D vessel-like structure of endothelial cells), cell–cell junctions and a polarised expression of influential proteins, but also reproduce the selective permeability, low fluid phase activity and transport processes and pathways of different substances by expressing the same enzymes, receptors, transporters and efflux transporters as those expressed in vivo [7]. The interaction between different cells is also an important factor, as it plays an important role in preserving tissue function, regeneration and repairing [8]. High transepithelial electrical resistance (TEER) values, high selective permeability to different molecules and shear stress are also envisioned, as these are characteristic of this barrier [7].

Several experimental BBB models have been developed during the last decades to study its function and anatomy, which may be grouped in in vivo and in vitro models. The first use consists on experimentation in living animals to closely mimic the complexity of the BBB microenvironment, since the experiments usually occur under natural conditions and with an intact membrane. The use of animal models by the industry, as tools for pharmacokinetic and pharmacodynamic studies, is still a requirement before the translation to human clinical trials. Nonetheless, there are some drawbacks to the use of these models, including the animal acquisition and the experimentation, which are both expensive and time consuming. Ethical concerns on the use and protection of laboratory animals for scientific purposes should also be considered, as well as the four Rs policy: replacement, responsibility, refinement and reduction [9]. Finally, the data obtained from animal experimentation is obtained from a different species, thus being considerate an approximation of the human environment. Therefore, there is commonly a lack of correlation between animal and human studies, which may be ascribed to differences in protein expression and physiology (cross-species differences) and poorly designed studies [10].

In vitro cellular BBB models include monolayer cultures, Transwell (co-)cultures, spheroids and microfluidic systems [11]. These approaches are based on cell culturing and provide some advantages over animal models, including a reduced cost and labour. Importantly, they may be developed using human cell cultures.

The use of endothelial cells alone or in combination with other components of the neurovascular units, in a controlled environment, is a frequently adopted strategy to yield a significant amount of data, with these models presenting a good reproducibility and high-throughput screening performance. To reproduce the physical barrier between the endothelial lumen and the brain tissue, cells are cultured over a microporous membrane, which separates the upper (luminal) compartment from the lower (abluminal) compartment. These are the Transwell models, the most common approach for BBB modelling. The simpler models rely on the use of endothelial cells over the membrane. However, these models do not take into consideration the communication between endothelial cells and other types of cells. A more trustworthy approach includes the co-culture of different types of cells, thus better reproducing the respective physiological interaction. While endothelial cells are cultured on the upper compartment, pericytes, astrocytes and/or neurons are cultured on the lower compartment [11].

Transwell BBB models are static systems, that is, they do not contemplate the free flow of fluids and the shear stress forces on the endothelial cells. In addition, most of the described models in the literature are incomplete co-culture models of the neurovascular unit. Altogether, these approaches do not fully replicate the microenvironment and physiological behaviour of the BBB. The use of microfluidic systems attempts to overtake these current limitations of the in vitro Transwell models. A brief comparison between in vivo and in vitro BBB modelling is presented in Table 12.1.

Table 12.1 Brief comparison between in vitro and in vivo BBB models

	In vivo	In vitro		
Properties	**Rodents**	**Monolayer cultures**	**Transwell cultures**	**Microfluidic systems**
Simulated microenvironment	Yes	No	Limited	Yes
Controlled microenvironment	No	Yes	Yes	Yes
Fluid flow system	Yes	No	No	Yes
Organ-level function	Yes	Limited	Limited	Potentially
Quantitative analysis of BBB properties	Limited	Limited	Limited	Yes
Real-time readouts	Limited	Limited	Limited	Yes
High-throughput screening	No	Yes	Yes	Potentially
PK/PD evaluation	Yes	No	No	Potentially
Human cell origin	No	Yes	Yes	Yes
Development of personalised medicine	No	Yes	Yes	Yes
Complexity	Moderate	Low	Low	High
Cost	High	Low	Low	Moderate

Source: Adapted with permission from Ref. [7], Copyright (2018), with permission from Elsevier.
BBB, blood–brain barrier; PK, pharmacokinetic; PD, pharmacodynamic.

12.2 Microfluidic BBB Models

The BBB-on-chip models are a new generation of in vitro approaches which emerged following the development of microfluidic technology and sensor engineering [12]. The geometrical, biochemical and mechanical features of these microsystems are finely tuned, thus promoting a close reproduction of the microenvironment of the BBB in vivo. In addition, these systems are highly regulated and are able to generate a good amount of physiological and pathological data in response of external stimuli [13, 14]. Similar to Transwell models, microfluidic BBB systems are also appropriate for the co-culture of several types of human cells which compose the microvascular unit. Yet, they present a major advantage over Transwell models: they take into consideration the dynamic flows and shear stress suffered by endothelial cells. Note that the integrity of the barrier is affected by shear stress forces, and in their absence, the membrane integrity is much lower. While TEER measurements in static models are usually lower than 200 Ω cm^2, microfluidic systems usually present higher values of resistance, with some of them closer to the 1500 to 8000 Ω cm^2 range of in vivo models [15–19].

Commonly, microfluidic models use a porous membrane to form structures in the chip, separating the endothelial from the remaining cells, with the membrane separating two microchannels, denoted as neural and vascular chambers (Fig. 12.1). These two microchannels promote the circulation of the culture medium, mimicking the movement of blood and extracellular fluids [20].

According to the design of microfluidic BBB models, they can be organised in four different categories: sandwich, parallel, 3D tubular structure and vasculogenesis design [21].

The sandwich design resembles the layout of Transwell models, with the co-culturing of endothelial and other cells being performed vertically, on the upper and lower side of the membrane, respectively. This evolved model uses polycarbonate or, more recently, polytetrafluoroethylene membranes to separate the chambers. The seeding configuration, the height of the channel and the opacity of the polycarbonate membranes makes difficult the interaction between cells and the real-time acquisition of high-resolution images, with the polytetrafluoroethylene membranes partially overcoming this imaging drawback [22].

In parallel design, the co-culturing occurs in a horizontal and parallel disposition, separated by an array of polydimethylsiloxane

(PDMS) microchannels. These devices are easier to assemble and promote a stronger cell–cell interaction and easier imaging [23]. Yet, the microchannels are typically thicker than the polycarbonate membranes (0.2–3 μm vs. 50 μm) [24]. To overcome this issue, ECM gel-based barriers, like collagen gels, have demonstrated good ability to simultaneously support astrocytes and neurons and to physically separate endothelial cells from the remaining, showing a more physiological thickness, protein composition and stiffness [17, 25].

The PDMS microchannels are usually manufactured with a rectangular cross section. This nonphysiological geometry promotes an irregular shear stress profile due to a non-uniform flow. As a consequence, the characteristics in terms of morphology and behaviour, of endothelial cells throughout the microchannels are also variable [26]. In 3D tubular structure designs, the microchannels are cylindrical, thus creating a constant shear stress along the inner walls [26]. These are generally achieved using ECM gel-derived matrices, as they are mouldable and can form cylindric hollow structures [27, 28]. However, they are not yet able to develop tight barriers with elevated TEER measurements [28].

Using different production strategies and materials, the scaffolds of the microvessels are first created and the endothelial cells are subsequently seeded to form the microvessels themselves. This is the basis of the formation of the microvessels in parallel and 3D tubular structure designs. In vasculogenesis designs, there are no previously formed scaffolds. Instead, endothelial cells are seeded next to a collagen matrix or fibrin hydrogel and allowed to sprout and form de novo microvessels [29, 30]. These more natural structures may better reproduce the interactions between the cells of the neurovascular units. Nevertheless, these models are more irregular and possess a higher variability and lower experimental reproducibility [21].

Microfluidic chips present unique advantages over other BBB models. The chips are easy to manufacture, include several functional units, present a moderate cost and can be tailor-made to meet specific needs. The integration of electrodes and the use of real-time high-resolution imaging, TEER measurements and data collection fit them for a wide range of applications (Fig. 12.1).

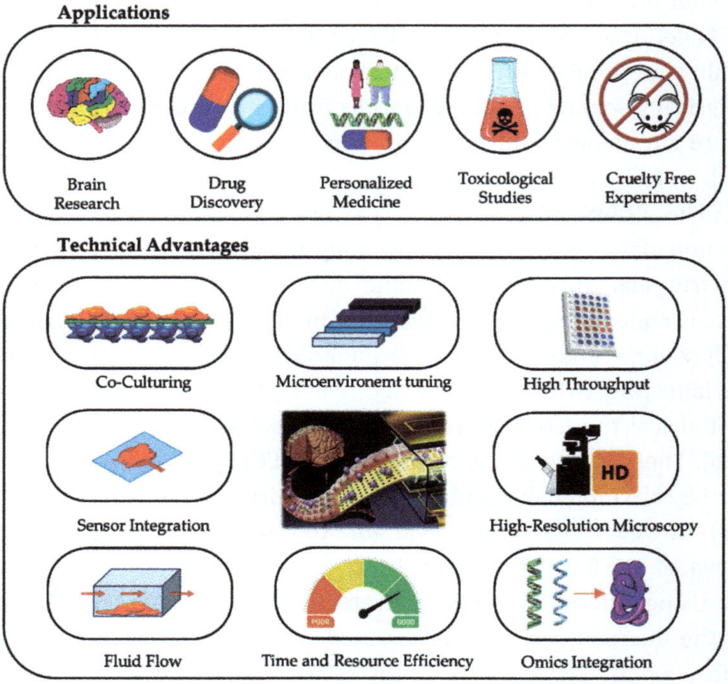

Figure 12.1 Applications and technical advantages of BBB-on-chip models. Microfluidic BBB models emerged from the development of microfluidics and sensor engineering and are a promising strategy to study the human BBB. These flexible devices may be used in fundamental brain research, as well as in the development of novel therapies, personalised medicine and toxicological studies. Additionally, they are a favourable alternative to in vivo animal testing. These time and resourceful approaches enable cell co-culturing, fluid flow and microenvironment tuning; are suitable for high-resolution microscopy, sensor and omics integration; and are a powerful tool for high-throughput screening of compounds. Reprinted from Ref. [21], Copyright (2019), with permission from Elsevier.

A brief analysis of microfluidic systems for BBB modelling is presented in Table 12.2.

Table 12.2 Brief overview of BBB microfluidic models

Specifications	Characterisation methods	Cells type	Main conclusions	Refs.
• Microfluidic BBB model to mimic drug delivery into the brain, assess drug permeability and cytotoxicity of CNS drug candidates • Resembles in vivo BBB and glioma microenvironments	• Structural integrity validated through immunostaining of tight junction proteins • Permeability analysis using two fluorescent tracers: sodium fluorescein (NaFL, $M_w = 376$) and FITC-dextran 70 kD (FD70, $M_w = 70$ kD) • TEER	• hCMEC/D3 • Glioblastoma cells (U-251)	• Better simulation of human cerebral microenvironment, adjusted flow rate to mimic in vivo BBB • Permeability of drug was highly correlated with literature-reported value • 48 h after treatment, the survival rate of U-251 cells cultured in 3D scaffolds was nearly 6% higher than that in 2D culture models	[31]
• Brain microchip able to culture human-derived cancer cells and to maintain the genetic fidelity of the primary tumours • A tool for oncologists to contribute for rapid response about patient-specific drug response • Use in early-stage testing of new drugs	• Immunofluorescence staining of glioblastoma with tumour-specific markers evaluated the impact on the expression of Nestin, VEGFR2 and GFAP	• Patient tumour specimens	• Drug administration displayed different drug responses between the three patients under evaluation • Temozolomide worked more effectively when used in combination with bevacizumab than temozolomide alone	[32]

(*Continued*)

Table 12.2 *(Continued)*

Specifications	Characterisation methods	Cells type	Main conclusions	Refs.
• Hydrogel microfluidic device for high-throughput screening 1. Multiple simultaneous drug administration 2. Massive parallel testing of drug response • A biocompatible 3D microenvironment	• Permeability analysis with FITC-dextran 70 kD (FD70, M_w = 70 kD) and eosin • Stability and leaking tested with Chicago blue	• Glioblastoma cells (U87)	• The fabrication of this hydrogel microfluidic chip takes less than two hours.	[33]
• Microfluidic model of GBM which mimics: 1. The dynamics of pseudopalisade formation 2. Hypoxia-driven phenomenon • The pseudopalisading process simulates a more aggressive behaviour of GBM cells.	• Glucose profile analysis using fluorescent glucose (2-NBDG) • Imaging analysis for cell distribution • Immunofluorescence staining with antibodies	• Glioblastoma cells (U-251, C6)	• C6 cells exhibited faster invasion than U-251 MG. • C6 cells have rapid metabolism, thus leading to accelerated invasion. • Nutrient and oxygen starvation triggers a strong migratory process, leading to pseudopalisade generation in vitro.	[34]

Specifications	Characterisation methods	Cells type	Main conclusions	Refs.
• The microvasculature-on-a-chip system can provide a functional perivascular niche to assess the dynamics of primary tumour cells.	• Permeability analysis with CY5-dextran, 70 kD • Immunofluorescent staining with antibodies • Imaging analysis	• Patient tumour specimens	• The microvascular tracks may serve as a path for tumour cell migration. • The co-localisation between tumour cells and microvessels depends on the patients. • The perivascular niche of single tumour cells can be associated with transcriptional subtype and correlates with interpatient heterogeneity.	[35]
• High-throughput microfluidic system which incorporates human brain endothelial cells, astrocytes and pericytes and which can be used for screening purposes	• Immunocytochemistry using antibodies (anti-claudin-5, anti-VE-cadherin, anti-PECAM-1, Alexa Fluor 488, Alexa Fluor 555, Alexa Fluor 647 and anti-human transferrin receptor) • Barrier integrity using FITC-dextran, 20 kDa • Analysis of cell surface binding of anti-human transferrin receptor MEM-189	• Human brain microvascular endothelial cells (TY10) • Human brain pericytes (hBPCT) • Human astrocytes (hAst)	• The TY10 brain endothelial cell line expresses relevant junctional markers and transporters. • Transferrin receptor: two-fold higher passage antibody targeting the hTfR receptor, across model compared to a control antibody.	[36]

(*Continued*)

Table 12.2 (*Continued*)

Specifications	Characterisation methods	Cells type	Main conclusions	Refs.
• Human BBB microfluidic containing human induced pluripotent stem cell–derived human brain microvascular endothelium interfaced with primary human pericytes and astrocytes	• Immunofluorescence microscopy with antibodies: Alexa Fluor 488, Alexa Fluor 555 and Alexa Fluor 647 • TEER • Apparent permeability with fluorescent labelled 10 kDa dextran and cetuximab • BBB opening using hypertonic solution • Metabolic barrier function regarding P-gp, MRP and BCRP functionality (verapamil, MK571 and Ko143 are the respective inhibitors)	• Induced pluripotent stem cell–derived human brain microvascular endothelium • Primary human brain astrocytes • Primary human brain pericytes	• The model express high levels of tight junctions, SLC and ABC proteins. • Suitable function of efflux proteins. • The model may improve brain therapies and advances in personalised medicine.	[37]
• Microfluidic BBB model which mimics: 1. In vivo BBB integrity 2. Compound permeability	• Immunofluorescence staining for zonula occludens protein-1 (ZO-1), claudin-5 and actin filaments (F-actin) • Permeability studies using fluorescein isothiocyanate (FITC)-dextrans of 70, 20 and 4 kDa, caffeine, cimetidine and doxorubicin • TEER	• Human induced pluripotent stem cells (hiPSCs) • Rat primary astrocytes	• Potential to be patient-specific shear stress is effective in establishing in vivo–like barrier properties. • High TEER levels can be sustained for up to at least 10 days on chip. • Oxygen and nutrient transportation provides sufficient nutrient and waste exchange.	[16]

Specifications	Characterisation methods	Cells type	Main conclusions	Refs.
• Microfluidic platform of the BBB: 1. Is suited to study barrier function in detail 2. Evaluates drug passage	• Mechanical function assessed by fluid shear stress • Biochemical function assessed by stimulation of necrosis factor alpha (TNF-α) • Fluorescent staining of cells using phalloidin-FITC, primary antibody ZO-1 and Alexa Fluor 488 • TEER	• Human brain endothelial cell line hCMEC/D3	• Platinum electrodes were integrated to evaluate TEER over time. • The BBB function was modulated by stimulation of shear stress and by exposure to the inflammation cytokine TNF-α.	[38]

12.3 Cell Cultures

The assembling of a microfluid BBB model involves the culturing of brain endothelial cells. These are not fenestrated and slightly overlap in a monolayer. They are also characterised by expressing tight junction proteins, such as claudins, occludins and junction adhesion molecules, and adherens junction proteins, including cadherin and vinculin [2]. Due to the specificity of these transmembrane proteins, they are often used as markers for a successful BBB formation [39]. As a consequence, these cells are close enough to one another to block paracellular diffusion of macromolecules, polar solutes and ions [2]. Furthermore, the expression of other membrane channels, transporters and enzymes also contributes to the formation of the physical and chemical barrier which secludes the CNS.

Although more accurate models rely on the additional culturing of astrocytes, pericytes and/or neurons, endothelial cells are mainly accountable for the formation of the physical barrier which separates blood from brain tissue.

Endothelial cells can be harvested from ex vivo brain samples, collected during surgical procedures from donors or animals [12, 17, 40]. As previously mentioned, the development of microfluidic BBB models is not restricted to the use of human cells, and it may include the use of mouse, rat, porcine or bovine endothelial cells. Once purified and isolated, primary cell cultures show encouraging characteristics, including a high phenotypic resemblance to those in vivo and a reduced extent of genotypic mutations. Yet, the use of these cells presents some important inconveniences: their extraction and purification is expensive and requires specialised technicians, there is a risk of cross-contamination with other cells during isolation and they can only be used with a low passage number due to changes in cell phenotype (loss of the expression of TJ proteins) [12, 41]. On the other hand, immortalised cell lines are pure and are known to a lower restriction in the number of passages. The hCMEC/D3, human brain microvascular endothelial cell (HBMEC) and human umbilical vein endothelial cell (HUVEC) lines are the most used human lines for modelling the BBB. The first is a well-characterised line and shows high expression of receptors, transporters and TJ proteins, whereas the HBMECs lead to the formation of tighter barriers in static and fluid shear models [42, 43]. Both lines are derived from human brain endothelial cells. As for HUVECs, their umbilical vein origin and the formation of leakier barriers are two causes against their use in these types of models [25].

Although the use of primary cells or cell lines counts for most of the manufactured microfluidic devices, pluripotent stem cells are a promising alternative. They can be differentiated into brain microvascular endothelial cells, with a good profile expression concerning TJ and other proteins which closely resemble the BBB [44]. Nonetheless, they also carry some drawbacks, such as the high cost, the complexity of protocols and the high sensitivity to external stimuli, which may impair the expected differentiation of the cells [44, 45]. These cells can be obtained from healthy or diseased subjects. Hence, these microchips may represent genetic neurological disorders, allowing to identify disease mechanisms and signalling pathways [46].

As previously mentioned, microfluidic models are extremely versatile and may also contemplate the culture of other cells of the neurovascular units, thus representing a more reliable physiological state. Astrocytes are star-shaped glial cells which perform different tasks in the CNS, including the biochemical support to the endothelial cells, the secretion of cellular growth substances (growth factors, cytokines and ECM proteins) for the BBB function and assistance in the transport regulation across the capillaries. The close contact with endothelial cells suggests that astrocytes are crucial for the development of BBB, and their differentiation is linked with the BBB maturation. Pericytes are found in the walls of the capillaries and are essential to the control of blood flow in cerebral vessels. Pericytes synthesise elements necessary for the differentiation of the BBB as beta-type platelet-derived growth factor receptor (PDGFRβ) and the proteoglycan neural/glial antigen 2 (NG2). Neurons are the main component of the brain and are in direct contact with endothelial cells and astrocytes. They are accountable for the degree of BBB permeability and the control of blood flow, as the presence of neurons increases the barrier effects. Microglia are innate immune cells in the CNS and have an important role in maintaining the function and the integrity of the BBB. For example, the activation of macrophages is one of the marks of an infected brain and suggests that the effectiveness of the barrier is compromised.

The use of cancer cell lines in the development of chip systems for BBB modelling is also a reality. In fact, this strategy proved to be suitable to understanding the behaviour of the BBB in the presence of a tumour. The treatment of glioblastoma and other brain tumours is limited due to the variability in patient response to treatment and highlights the need for the development of these types of systems. The representation on a chip of the vasculature, limited supply of oxygen and nutrients, recognition by nearby cell types and the protumourigenic state within the microenvironment also helps to better characterise the behaviour of the tumour during the treatment. As a consequence, this kind of approach may identify new therapeutic opportunities to target the metabolic heterogeneity observed in patients. Thus, personalised information is obtained regarding the efficacy of multiple treatment options in a clinical setting [47].

12.4 Model Assessment

Taking into account the importance of the performance of the models, it is necessary to evaluate some parameters. Shear stress, barrier permeability and TEER are the most frequent evaluated parameters, regardless of the microfluid models. Depending on the cells used in the design of the systems, other parameters, such as the interneuronal signalling, the release of neurotransmitters (type and amount), voltage and calcium indicators, are also assessed. Cell adhesion and growth is another important parameter, due to the formation of tight and adherens junction molecules which maintain barrier integrity. Immunofluorescence or western blot methods can be used to observe the expression of specific markers.

12.4.1 Shear Stress

Shear stress, a mechanical stimulus, is the tangential force generated by flow across the apical surface of vascular endothelium which plays a major role in microfluidic devices. Several studies have highlighted the importance of physiological levels of shear stress on brain microvascular endothelial cells, with impact on their function, including the induction/suppression of genes, tight junctions formation, cell division and the expression of multidrug-resistant transporters [48].

A recent study suggests that at low shear stress conditions, the HBMEC monolayers become extremely compact and overgrowth. On the contrary, at higher shear stress settings, the monolayer is distinctly less dense and present much less overgrowth. Thus, HBMECs are programmed to resist elongation and alignment under shear stress [49]. At the same time, this parameter is associated with fluid viscosity, flow rates, channel geometry, and flow profile. Typically, in the physiological state, shear stress for brain capillaries is around 0.3-2 Pa [38]. For these reasons, the evaluation of shear stress is microfluidic technology is commonly conducted.

12.4.2 Barrier Permeability

The BBB is a mechanical barrier highly selective to the passage of molecules. The permeability assessment is important since it provides direct information about the barrier integrity and should agree with physiological levels.

Passive transport (diffusion) across the barrier can be quantified pertaining to the permeability coefficient (cm/s). The permeability coefficient is a common measure which is independent of the microdevice design, thus being an acceptable parameter for model comparison. However, it should be noted that other modes of transport than diffusion or active transport may also contribute to the measurement of the permeability coefficient. For this reason, it is necessary to control the solute concentration and the pressure in the microchannels during the experiments. Fluorescent compounds (which should be inert and without affecting the physiology and function of the BBB) are a good approach to confirm the barrier integrity [23, 50–53].

12.4.3 Transepithelial Electrical Resistance

TEER is a common parameter which allows to predict if endothelial cells in BBB models form tight junction complexes. During endothelial cell growth, tight junctions are formed between adjacent cells and the intercellular spaces are blocked, thus leading to a higher resistance to the electrical current and, consequently, to higher TEER values. To allow a comparison between models of microdevices, TEER is generally described according to the membrane area and measured in $\Omega\ cm^2$

$$\text{TEER}\ (\Omega\ \text{cm}^2) = \text{Resistance}\ (\Omega) \times \text{Cell culture area}\ (\text{cm}^2)$$

In the design of microfluidic devices, it is possible to integrate sensors which monitor the TEER, using a low electrical current across the cellular layer [53]. This method is quick, non-invasive and records data in real-time. BBB in vitro models should reach TEER values above 150–200 $\Omega\ cm^2$ to be considered acceptable models, although in vivo TEER values are substantially higher [54]. Finally, suitably measured and calculated TEER values can also be compared between devices.

12.5 Concluding Remarks

Studies on BBB structure and function are extensive to both academia and pharmaceutical industries. Among the different strategies, microfluidic models are standing out due to their advantages over traditional models.

In fact, this technology is a promising approach, not only to study the physiology of the BBB, but also to identify novel drugs with potential activity against several CNS disorders, by measuring the efficacy of drug transport into brain tissue and determining the contribution of the BBB in the progression of these diseases.

This new technology is also suitable for high-throughput screening and for the understanding of drug transport mechanisms. Furthermore, the incorporation of stem or patient-derived cells improves the physiological relevance of current BBB-on-chip systems and contributes to more realistic and patient-specific disease models.

The simulation of the BBB on a plate or a chip is highly challenging. Although the presence of a thin ECM and the interactions between the different components of the neurovascular units are difficult to simulate, efforts are being made to overcome these issues. Additional characteristics which require special attention include the type and origin of the cells, their spatial disposition and the shear stress promoted by fluid flow.

Considering the higher complexity and wide range of designs, there is a need to standardise the experiments and parameters, since it can be difficult to compare the results obtained between different chip systems and with other conventional assays (2D or 3D models). Also, these results should be compared with in vivo models data to obtain stronger and authentic results.

Overall, microfluidics holds great promise in disease intelligence and management, and may be paving its way to replace in vivo and other in vitro models of the BBB in the future.

Acknowledgements

The authors acknowledge Fundação para a Ciência e a Tecnologia (FCT), the Portuguese Agency for Scientific Research, for financial support through the Research Project no. 016648 (Ref. POCI-01-0145-FEDER- 016648), the project PEst-UID/NEU/04539/2013, and COMPETE (Ref. POCI-01-0145-FEDER-007440). The Coimbra Chemistry Centre is supported by FCT, through the Project PEst-OE/QUI/UI0313/2014 and POCI-01-0145-FEDER-007630. João Basso and Maria Mendes acknowledge the PhD research grants SFRH/BD/149138/2019 and SFRH/BD/133996/2017 assigned by FCT.

References

1. Davson, H. (1989). In *Implications of the Blood-Brain Barrier and Its Manipulation: Volume 1 Basic Science Aspects*, Neuwelt, E. A., ed., Springer US, pp. 27–52.
2. Hawkins, B. T., Davis, T. P. (2005). The blood-brain barrier/neurovascular unit in health and disease. *Pharmacol. Rev.*, **57**, 173–185.
3. Rosenberg, G. A. (2012). Neurological diseases in relation to the blood–brain barrier. *J. Cereb. Blood Flow Metab.*, **32**, 1139–1151.
4. Erdő, F., Denes, L., de Lange, E. (2017). Age-associated physiological and pathological changes at the blood–brain barrier: a review. *J. Cereb. Blood Flow Metab.*, **37**, 4–24.
5. Stamatovic, S. M., Johnson, A. M., Keep, R. F., Andjelkovic, A. V. (2016). Junctional proteins of the blood-brain barrier: new insights into function and dysfunction. *Tissue Barriers*, **4**, e1154641.

6. Carroll, W. M. (2019). The global burden of neurological disorders. *Lancet Neurol.*, **18**, 418–419.
7. Chin, E., Goh, E. (2018). Blood-brain barrier on a chip. *Methods Cell Biol.*, **146**, 159–182.
8. Abbott, N. J., Rönnbäck, L., Hansson, E. (2006). Astrocyte–endothelial interactions at the blood–brain barrier. *Nat. Rev. Neurosci.*, **7**, 41.
9. Arora, T., et al. (2011). Substitute of animals in drug research: an approach towards fulfillment of 4R's. *Indian J. Pharm. Sci.*, **73**, 1.
10. Perrin, S. (2014). Preclinical research: make mouse studies work. *Nat. News*, **507**, 423.
11. Stone, N. L., England, T. J., O'Sullivan, S. E. (2019). A novel transwell blood brain barrier model using primary human cells. *Front. Cell. Neurosci.*, **13**, 230.
12. Kaisar, M. A., et al. (2017). New experimental models of the blood-brain barrier for CNS drug discovery. *Expert Opin. Drug Discov.*, **12**, 89–103.
13. Huh, D., et al. (2013). Microfabrication of human organs-on-chips. *Nat. Protoc.*, **8**, 2135.
14. Osaki, T., Shin, Y., Sivathanu, V., Campisi, M., Kamm, R. D. (2018). In vitro microfluidic models for neurodegenerative disorders. *Adv. Healthcare Mater.*, **7**, 1700489.
15. Wolff, A., Antfolk, M., Brodin, B., Tenje, M. (2015). In vitro blood–brain barrier models: an overview of established models and new microfluidic approaches. *J. Pharm. Sci.*, **104**, 2727–2746.
16. Wang, Y. I., Abaci, H. E., Shuler, M. L. (2017). Microfluidic blood–brain barrier model provides in vivo-like barrier properties for drug permeability screening. *Biotechnol. Bioeng.*, **114**, 184–194.
17. Xu, H., et al. (2016). A dynamic in vivo-like organotypic blood-brain barrier model to probe metastatic brain tumors. *Sci. Rep.*, **6**, 36670.
18. Falanga, A. P., et al. (2017). Shuttle-mediated nanoparticle transport across an in vitro brain endothelium under flow conditions. *Biotechnol. Bioeng.*, **114**, 1087–1095.
19. Partyka, P. P., et al. (2017). Mechanical stress regulates transport in a compliant 3D model of the blood-brain barrier. *Biomaterials*, **115**, 30–39.
20. Wilhelm, I., Krizbai, I. A. (2014). In vitro models of the blood–brain barrier for the study of drug delivery to the brain. *Mol. Pharmaceutics*, **11**, 1949–1963.

21. Oddo, A., et al. (2019). Advances in microfluidic blood–brain barrier (BBB) models. *Trends Biotechnol.*, **37**, 1295–1314.

22. Sellgren, K. L., Hawkins, B. T., Grego, S. (2015). An optically transparent membrane supports shear stress studies in a three-dimensional microfluidic neurovascular unit model. *Biomicrofluidics*, **9**, 061102.

23. Deosarkar, S. P., et al. (2015). A novel dynamic neonatal blood-brain barrier on a chip. *PLoS One*, **10**, e0142725.

24. Prabhakarpandian, B., et al. (2013). SyM-BBB: a microfluidic blood brain barrier model. *Lab Chip*, **13**, 1093–1101.

25. Adriani, G., Ma, D., Pavesi, A., Kamm, R. D., Goh, E. L. (2017). A 3D neurovascular microfluidic model consisting of neurons, astrocytes and cerebral endothelial cells as a blood–brain barrier. *Lab Chip*, **17**, 448–459.

26. van Der Helm, M. W., Van Der Meer, A. D., Eijkel, J. C., van den Berg, A., Segerink, L. I. (2016). Microfluidic organ-on-chip technology for blood-brain barrier research. *Tissue Barriers*, **4**, e1142493.

27. Kim, J. A., et al. (2015). Collagen-based brain microvasculature model in vitro using three-dimensional printed template. *Biomicrofluidics*, **9**, 024115.

28. Herland, A., et al. (2016). Distinct contributions of astrocytes and pericytes to neuroinflammation identified in a 3D human blood-brain barrier on a chip. *PLoS One*, **11**, e0150360.

29. Song, J. W., Munn, L. L. (2011). Fluid forces control endothelial sprouting. *Proc. Natl. Acad. Sci.*, **108**, 15342–15347.

30. Bang, S., et al. (2017). A low permeability microfluidic blood-brain barrier platform with direct contact between perfusable vascular network and astrocytes. *Sci. Rep.*, **7**, 8083.

31. Shao, X., et al. (2016). Development of a blood-brain barrier model in a membrane-based microchip for characterization of drug permeability and cytotoxicity for drug screening. *Anal. Chim. Acta*, **934**, 186–193.

32. Akay, M., et al. (2018). Drug screening of human GBM spheroids in brain cancer chip. *Sci. Rep.*, **8**, 15423.

33. Fan, Y., Nguyen, D. T., Akay, Y., Xu, F., Akay, M. (2016). Engineering a brain cancer chip for high-throughput drug screening. *Sci. Rep.*, **6**, 25062.

34. Ayuso, J. M., et al. (2017). Glioblastoma on a microfluidic chip: generating pseudopalisades and enhancing aggressiveness through blood vessel obstruction events. *Neuro-Oncol.*, **19**, 503–513.

35. Xiao, Y., et al. (2019). Ex vivo dynamics of human glioblastoma cells in a microvasculature-on-a-chip system correlates with tumor heterogeneity and subtypes. *Adv. Sci.*, **6**, 1801531.
36. Wevers, N. R., et al. (2018). A perfused human blood–brain barrier on-a-chip for high-throughput assessment of barrier function and antibody transport. *Fluids Barriers CNS*, **15**, 23.
37. Park, T.-E., et al. (2019). Hypoxia-enhanced blood-brain barrier chip recapitulates human barrier function and shuttling of drugs and antibodies. *Nat. Commun.*, **10**, 2621.
38. Griep, L., et al. (2013). BBB on chip: microfluidic platform to mechanically and biochemically modulate blood-brain barrier function. *Biomed. Microdevices*, **15**, 145–150.
39. Maiuolo, J., et al. (2018). The "Frail" brain blood barrier in neurodegenerative diseases: role of early disruption of endothelial cell-to-cell connections. *Int. J. Mol. Sci.*, **19**, 2693.
40. Jeong, S., et al. (2017). A three-dimensional arrayed microfluidic blood–brain barrier model with integrated electrical sensor array. *IEEE Trans. Biomed. Eng.*, **65**, 431–439.
41. Shawahna, R., Declèves, X., Scherrmann, J.-M. (2013). Hurdles with using in vitro models to predict human blood-brain barrier drug permeability: a special focus on transporters and metabolizing enzymes. *Curr. Drug Metab.*, **14**, 120–136.
42. Cucullo, L., et al. (2008). Immortalized human brain endothelial cells and flow-based vascular modeling: a marriage of convenience for rational neurovascular studies. *J. Cerebral Blood Flow Metab.*, **28**, 312–328.
43. Eigenmann, D. E., et al. (2013). Comparative study of four immortalized human brain capillary endothelial cell lines, hCMEC/D3, hBMEC, TY10, and BB19, and optimization of culture conditions, for an in vitro blood–brain barrier model for drug permeability studies. *Fluids Barriers CNS*, **10**, 33.
44. Aday, S., Cecchelli, R., Hallier-Vanuxeem, D., Dehouck, M., Ferreira, L. (2016). Stem cell-based human blood–brain barrier models for drug discovery and delivery. *Trends Biotechnol.*, **34**, 382–393.
45. Chen, K. G., Mallon, B. S., McKay, R. D., Robey, P. G. (2014). Human pluripotent stem cell culture: considerations for maintenance, expansion, and therapeutics. *Cell Stem Cell*, **14**, 13–26.
46. Vatine, G. D., et al. (2019). Human iPSC-derived blood-brain barrier chips enable disease modeling and personalized medicine applications. *Cell Stem Cell*, **24**, 995–1005.e6.

47. Yi, H.-G., et al. (2019). A bioprinted human-glioblastoma-on-a-chip for the identification of patient-specific responses to chemoradiotherapy. *Nat. Biomed. Eng.*, **3**, 509–519.

48. Cucullo, L., Hossain, M., Puvenna, V., Marchi, N., Janigro, D. (2011). The role of shear stress in Blood-Brain Barrier endothelial physiology. *BMC Neurosci.*, **12**, 40.

49. Reinitz, A., DeStefano, J., Ye, M., Wong, A. D., Searson, P. C. (2015). Human brain microvascular endothelial cells resist elongation due to shear stress. *Microvasc. Res.*, **99**, 8–18.

50. Booth, R., Kim, H. (2014). Permeability analysis of neuroactive drugs through a dynamic microfluidic in vitro blood–brain barrier model. *Ann. Biomed. Eng.*, **42**, 2379–2391 (2014).

51. Booth, R., Kim, H. (2012). Characterization of a microfluidic in vitro model of the blood-brain barrier (μBBB). *Lab Chip*, **12**, 1784–1792.

52. Cho, H., et al. (2015). Three-dimensional blood-brain barrier model for in vitro studies of neurovascular pathology. *Sci. Rep.*, **5**, 15222.

53. Wang, Y. I., Abaci, H. E., Shuler, M. L. (2017). Microfluidic blood-brain barrier model provides in vivo-like barrier properties for drug permeability screening. *Biotechnol. Bioeng.*, **114**, 184–194.

54. Reichel, A., Begley, D. J., Abbott, N. J. (2003). In *The Blood-Brain Barrier*, Springer, pp. 307–324.

Chapter 13

Current in vivo Models for Brain Disorders

Marta Guerra-Rebollo[a] and Cristina Garrido[b]
[a]*Department of Bioengineering, Institut Químic de Sarrià (IQS), Via Augusta 390, 08017 Barcelona, Spain*
[b]*Biomaterials for Regenerative Therapies, Institute for Bioengineering of Catalonia (IBEC), Barcelona, Spain*
marta.guerra@iqs.edu, cpfarm@hotmail.com

Neurological disorders are considered a major strike on the human health of developing countries and constitute 12% of total deaths globally. Although numerous efforts have been made to treat these disorders, many drugs fail on effectively deliver their effect into the central nervous system due to their impossibility of across the blood–brain barrier. In this chapter, it is described some of the animal models commonly used to study relevant brain disorders, all of them essentials to solve one of the major problems in the treatment of these diseases which is crossing the blood–brain barrier. It is also explained some relevant imaging techniques for the use of nanoparticles in diagnosis and treatment focusing on the use of bioluminescence to monitor brain tumour growth.

Nanoparticles for Brain Drug Delivery
Edited by Carla Vitorino, Andreia Jorge and Alberto Pais

ISBN 978-981-4877-31-2 (Hardcover), 978-1-003-11932-6 (eBook)
www.jennystanford.com

13.1 Introduction to Animal Models

Neurological disorders involve damage to the central nervous system (CNS). They are considered a major strike on the human health of developing countries and constitute 12% of total deaths globally. Moreover, CNS disorders affect 1.5 million people worldwide and it is responsible for 1% of deaths [1]. Pathological CNS disorders include from neurodegeneration (e.g. amyotrophic lateral sclerosis [ALS], multiple sclerosis [MS], Alzheimer's disease [AD], Parkinson's disease [PD], Huntington's disease [HD]) to brain cancers (e.g. glioblastoma [GB]) or cerebrovascular accidents (ischaemic stroke). This compendium of diseases has many differences in their causes and pathology which require different strategies of therapeutic approach but even though, all of them share a common difficulty, crossing the blood–brain barrier (BBB). Consequently, although numerous efforts have been made to treat these disorders, many drugs fail on effectively deliver their effect into the CNS due to their impossibility of across the BBB. Nanotechnology has born as an exciting and promising platform to deliver drugs to the brain across the BBB [2].

13.2 Neurological Disease Animal Models

Actually, animal modelling of human disease is the most trustworthy technique to basic scientific studies of disease mechanisms and progression, as well as preclinical studies of potential therapies. Much progress has been accomplished in animal modelling and has led to advancements in the understanding of fundamental disease mechanisms of many CNS disorders (e.g. initial cell death and later repair in stroke, motor and nonmotor pathologies in PD). This experimental platform has allowed understanding basic insights in neurological disease, as well as the development of preclinical trials of novel therapies [3].

Yet, controversy and challenges continue to occur as failures in the application of an animal model to preclinical testing of candidate treatment molecules. Many tested drugs which presented curative results in animals failed when they were translated to clinical trials with human patients, and a few of them finally emerged as newly approved therapies [4]. For example, in the field of ALS, only one therapy (riluzole) emerges as a new approval therapy into clinical practice in the past years, and with a modest functional benefit, while hundreds of candidates have been tested. Importantly, many of these failures in animal models may relate to experimental design and data analysis rather than to the models themselves. It is important to identify the most critical biological variables and parameters to subsequently institute an optimal study design [5]. Animal studies not reporting quality items like randomisation, concealment of treatment allocation, and blinded outcome assessment gave substantially higher estimates of efficacy than did higher-quality studies, which explains the neutral results and the difficulties of translating neuroprotective efficacy to clinical trials [6]. As animal models came to be incorporated in preclinical testing and the translational process of neuroprotective drug development, it is becoming increasingly necessary a careful study of animal modelling.

Mice are one of the most commonly used animal models for the study of neurological diseases, they present several advantages including that genetic manipulation can be routinely carried out in the mouse genome. But most importantly, mice and humans share the same mammalian genes, have many similar biochemical pathways and present the same diseases [7]. However, the issue of brain size and complexity, as well as neuroanatomical differences between humans and rodents is a recurring topic which makes modelling some CNS diseases difficult [8]. Large animal models of human CNS disease require substantial resources and dedicated time and personnel. Even so, the benefits in modelling biodistribution and mimicking the anatomical complexity of the human brain and spinal cord may justify such expense [9].

At present, there is a large spectrum of brain disorders which can be classified into: neurodegenerative diseases (NDs), brain tumours or ischaemic stroke. These deficits are the results of intrinsic brain dysfunction or environmental interaction with the brain. The pathological nature of the CNS disease determines the animal model used to mimic that disorder (Table 13.1).

Table 13.1 Types of CNS disorders and strategies to generate an animal model, with some examples

Type of CNS disorder	Strategies to generate a model and examples of models	
Neurodegenerative diseases	Reproducing gene mutations	AD model: mutants of the amyloid precursor protein, presenilin protein, tau protein or the double-triple mutants PD model: reversible (reserpine) and irreversible (MPTP, 6-OHDA, paraquat, rotenone) PD-related pathology
	Phenotype-driven approach	
	Environmental toxins causing the disorder	
Brain tumours	Xenografts models	Altering key signalling pathways Inoculation of established cell lines or human brain tumour primary cells subcutaneously or orthotopically
	Genetically engineered mouse models	
	Chemically induced	
Stroke	Intraluminal suture of the middle cerebral artery	
	Photothrombotic stroke intravascular photo-oxidation	
	Endothelin-1 (ET-1) focal stroke model: application of ET-1, a potent vasoconstrictive peptide	
	Embolic stroke models: microsphere or macrosphere inserted into the MCA or the internal carotid artery	

13.2.1 Neurodegenerative Diseases

NDs represent a large group of neurological disorders with heterogeneous clinical and pathological expressions affecting specific subsets of neurons in specific functional anatomic systems. Some of the most studied diseases are PD, AD, HD, frontotemporal lobar degeneration (FTLD) and ALS among others. The pathology associated with NDs only affects particular neurons which are known as a selective neuronal vulnerability [10]. Mouse models which reproduce spatial and temporal features of the pathology have helped to shed some light on the fundamental features of NDs.

ND models should reproduce the clinical manifestations characteristic of a specific disorder or the loss of specific neural populations. For example, PD pathophysiology is characterised by the loss of some but not all dopaminergic neurons, a loss of some nondopaminergic neurons, and alpha-synuclein-positive inclusions resembling Lewy bodies. To develop animal models of human NDs there are different approaches based on the aetiology of the disease: (a) reproducing animal mutations based on the altered genotype in inherited forms, (b) phenotype-driven approach which uses gene-mapping and cloning techniques to identify the causal genetic change in an interesting phenotype or (c) intoxicating animals with environmental toxins causing the disorder [11, 12]. In AD it has been developed many experimental models which aim to replicate the symptoms, the lesions or the cause. There are AD models based on transgenic mice which overexpress the wild-type or the mutant form of the amyloid precursor protein, the Presenilin protein, the tau protein or the double-triple mutants which develop the lesions earlier [13]. While toxic models represent the classic experimental PD animal models which are able to replicate most of the pathological and phenotypic features of PD in mammals. They can be divided into those using neurotoxins which produce both reversible (reserpine) and irreversible (MPTP, 6-OHDA, paraquat, rotenone) PD-related pathology and symptomatology. However, the recent identification of different genetic mutations has led to the development of more elegant genetic models of PD which are useful to investigate molecular mechanisms of PD pathogenesis [14, 15].

13.2.2 Brain Tumours

GB is the most common and aggressive brain tumour with a median survival of 15 months for GB patients. GB tumours are resistant to conventional radiation and cytotoxic chemotherapies. One reason for the clinical failure of GB therapies is the inability of the drugs crossing the blood–brain tumour barrier (BBTB) and achieving effective concentrations in the bulk tumour and invasive regions.

Brain tumour models can be categorised in xenografts models, genetically engineered mouse (GEM) models or chemically induced models. Such models have provided important insight into our understanding of the mechanisms related to brain tumour initiation and progression, providing an experimental system to discover and test novel therapeutic agents [16, 17]. Xenografts models refer to the implantation of human brain tumour primary cells or the inoculation of established cell lines subcutaneously (s.c.) or orthotopically (into the brain) of immunodeficient mice. Xenograft tumours are characterised by synchrony and reproducibility of tumour formation and rapid tumour development but rarely recapitulate original tumour phenotype and many xenograft tumours growth well circumscribed (not brain infiltrating morphology). Moreover, antitumour immune effects are not present in immunocompromised mice [18].

GEM models are based on specific genetic alterations observed in human tumours. GEM models have been established by regulating gene expression or by altering key signalling pathways known to be disrupted in human GB [19]. Spontaneous tumours recapitulate complex processes which address specific molecular events responsible for tumour initiation and progression [20]. GEM models present a specific dysfunctional cancer-related pathway in a controlled manner and can provide invaluable insights into the efficacy of single- or multiple-drug treatment [21]. However, their use in therapeutic studies is often difficult because of tumour initiation cannot be controlled and they characterised by poor reproducibility [22, 23].

13.2.3 Ischaemic Stroke

Stroke still represents one of the most common causes of death and disability worldwide. Acute ischaemic stroke (AIS), caused by brain arterial occlusion resulting from a thrombus or embolus, is the most common form of stroke.

The most frequently used ischaemic stroke models are as follows:

- The middle cerebral artery (MCA) stroke model which can be divided into the intraluminal suture MCA model where the MCA is occluded [24] or the craniectomy model where a craniectomy and the section of the dura mater to expose the MCA is required. Cerebral ischaemia induced by this method compromises most of the frontal, parietal, temporal and rostral occipital cortices; the underlying white matter; and a marginal part of the striatum. This technique avoids the thalamic, hypothalamic, hippocampal and midbrain damage seen in the suture MCA model. Compared to the suture MCA model, this procedure induces smaller infarcts [25].

- The photothrombotic stroke model is based on intravascular photo-oxidation. A photoactive dye is injected intraperitoneally (mice) or intravenously (rats) and the skull is irradiated by a light beam at a specific wavelength [26, 27].
- The endothelin-1 (ET-1) focal stroke model is based on the application of ET-1, a potent vasoconstrictive peptide. ET-1 could be applied directly onto the exposed MCA, as an intracerebral injection or onto the cortical surface [28].
- The embolic stroke models can be divided into the micro-/macrosphere-induced stroke models and the thromboembolic clot models. Microspheres (diameter of 20–50 μm) are inserted into the MCA or the internal carotid artery (ICA) via the external carotid artery (ECA) using a microcatheter, resulting in multifocal and heterogeneous infarcts, while macrospheres (diameter of 100–400 μm) are instilled into the ICA providing reproducible occlusion of the MCA main stem which results in focal ischaemic lesions which are comparable to the suture MCA model [29]. The thromboembolic clot model is based on the application of spontaneously formed clots or thrombin-induced clots from autologous blood [30].

13.3 Animal Trials in the Development of Nanoparticles for CNS Disorders

Impressive advancements have been made in the knowledge of cellular and molecular neurological pathologies, which offered new approaches and innovative potential drug development for neurological disorders and brain tumours. Unfortunately, their efficacy is still moderate and clinical trials have produced disappointing results, in part due to the lack of successful drug delivery across the BBB. Conventional drug delivery strategies are associated with alterations in the BBB which allow the drug crossing into the brain, but they are unable to restore cytoarchitecture and connection patterns in CNS disorders.

Nanotechnology-based drug delivery methods mean a powerful tool to overcome this drawback. The small size of nanoparticles (NPs) and the possibility of biofunctionalisation facilitate their penetration through the barrier. In recent years, nanotechnology had patented new formulations (see some examples in Table 13.2), especially for NDs, where genetically engineered cells can be used to deliver specific growth factors to target cells [31]. Nevertheless, a major understanding of the toxicity, as well as optimisation and standardisation of their use, is a long way to go. The knowledge of efficacy and toxicity for these new approaches is based on the scientific evidence, and require animals' preclinical trials before reaching human therapy [32].

Furthermore, in brain tumours, the clinical failure of these novel therapies can be the inability of the drugs to achieve effective concentrations in both the tumour core and infiltrative regions by delivering drugs through the BBTB [33].

One successful example is the use of a polyethylene glycol (PEG)ylated nanoliposome (Stealth® liposomal drugs) loaded with doxorubicin (Caelyx®). Stealth® liposome-encapsulated doxorubicin demonstrated a major accumulation in brain tumour model than injections of free doxorubicin [34]. The experimentation was performed using a rat model of brain metastatic osteosarcoma in Fischer rats, where tumour cells were inoculated in the right brain parietal through a craniotomy. Biodistribution of doxorubicin and its aglycone metabolites were analysed after intravenous inoculation of free versus encapsulated version in plasma, tumour mass, adjacent brain and contralateral hemisphere, and cerebrospinal fluid by high-performance liquid chromatography analysis. These results encourage to investigate the accumulation of radiolabelled Stealth® liposomal doxorubicin in patients with GBs and with metastatic brain tumours undergoing radiotherapy. Results demonstrated a successful radioactivity accumulation of encapsulated doxorubicin 13–19 times higher in the GBs and 7–13 times higher in the metastatic lesions, as compared to the normal brain. Moreover, 4 of 10 patients with metastatic lesions showed a complete response in

CT-scan performed 2 months following therapy, and there was no severe toxicity related to radiotherapy or to chemotherapy noted [35].

Table 13.2 Examples of nanomedicines for CNS disorders and their activity

Alzheimer's disease	Cerium oxide nanoparticles, tempol-loaded PLGA nanoparticles [39]	Inhibits oxidative stress and cell death
	Thioflavin-T (ThT), charged and fluorescent biomarker-encapsulated polymerised	Detects Aβ in senile plaques by TEM analysis [40]
	Curcumin nanoparticles	AD treatment [41]
Parkinson's disease	Nerve growth factor bound poly-butyl cyanoacrylate nanoparticles [42] and L-Dopa-encapsulated nanoparticles [43]	Crosses the BBB and reduces basic symptoms of Parkinson's disease
	Coumarin-6-loaded lactoferrin-conjugated PEG-PLGA nanoparticle	Neuroprotection in Parkinson's disease [44]
Brain tumour (e.g. GB)	DOX-loaded nanodiamond	Biocompatibility and apoptosis of glioma cell lines [45]
	Multiwall carbon nanotubes (MWCNTs)	Internalisation in microglial cells, cancer immunotherapy [46]
NeuroAIDS	Indinavir NP-loaded murine bone marrow macrophages	Reduce HIV-1 replication in neuroAIDS [36]
	Antiretroviral drugs nanoformulations with methylmethacrylate-sulphopropyl-methacrylate, polybutylcyanoacrylate and polylactide	Increases BBP 10–20-fold [47]

(Continued)

Table 13.2 (*Continued*)

Stroke	Platinum nanoparticles	Antioxidant property, improve motor function [48]
	Irreversible caspase-3 inhibitor–loaded transferrin-targeted nanospheres	Reduction in infarct volume in ischaemic brain [49]
	Transferrin-coupled liposomes	Promote vascular regeneration and neuroprotection [50]
Cerebral palsy	PAMAM dendrimers and dendrimer-based N-acetyl-L-cysteine administration	Suppress neuroinflammation and motor dysfunction [51]
Multiple sclerosis	Ultrasized cerium oxide nanoparticles	Declines oxidative stress and alleviates motor deficits [52]

Nanotechnology has also offered the first rays of hope in the treatment for neuroAIDS, which until the date has no effective vaccines or specific drug therapy. Dou et al. have developed a macrophage-based NP platform for antiretroviral drug delivery [36]. They designed a novel bone marrow–derived macrophage (BMM) pharmacologic NP delivery system. Hypothesising that the system will improve drug distribution to areas of active viral replication, and extend dosing intervals and this way achieving therapeutic efficacy. Their model was based on loading indinavir (antiretroviral drug) nanosuspension into BMMs (NP-IDV-BMMs) and administered intravenously into naive mice or NOD/SCID mice humanised with human peripheral blood lymphocytes reconstitution infected with human immunodeficiency virus 1 (HIV-1). Cell tissue distribution was tracked by single-photon emission computed tomography (SPECT) and magnetic resonance imaging (MRI) of radio- and superparamagnetic iron oxide (SPIO; Feridex)-labelled BMMs, and confirmed by histology. Antiretroviral therapeutic responses and immune response were studied in humanised infected mice.

Interestingly the used animal models have already demonstrated bench-to-bedside translational potential in antiretroviral and adjunctive therapies for HIV-1 infection and virus-associated dementia [37, 38]. Their results showed that NP-IDV-BMMs target disease sites where active HIV-1 replication occurs and enhances the amount of drug present at sites of active disease affecting bioavailability and tissue distribution. NP-IDV-BMM formulations promoted sustained "local" drug release in HIV-1 target tissues positively affecting therapeutic outcomes. And the toxicities were not evident in animal behaviour, histopathology, weight, or immune function. Promising results have allowed this group to plan a nanoformulation trial for HIV-1-infected patients who have failed conventional therapy or in whom oral administration cannot be administered or absorbed adequately.

These two examples of successful projects of nanotechnology development share the election of a delivery system based on the pathological cellular and molecular mechanism of the disease they want to address.

13.4 Imaging Techniques for Nanoparticles: Diagnosis and Treatment

The use of nanotechnology in combination with multiple imaging techniques has an important role in the theranostics of the CNS. These techniques include anatomical imaging modalities, such as MRI, ultrasound (US), X-ray CT, positron emission tomography (PET), SPECT, electron microscopy, autoradiography, inductively coupled plasma mass spectrometry (ICP-MS), neutron activation and optical imaging, as well as thermal images [53, 54].

Real-time monitoring of NPs allows studying their biodistribution and pharmacokinetics, helping to understand the organs they target and their metabolism routes explaining their desire effects and their toxicity.

In vivo models are essential to visualise NP transport across the BBB, and it is necessary a quantification to monitor NP transport into the brain.

The selection of the best quantification methods depends on several factors such as the nature of the NP, for example, gold NPs are easily quantifiable by ICP-MS and transmission electron microscopy (TEM) [55], or polymer-coated magnetic NPs allow magnetic resonance image-guided focused ultrasound [53]. Another important factor is the cargo, NPs can be loaded with fluorescent probes and detected by fluorescent in vivo imaging or ex vivo by immunohistochemistry [56]. Cationic liposomes are very positively charged and are used to deliver genetic material, negatively charged as DNA. They can be loaded with DNA vectors of luciferases to transfect cells of interest, which are later detected by in vivo bioluminescent imaging (BLI).

In the specific case of brain tumours, one of the most utilised techniques to visualise drug delivery into the tumour is using BLI. The firefly luciferase (FLuc) can be used as a reporter gene and d-luciferin as a substrate. FLuc catalyses d-luciferin oxidation in the presence of adenosine triphosphate (ATP) and coenzyme A (CoA) producing O_2 and photons which can be detected in vivo. Recording of the emitted light by photodetectors, capable of linear response allows for real-time measurements [57, 58]. This technique is based on the stable expression of luciferase by the brain tumour cell line selected for the experiment. Once the cells are implanted into the mouse brain, d-luciferin could be injected intraperitoneally into the host mice, where it is distributed throughout the mouse body and crosses the BBB. The intensity of the emitted light correlates to the size of the tumour and allows comparisons of tumours size across different animals but also within the same animal in different time points (Fig. 13.1) [59].

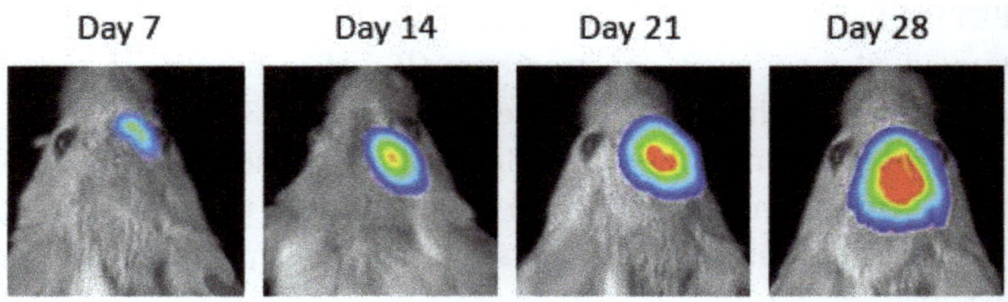

Figure 13.1 The U87 glioblastoma cell line stably expressing FLuc was injected in a CB17/SCID mouse, and tumour growth was monitored over time. The increase in the light signal corresponds with tumour growth.

One study recently published that use BLI to monitor drug delivery into the brain was the performed by Fornaguera et al. [60]. In this study polymeric NPs were designed to treat GB via the encapsulation of paclitaxel (PTX), which is one of the most effective chemotherapeutic agents known [61]. However, it also has many problems such as the low solubility in aqueous solvents, a thing which limits the possible dose to be administered or their moderate activity treating brain tumours due to the low BBB permeability. Moreover, PTX is actively excreted by the P-glycoprotein (P-gp) pump not being able to produce a therapeutic effect on the brain. To overcome these difficulties Fornaguera et al. functionalise polymeric NPs with the Seq12 Sagetis proprietary peptide [62] which targets specific receptors of the BBB avoiding being substrate of the P-gp pump. In order to test the in vivo therapeutic efficacy of this strategy, a luciferase-expressing U87 GB tumour model was used. Plots of total lights events were measured and they show how tumours in control animals (empty NPs) grew faster compared with those treated with NP-PTX.

NPs have been greatly studied for tumour imaging and diagnostics [63, 64] but fewer efforts are made on brain imaging for CNS diseases. Development of imaging technologies, especially MRI and CT has improved the control and prognosis of NDs. An example of these advances is the use of dynamic contrast-enhanced MRI (DCE-MRI) to quantify the BBB disruption in ischaemic stroke patients [65]. Multimodal MRI could also be used to follow the progression of the injury and the BBB disruption after intracerebral haemorrhage [66].

What is more important, brain imaging using CT and MRI could be applied to assess patients for brain diseases. The principal treatment for patients with acute stroke is the tissue plasminogen activator (tPA), but this treatment could induce haemorrhage. Studies using CT angiography show that the haemorrhage transformation was correlated with an increase of the BBB permeability so CT could be used to evaluate the risk of haemorrhage before tPA treatment [67]. Another example is the use of Gd-micelles, which were elaborate as an MRI contrast agent for tumour imaging [68] and they could also be used to examine BBB permeability. MRI images with Gd-micelles show a significant contrast area in the ischaemic hemisphere, indicating BBB permeability for macromolecules.

These NPs have been developed to intensify CT or MRI images for tumour diagnosis. Due to the BBB leakiness under certain disease conditions, it is possible to apply tumour diagnostic NPs for other brain diseases [69].

References

1. Soni, S., Ruhela, R. K., Medhi, B. (2016). Nanomedicine in central nervous system (CNS) disorders: a present and future prospective. *Adv. Pharm. Bull.*, **6**(3), 319–335.
2. Masserini, M. (2013). Nanoparticles for brain drug delivery. *ISRN Biochem.*, **2013**, 238428.
3. Chesselet, M. F., Carmichael, S. T. (2012). Animal models of neurological disorders. *Neurotherapeutics*, **9**(2), 241–244.
4. O'Collins, V. E., et al. (2006). 1,026 experimental treatments in acute stroke. *Ann. Neurol.*, **59**(3), 467–477.
5. Scott, S., et al. (2008). Design, power, and interpretation of studies in the standard murine model of ALS. *Amyotroph. Lateral Scler.*, **9**(1), 4–15.
6. Macleod, M. R., et al. (2008). Evidence for the efficacy of NXY-059 in experimental focal cerebral ischaemia is confounded by study quality. *Stroke*, **39**(10), 2824–2829.
7. Hafezparast, M., et al. (2002). Mouse models for neurological disease. *Lancet Neurol.*, **1**(4), 215–224.
8. Courtine, G., et al. (2007). Can experiments in nonhuman primates expedite the translation of treatments for spinal cord injury in humans? *Nat. Med.*, **13**(5), 561–566.
9. Cook, D. J., Tymianski, M. (2012). Nonhuman primate models of stroke for translational neuroprotection research. *Neurotherapeutics*, **9**(2), 371–379.
10. Fu, H., Hardy, J., Duff, K. E. (2018). Selective vulnerability in neurodegenerative diseases. *Nat. Neurosci.*, **21**(10), 1350–1358.
11. Dominguez, A., Suarez-Merino, B., Goni-de-Cerio, F. (2014). Nanoparticles and blood-brain barrier: the key to central nervous system diseases. *J. Nanosci. Nanotechnol.*, **14**(1), 766–779.
12. Hirsch, E. C. (2007). Animal models in neurodegenerative diseases. *J. Neural. Transm. Suppl.*, (72), 87–90.
13. Manzano, S., et al. (2009). [Experimental models in Alzheimer's disease]. *Neurologia*, **24**(4), 255–262.
14. Blesa, J., et al. (2012). Classic and new animal models of Parkinson's disease. *J. Biomed. Biotechnol.*, **2012**, 845618.

15. Blandini, F., Armentero, M. T. (2012). Animal models of Parkinson's disease. *FEBS J.*, **279**(7), 1156–1166.
16. Huszthy, P. C., et al. (2012). In vivo models of primary brain tumors: pitfalls and perspectives. *Neuro Oncol.*, **14**(8), 979–993.
17. Holland, E. C. (2004). Mouse models of human cancer as tools in drug development. *Cancer Cell*, **6**(3), 197–198.
18. Fomchenko, E. I., Holland, E. C. (2006). Mouse models of brain tumors and their applications in preclinical trials. *Clin. Cancer Res.*, **12**(18), 5288–5297.
19. Hambardzumyan, D., et al. (2011). Genetic modeling of gliomas in mice: new tools to tackle old problems. *Glia*, **59**(8), 1155–1168.
20. Hesselager, G., Holland, E. C. (2003). Using mice to decipher the molecular genetics of brain tumors. *Neurosurgery*, **53**(3), 685–694; discussion 695.
21. Huse, J. T., Holland, E. C. (2009). Genetically engineered mouse models of brain cancer and the promise of preclinical testing. *Brain Pathol.*, **19**(1), 132–143.
22. Huse, J. T., Holland, E. C. (2010). Targeting brain cancer: advances in the molecular pathology of malignant glioma and medulloblastoma. *Nat. Rev. Cancer*, **10**(5), 319–331.
23. Simeonova, I., Huillard, E. (2014). In vivo models of brain tumors: roles of genetically engineered mouse models in understanding tumor biology and use in preclinical studies. *Cell Mol. Life Sci.*, **71**(20), 4007–4026.
24. Howells, D. W., et al. (2010). Different strokes for different folks: the rich diversity of animal models of focal cerebral ischemia. *J. Cereb. Blood Flow Metab.*, **30**(8), 1412–1431.
25. Buchan, A. M., Xue, D., Slivka, A. (1992). A new model of temporary focal neocortical ischemia in the rat. *Stroke*, **23**(2), 273–279.
26. Kleinschnitz, C., et al. (2008). Blocking of platelets or intrinsic coagulation pathway-driven thrombosis does not prevent cerebral infarctions induced by photothrombosis. *Stroke*, **39**(4), 1262–1268.
27. Watson, B. D., et al. (1985). Induction of reproducible brain infarction by photochemically initiated thrombosis. *Ann. Neurol.*, **17**(5), 497–504.
28. Carmichael, S. T. (2005). Rodent models of focal stroke: size, mechanism, and purpose. *NeuroRx*, **2**(3), 396–409.
29. Hossmann, K. A. (2008). Cerebral ischemia: models, methods and outcomes. *Neuropharmacology*, **55**(3), 257–270.

30. Overgaard, K., et al. (1992). A rat model of reproducible cerebral infarction using thrombotic blood clot emboli. *J. Cereb. Blood Flow Metab.*, **12**(3), 484–490.

31. Spuch, C., Saida, O., Navarro, C. (2012). Advances in the treatment of neurodegenerative disorders employing nanoparticles. *Recent Pat. Drug Deliv. Formul.*, **6**(1), 2–18.

32. van Tellingen, O., et al. (2015). Overcoming the blood-brain tumor barrier for effective glioblastoma treatment. *Drug Resist. Updat.*, **19**, 1–12.

33. Oberoi, R. K., et al. (2016). Strategies to improve delivery of anticancer drugs across the blood-brain barrier to treat glioblastoma. *Neuro Oncol.*, **18**(1), 27–36.

34. Siegal, T., Horowitz, A., Gabizon, A. (1995). Doxorubicin encapsulated in sterically stabilized liposomes for the treatment of a brain tumor model: biodistribution and therapeutic efficacy. *J. Neurosurg.*, **83**(6), 1029–1037.

35. Koukourakis, M. I., et al. (2000). High intratumoural accumulation of stealth liposomal doxorubicin (Caelyx) in glioblastomas and in metastatic brain tumours. *Br. J. Cancer*, **83**(10), 1281–1286.

36. Dou, H., et al. (2006). Development of a macrophage-based nanoparticle platform for antiretroviral drug delivery. *Blood*, **108**(8), 2827–2835.

37. Poluektova, L. Y., et al. (2002). Generation of cytotoxic T cells against virus-infected human brain macrophages in a murine model of HIV-1 encephalitis. *J. Immunol.*, **168**(8), 3941–3949.

38. Gorantla, S., et al. (2005). Human dendritic cells transduced with herpes simplex virus amplicons encoding human immunodeficiency virus type 1 (HIV-1) gp120 elicit adaptive immune responses from human cells engrafted into NOD/SCID mice and confer partial protection against HIV-1 challenge. *J. Virol.*, **79**(4), 2124–2132.

39. Carroll, R. T., et al. (2010). Brain-targeted delivery of Tempol-loaded nanoparticles for neurological disorders. *J. Drug Targeting*, **18**(9), 665–674.

40. Hartig, W., et al. (2003). Electron microscopic analysis of nanoparticles delivering thioflavin-T after intrahippocampal injection in mouse: implications for targeting beta-amyloid in Alzheimer's disease. *Neurosci. Lett.*, **338**(2), 174–176.

41. Cheng, K. K., et al. (2013). Highly stabilized curcumin nanoparticles tested in an in vitro blood-brain barrier model and in Alzheimer's disease Tg2576 mice. *AAPS J.*, **15**(2), 324–336.

42. Kurakhmaeva, K. B., et al. (2009). Brain targeting of nerve growth factor using poly(butyl cyanoacrylate) nanoparticles. *J. Drug Targeting*, **17**(8), 564–574.

43. Mohanraj, K., Sethuraman, S., Krishnan, U. M. (2013). Development of poly(butylene succinate) microspheres for delivery of levodopa in the treatment of Parkinson's disease. *J. Biomed. Mater. Res. Part B*, **101**(5), 840–847.

44. Hu, K., et al. (2011). Lactoferrin conjugated PEG-PLGA nanoparticles for brain delivery: preparation, characterization and efficacy in Parkinson's disease. *Int. J. Pharm.*, **415**(1–2), 273–283.

45. Xi, G., et al. (2014). Convection-enhanced delivery of nanodiamond drug delivery platforms for intracranial tumor treatment. *Nanomedicine*, **10**(2), 381–391.

46. Kateb, B., et al. (2007). Internalization of MWCNTs by microglia: possible application in immunotherapy of brain tumors. *Neuroimage*, **37**(Suppl 1), S9–S17.

47. Kuo, Y. C., Su, F. L. (2007). Transport of stavudine, delavirdine, and saquinavir across the blood-brain barrier by polybutylcyanoacrylate, methylmethacrylate-sulfopropylmethacrylate, and solid lipid nanoparticles. *Int. J. Pharm.*, **340**(1–2), 143–152.

48. Takamiya, M., et al. (2012). Strong neuroprotection with a novel platinum nanoparticle against ischemic stroke- and tissue plasminogen activator-related brain damages in mice. *Neuroscience*, **221**, 47–55.

49. Karatas, H., et al. (2009). A nanomedicine transports a peptide caspase-3 inhibitor across the blood-brain barrier and provides neuroprotection. *J. Neurosci.*, **29**(44), 13761–13769.

50. Zhao, H., et al. (2011). Postacute ischemia vascular endothelial growth factor transfer by transferrin-targeted liposomes attenuates ischemic brain injury after experimental stroke in rats. *Hum. Gene Ther.*, **22**(2), 207–215.

51. Kannan, S., et al. (2012). Dendrimer-based postnatal therapy for neuroinflammation and cerebral palsy in a rabbit model. *Sci. Transl. Med.*, **4**(130), 130ra46.

52. Heckman, K. L., et al. (2013). Custom cerium oxide nanoparticles protect against a free radical mediated autoimmune degenerative disease in the brain. *ACS Nano*, **7**(12), 10582–10596.

53. Ding, H., Wu, F., Nair, M. P. (2013). Image-guided drug delivery to the brain using nanotechnology. *Drug Discov. Today*, **18**(21–22), 1074–1080.

54. Saraiva, C., et al. (2016). Nanoparticle-mediated brain drug delivery: overcoming blood-brain barrier to treat neurodegenerative diseases. *J. Control. Release*, **235**, 34–47.
55. Etame, A. B., et al. (2011). Design and potential application of PEGylated gold nanoparticles with size-dependent permeation through brain microvasculature. *Nanomedicine*, **7**(6), 992–1000.
56. Zhang, C., et al. (2017). Direct macromolecular drug delivery to cerebral ischemia area using neutrophil-mediated nanoparticles. *Theranostics*, **7**(13), 3260–3275.
57. Genevois, C., Loiseau, H., Couillaud, F. (2016). In vivo follow-up of brain tumor growth via bioluminescence imaging and fluorescence tomography. *Int. J. Mol. Sci.*, **17**(11), 1815.
58. El Hilali, N., Rubio, N., Blanco, J. (2005). Different effect of paclitaxel on primary tumor mass, tumor cell contents, and metastases for four experimental human prostate tumors expressing luciferase. *Clin. Cancer Res.*, **11**(3), 1253–1258.
59. Frenster, J. D., Placantonakis, D. G. (2018). Bioluminescent in vivo imaging of orthotopic glioblastoma xenografts in mice. *Methods Mol. Biol.*, **1741**, 191–198.
60. Fornaguera, C., et al. (2018). Application of an assay Cascade methodology for a deep preclinical characterization of polymeric nanoparticles as a treatment for gliomas. *Drug Deliv.*, **25**(1), 472–483.
61. Crown, J., O'Leary, M., Ooi, W. S. (2004). Docetaxel and paclitaxel in the treatment of breast cancer: a review of clinical experience. *Oncologist*, **9**(Suppl 2), 24–32.
62. Borrós, G. S., Rivero, M. F. X., Cascante, C. A. (2014). Polypeptides for blood-brain barrier transport. *Google Patents, WO2014076655A1*.
63. Meola, A., et al. (2018). Gold nanoparticles for brain tumor imaging: a systematic review. *Front. Neurol.*, **9**, 328.
64. Meyers, J. D., et al. (2013). Nanoparticles for imaging and treating brain cancer. *Nanomedicine (Lond)*, **8**(1), 123–143.
65. Heye, A. K., et al. (2014). Assessment of blood-brain barrier disruption using dynamic contrast-enhanced MRI. A systematic review. *Neuroimage Clin.*, **6**, 262–274.
66. Yang, J., et al. (2017). Multimodality MRI assessment of grey and white matter injury and blood-brain barrier disruption after intracerebral haemorrhage in mice. *Sci. Rep.*, **7**, 40358.
67. Scalzo, F., et al. (2013). Multi-center prediction of hemorrhagic transformation in acute ischemic stroke using permeability imaging features. *Magn. Reson. Imaging*, **31**(6), 961–969.

68. Zhou, Z., Lu, Z. R. (2013). Gadolinium-based contrast agents for magnetic resonance cancer imaging. *Wiley Interdiscip. Rev. Nanomed. Nanobiotechnol.*, **5**(1), 1–18.
69. Dong, X. (2018). Current strategies for brain drug delivery. *Theranostics*, **8**(6), 1481–1493.

Chapter 14

Modelling and Simulation of Nanosystems for Delivering Drugs to the Brain

Tânia F. G. G. Cova and Sandra C.C. Nunes
CQC, Department of Chemistry, Faculty of Sciences and Technology, University of Coimbra, Rua Larga, 3004-535 Coimbra, Portugal
tfirmino@qui.uc.pt, snunes@qui.uc.pt

The design of brain drug delivery systems involves multiple factors and cooperative effects which govern the success of targeting, delivery and efficacy of therapeutics in brain-related diseases. The ability to modulate the transport of therapeutics, including those with antitumour activity, and predict drug permeability across the blood–brain barrier (BBB) faces critical challenges, such as (i) the access to the brain by circumventing the anatomical/physiological aspects of BBB, (ii) the biophysical aspects of drug carrying and transport and cellular uptake and (iii) the complex synergy among the intrinsic properties of tumours.

Recent progress has been made on the use of nanocarriers for transporting drugs to the brain together with the design of cost-effective computational methods and models, that is, approximations

Nanoparticles for Brain Drug Delivery
Edited by Carla Vitorino, Andreia Jorge and Alberto Pais

ISBN 978-981-4877-31-2 (Hardcover), 978-1-003-11932-6 (eBook)
www.jennystanford.com

which represent the target system or process, which are invaluable for dealing with BBB-related features, interactions and conditions at the molecular, cellular, tissue, and organ levels.

Molecular simulations (atomistic and coarse-grained) have allowed describing, at the molecular and cellular levels, the underlying energy contributions, affinity, type and strength of interactions, associated, for example, to BBB transporters, mutated proteins and receptors. At the tissue and organ levels, several mechanistic/pharmacokinetic models and pathway analyses have been reinforced with complementary data obtained from different sources including in vitro, in vivo, and histopathological, omics and imaging patterns.

Machine learning approaches, including classical and deep learning schemes, have supplied promising alternatives for developing computational models able to handle nonlinear relationships and have provided new insights on the complex nature of BBB, by selecting the best targets, identifying the most relevant predictive features, and also displaying high predictive capability on BBB permeation.

Could drug delivery to the brain and the respective efficacy be rationalised and predicted in silico? How have computational approaches enlightened relevant interaction patterns in nanosystems for delivering drugs to the brain? This chapter present a brief but timely overview of the most recent computational methods and models used to (i) construct optimal brain drug delivery systems with special focus on nanoparticle-mediated drug delivery and (ii) investigate the mechanistic details of different brain drug delivery routes and processes, including drug transport, BBB permeability, disruption and diffusion, release and efficacy. The critical role of computational modelling in the development and optimisation of nanotherapeutic brain delivery systems is also highlighted.

14.1 Impact of Computational Approaches in the Design and Optimisation of Nanocarriers

The computational investigation of drug delivery to the brain has been addressed using a huge variety of models and methods, such as mechanistic and pharmacokinetic/pharmacodynamics models, molecular docking and molecular dynamics simulations or neural networks models among many others, with the aim of exploring different aspects at different levels of complexity [1–3].

Some models focus on the delivery systems while others focus on tumour features, either considering only tumour growth or, those of increased complexity, including genetic and proteomic parameters involved in the development of brain tumours. Also relevant for the construction of reliable models is the inclusion of parameters which affect drug distribution into the brain, such as plasma pharmacokinetics, plasma protein binding, passive and active transport across the blood–brain barrier (BBB) extracellular fluid (ECF) bulk flow, diffusion, passive and active extracellular–intracellular exchange and human cerebrospinal fluid (CSF) turnover [1]. The importance of exploring and understanding brain functions and of the use of patient-specific multiscale mechanistic models to predict treatment response has been duly addressed in Ref. [3].

In terms of molecular modelling, simulations have been used to explore different types of materials to be used as drug carriers, to optimise already known nanocarriers (nanoparticles) and to understand nanocarrier–BBB interaction, disruption effects, permeation and nanocarrier toxicity, just to mention a few [4]. Computational modelling is especially useful to understand how physicochemical properties of nanoparticles, such as shape and binding properties affect therapeutic delivery and efficacy in order to optimise brain treatments [5].

Bramini et al. [6] addressed the potential and advantages of using graphene and graphene-based materials to develop nanocarriers to cross the BBB, through appropriate functionalisation of the respective surface to delivery molecules to the brain. The main contribution of computational methods to providing details on the interaction between graphene-based materials and biomolecules is also addressed.

Alternative routes of administration such as the direct nose-to-brain delivery have also been explored as a strategy to circumvent the problems associated with BBB permeability. A recent review on the computational approaches related to the nose-to-brain delivery of pharmaceutics can be found in Ref. [7].

The use for nanoparticles (NPs) for powering the treatment of brain disorders, including brain tumours, Alzheimer's disease,

Parkinson's disease and multiple sclerosis, has known an increasing success in the past few years, together with the integration of computational methods for modelling the key processes underlying the most effective and sustainable therapies [8–17]. In comparison to conventional therapeutic alternatives, the unique features of NPs discussed in Chapter 5, including composition and nature, suitability, biocompatibility and mitigation of side effects, have accelerated the results associated to the targeted delivery of optimised therapies. However, critical challenges encompassing the proper characterisation of the respective physicochemical properties (e.g. size, shape, surface charge and functionalisation), distribution, tissue penetration and the complex interactions between the NP surface and target biomacromolecules [18], as well as the understanding of the drug delivery process, drug accumulation, loss of targeting ability or inappropriate tissue penetration of NPs, together with the translation of NP formulations to clinical scenarios, constitute issues still to be resolved [19].

During the past 10 years, nanocarriers have emerged as promising targeted carriers of therapeutic agents through the BBB, enhancing drug delivery to the brain. However, the disparity in the type of material, morphology, size and targeting agents has made difficult the establishment of a definite design basis and a general library of carrier descriptors [8].

Another critical challenge is related to the evaluation of the anatomical and physiological features of the blood–brain barrier (BBB) which conditions the access of conventional drugs to the brain [20] and also the design of suitable strategies for drug delivery (e.g. barrier disruptions, receptor mediated transport, intracerebral delivery, intranasal delivery, prodrugs).

Computational modelling and simulation, with proper method and model validation, have provided a deeper understanding of transport processes in blood, across the BBB and within the tissue, and have enabled the optimal design of nanosystems with improved and tailored properties, allowing to (i) investigate systematically how nanocarrier physical features and tissue characteristics influence the therapeutic performance; (ii) enlarge fundamental knowledge on the complex interactions, behaviour and impact of such systems; and also (iii) maximise efficacy and minimise safety concerns.

14.2 Understanding BBB Permeability

The BBB is a complex and dynamic cell-based protective barrier which prevents the entry of bio/chemical compounds and the respective carriers into the central nervous system (CNS), hampering most therapeutics (based on drugs, proteins, nucleic acids) from reaching their specific targets [5, 17, 21–23]. Improving BBB permeability and delivery of such compounds and nanomaterials is still a critical challenge generally accompanied by exhausting trial-and-error efforts [17, 19, 24].

Different forms of nanomaterials, including solid lipid, polymeric and inorganic nanoparticles; liposomes; micelles; dendrimers; polymersomes and exosomes; quantum dots; and nanogels have been developed and are summarised in Refs. [10, 14, 17, 23, 25, 26]. Specifically, a wide range of delivery systems based on nanoparticles have been designed with the aim of targeting therapeutics to the brain following administration by several routes (see Refs. [10, 13, 17, 21, 22, 27] for a full description of these brain nanodelivery systems).

The most recent computational studies have focused on nanoparticle-mediated drug delivery (e.g. using lipid and magnetic nanoparticles) and have been in the genesis of cost-effective strategies for rational design, connecting physical and biological aspects of the BBB structure and developing predictive models of BBB permeability [12].

Although significant progress has been made in the molecular modelling of drug permeation and delivery through BBB, it is still premature to propose the designed black-box type models [5].

Pogocki and co-workers [5] have provided an extensive and timely summary of the fundamental concepts supporting the implementation of computational modelling and simulation to the BBB-nanodelivery design. These include the thermodynamics basis applied for medium-sized drug-like molecules and the molecular modelling of nanoparticles, cell internalisation and endocytosis, as well as the models for describing the dynamics of transport between compartments of the CNS and the affinity of nanoparticles-surface ligands to the membrane transport receptors.

The main driving forces underlying nanoparticle-membrane interactions, and the factors affecting delivery (e.g. concentration of nanoparticles, size, shape, surface chemistry and the mechanical properties of nanoparticles and membranes) have raised increasing attention [28, 29].

Surface chemistry deals with nanoparticles' hydrophobicity, charge density and charge distribution and also refers to the length and nature of coating ligands, grafting density and distribution, rigidity and affinity to receptors.

Following a quality-by-design approach, our group [15] recently modified the surface of ultrasmall nanostructured lipid carriers by introducing positive charge via grafting of serine-derived surfactants to overcome the biological barrier and promote the site-specific drug delivery for glioblastoma multiforme treatment. A more effective interaction with negatively charged lipid bilayers, including the BBB, facilitates the nanoparticle access to the brain.

Relevant mathematical concepts and innovative algorithms have been introduced or improved for specific nanoparticle-membrane transport purposes, as highlighted in Ref. [5].

Soft matter nanomaterials including those for drug delivery applications are affected by a delicate balance between enthalpic and entropic contributions, requiring specific computational methods to predict their behaviour. Computational simulations are thus invaluable for solving these type of issues which are prohibitive for experimental validation [5]. Molecular dynamics (MD), in particular, has provided the means to systematically sample the conformational ensemble of complex systems [19, 30–32]. High-throughput screening based on MD involves one simulation per molecule, remaining computationally expensive in atomistic resolution. The use of coarse-grained models has been adopted as an alternative for establishing high-throughput schemes, allowing to agglomerate multiple atoms into one bead in order to reduce the number of degrees of freedom, accelerate sampling of conformational space, and reduce the size of chemical space. MD based on coarse-grained force fields has been particularly useful to explore the permeability of drugs through the BBB by inducing structural changes and controlling the opening of tight junctions caused by a shock wave–induced microbubble implosion [33–35].

Other strategies for establishing the bridge between models which describe the BBB structure and behaviour at nano- and microscales are much needed. For instance, Shamloo et al. [36] performed steered molecular dynamics (SMD) simulations of the BBB-crossing process with the aim of explaining, at the molecular level, the interactions between nanoparticles and the membranes of endothelial cells present in the BBB. The force profile required to overcome the barrier, that is, the force required to be applied to gold nanoparticles to promote the respective crossing though the BBB has been estimated from the simulations. For that purpose, the authors have developed an atomistic model of the BBB, represented by two different lipid membranes, 1-palmitoyl-2-oleoylphosphatidylcholine (POPC) and dipalmitoylphosphatidylcholine (DMPC). An average value of 45.6 A^2/ns for the diffusion coefficient was determined based on the proposed model. Computation of the diffusion coefficient requires a method compatible with this parameter, and there are several traditional biasing approaches such as umbrella sampling suitable for this purpose [19]. Such an approach provided a transfer function model and described the diffusion coefficient through the barrier, confirming its critical role in the evaluation of potential organic coatings for enhancing the brain permeability to nanocarriers upon the magnetic force-driven delivery.

Ghafar-Zadeh and co-workers [37] proposed a non-invasive or minimally invasive technique to deliver drugs or nanoparticles into the brain by exploring the effect of the magnetic field to deliver the superparamagnetic nanoparticles (SPMNs) composed of a core/shell (Fe_2O_3)Au structure (2 nm diameter) through the BBB. This prompted the modelling and simulation of the MD SPMNs in the crossing process through the endothelial membrane under a magnetic field. It was shown that the nanoparticles were able to cross the cell membrane under very weak mechanical forces. A magnetic field in the range of 0.6 T to 2.5 T was established. The maximum magnetic force varied from 4000 pN to 5000 pN, depending on the size of the nanoparticle (5 nm and 45 nm, respectively). The force profile allowed extracting the crossing time, which was controlled by varying the magnetic pattern and the strength of the magnetic field.

Figure 14.1 illustrates the proposed computational model for describing SPMNs and the crossing mechanism through the BBB, based on the applied magnetic field [37].

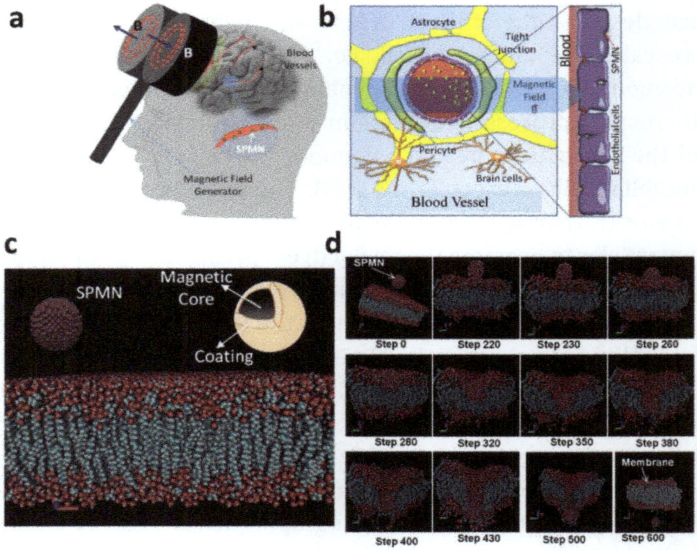

Figure 14.1 (Top) Schematic illustration of the delivery process to the brain involving magnetic SPMNs, including (a) a portable magnetic stimulator and (b) the mechanism of crossing the BBB based on the applied magnetic field. (Bottom) Computational model of (c) a 100 × 100 membrane and a core/shell magnetic nanoparticle (NP). (d) Representative configurations obtained after MD simulation reflecting multiple steps of the NP-crossing process through the BBB [37].

In the context of glioblastoma treatment, the major progress pertaining to computational modelling has been recently reviewed by Miranda et al. [19]. A wide range of MD simulations applied to glioblastoma-related systems and aimed at studying both the integrity and permeability of the BBB are summarised in Ref. [19].

Another innovative strategy which has benefitted from computational modelling consists on the intranasal administration which offers a bypass for BBB, safer and faster brain delivery, enhanced targeting and reduced systemic side effects. This requires the rational design of nanosystems for nose-to-brain drug delivery [5]. In this context, the low maximal dosing volume for nasal administration (ca. 0.4 cm^3) implies designing nanocarries with a high loading capacity.

Several advanced methodologies based on supervised learning approaches have been proposed in recent years [38], as robust and accurate alternatives to conventional physical and chemical methods for predicting drug permeation and delivery through the BBB [39]. These alternatives have adopted physical or chemical features to train prediction models and have included the support vector machine (SVM) [40], decision trees (DTs) [41] and *K*-nearest neighbours (KNNs) [42].

For example, Winkler and Burden modelled BBB partitioning of more than 100 compounds using the Bayesian regularised neural network (BRNN) [43]. The authors combined three families of molecular descriptors to model the partitioning of several drugs across the BBB. The relative significance of the molecular descriptors for the best-predictive BBB model was estimated and compared with other descriptors from literature models of BBB partitioning. It was shown that BRNN was robust, without a tendency to overfitting, and not strongly affected by poor data ($R2 = 0.81$ and $Q2 = 0.65$). The parameters log*P* and polar surface area (PSA) were identified as relevant in the description.

In a different perspective, Hemmateenejad [44] have used hybrid approaches based on principal component analysis to reduce the dimensionality of the data, and different variables extracted from correlation-ranking, genetic algorithms, and backpropagation neural networks, which allowed estimating logBB. The genetic neural network was used to model quantum chemical descriptors, topological indices and log*P*. Final predictions of the three best models were 0.904, 0.943 and 0.979. Other simplified approaches [45] have also been proposed based on linear and nonlinear regression analysis applied for partitioning of many tissues.

Common machine learning methods can only be used for predicting data pertaining to small molecules which penetrate the BBB via passive diffusion. However, for molecules which cross BBB through more complex mechanisms (e.g. glucose) it is necessary to adopt more elaborated solutions, such as the drug prediction model proposed by Gao et al. [39, 46]. This model was constructed based on drug side effects and drug features. The authors have contributed to the challenge of drug permeation using a multicore SVM method (displaying an accuracy of only 0.76, area under the curve [AUC] of 0.739 and an f_1 score of 0.76) but without performing comparisons of the results with other methods.

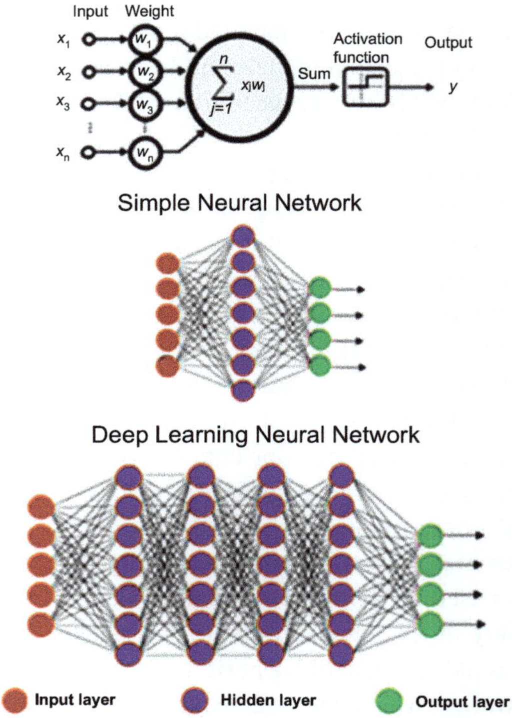

Figure 14.2 Schematic representation of an artificial neuron (top) and a simple neural network composed of three basic elements: input, hidden and output layers (middle). A deep neural network displaying at least three hidden layers, or nodes (bottom).

Liang and co-workers [39] proposed a deep learning (DL) method for predicting the drug permeability of BBB, based on clinical features. The ability of DL to establish the relevant crossing/delivery phenomena, predict structural and biochemical properties, solve critical analytical uncertainties and reduce costs and resources, is invaluable in nanotechnology [47]. The majority of DL algorithms currently developed are based on artificial neural networks (ANN) [48]. Similarly to ANNs, deep learning networks (DLNs) are produced to resemble the brain, in which the information passes through a series of interconnected nodes mimicking neurons [48]. Each node evaluates segments of data and transfer that data to adjacent nodes (see Fig. 14.2). The calculation is performed through the connections, which contain the input data, the preassigned weights and the paths defined by the activation function. The accuracy of the results is tested and improved by recalibrating the weights of the connections.

Specifically, the computational model consists of multiple hidden layers which confer the ability of DLNs to learn from highly complex data and perform correlation and reduction, that is, the algorithm discovers correlated data, while discarding irrelevant data. Each layer combines data collected from the previous layer, and subsequently infers on the respective significance and send the relevant data to the next layer. The process allows constructing increasingly complex and abstract features, by adding layers and/or increasing the number of neurons per layer. A complete description of the main core concepts and architecture of deep learning is given in Refs. [49, 50].

The use of DL methods in the field of drug delivery prediction have achieved promising outputs [51, 52] but is still very sparse in the case of the BBB.

Liang and co-workers [39] evaluated the efficiency of the proposed four-layer DL method in the prediction of drug permeation in BBB, based on clinical phenotypes. The average prediction accuracy, the average AUC and the f_1 score were 0.97, 0.98 and 0.9, respectively. These results outperformed the multicore SVM, DT and KNN methods by more than 15% [39].

ML algorithms have also been introduced by Tang and co-workers [53] for constructing a series of single models and a consensus model (combining several top models and predictors of different nature) to estimate the BBB permeability of chemical compounds. The authors have developed an imbalance learning method and used feature selection strategies for circumventing the initial imbalanced samples of the BBB dataset. It was found (using a 10-fold cross-validation) that the selected molecular access system (MACCS) fingerprint was the best molecular feature for model construction. The consensus model was built by combining the best models constructed based on MACCS fingerprints and 2 D molecular descriptors.

To define the applicability domain of the model and analyse the significance of descriptors in the mechanism of BBB permeation, three molecular descriptors associated to logBB were applied. An accuracy of 0.956 was predicted in the best domain, and the SE and SP values were 0.972 and 0.889, respectively. After using an external validation set containing 92 CNS+ chemicals the accuracy increased to 0.966 [53]. The information gain method used to identify privileged substructures of both BBB+ and BBB@ and the established substructure provided relevant information for discovering potential BBB+ compounds and modify/discard compounds with poor BBB permeability.

The computational methods and models employed for studying the BBB pathology, at different levels of complexity (molecular, cellular, tissue and organ levels), have also been duly discussed by Shityakov and Förster [2], providing a deeper understanding of BBB-related neuropathological events and some future directions for diagnosis and treatment improvement.

For instance, BBB permeation of different drugs, drug-like molecules, nanoparticles and formulation agents could be potentially harmful to the endothelial cell causing necrotic and apoptotic changes [2]. Using all-atom MD simulations, the authors have enlightened the possible cytotoxic potential of cyclodextrin-based drug excipients and hydrophobic carbon nanoparticles (e.g. carbon nanotubes) due to membrane cholesterol depletion or aggregation mechanisms [20].

14.3 Predicting Treatment Efficacy

Several mathematical and computational models have been developed to represent and describe tumour responses to different treatments. These models and tools range from simplistic ones, describing only tumour growth, to more complex models which include environment features and genetic or proteomic aspects related to the tumour development.

In general, the numerical models focus on tumour vascularisation and invasion capacity and on drug diffusion based on mass transport phenomena. An extensive review on the different therapies for brain tumour together with a compilation of the experimental and computational approaches developed to enhance the targeted delivery of nanoparticles to glioblastoma through the BBB has been made recently by Ozdemir-Kaynak et al. [54]. In the final part of the paper the authors carefully exemplify how mathematical analysis can be used to inspect the advantage of encapsulating in nanoparticles a high potential anticancer molecule, delphinidin, to cross the BBB.

Wijeratne and Vavourakis [55] recently presented an in silico dynamic model for describing tumour growth, angiogenesis and drug delivery. By explicitly including drug properties, such as size and binding affinity, the interaction between the changing tumour and the drug and nanocarrier delivery efficacy and distribution were detailed. The model was able to follow tumour–host environment changes as a function of time and thus allows to predict drug and nanoparticle distribution in the posttreatment period. The proposed model comprises three interconnected compartments accounting for the tumour and fluid biomechanical and biochemical factors, drug delivery and microvasculature and angiogenesis issues (see Fig. 1 in Ref. [55]).

By quantitatively simulating the administration, in an animal model, of anticancer drugs of variable size and with different half-times to a dynamically changing tumour–host environment, the model allowed to predict the tumour regression as a function of drug and of the nanoparticles distribution, which in the latter case depends on the porosity of the extracellular matrix. The authors also found that there is a regime where cytotoxics are effective but not the nanoparticles.

With the aim of assisting in the design of new drug carriers to overcome the problems associated with brain delivery, Dutta and co-workers [56] successfully predicted the transport of polymeric nanoparticles through the BBB by a mathematical model based on mass action laws. The kinetic rate parameters for transcytosis of polymeric nanoparticles through an in vitro BBB were obtained by an ANN model consisting of one input, one hidden and one output layer. Besides the good performance of the model, which was able to capture the nonlinear behaviour of nanoparticle uptake, accumulation and transport across the BBB, the results suggested that exocytosis of nanoparticles (considerably slower than the endocytosis) define the overall transcytosis process.

Arvanitis and co-workers [57] combined mathematical modelling with high-resolution imaging techniques to explore drug transport after disruption of BBB/brain–tumour barrier (BTB) mediated by focused ultrasound (FUS). The authors demonstrated that FUS-induced BBB/BTB disruption enhances the interstitial convective transport in solid tumours, improving the penetration of both nontargeted and antibody targeted chemotherapies.

Doxorubicin (as a model nontargeted drug) and adotrastuzumabemtansine, T-DM1 (as targeted chemotherapy drug), were used. Parameters such as BBB/BTB diffusive permeability, interstitium diffusion coefficient, hydraulic conductivity, vessel and interstitium porosity, cellular binding and transmembrane kinetics and uptake were considered [57] to determine their influence on interstitial drug transport after FUS-BBB/BTB disruption. The proposed model supports the effects of FUS on drug delivery and tumour tissue penetration, providing a quantitative framework for the development of therapeutic protocols based on FUS–drug combinations to maximise drug uptake in brain by altering the drug delivery towards convective transport.

Woodworth [58] also resorted to magnetic resonance imaging (MRI)-guided focused ultrasounds to check the possibility of safely enlarge the interstitial spaces of the brain in order to increase the uptake of large therapeutic entities such as particulate drug carriers or modified viruses. Computer simulations were employed to assist treatment planning, evaluate magnetic resonance acoustic radiation force impulse imaging for target validation and examine treatment response by monitoring the electrophysiological and histopathological changes during the administration of a small molecule, Evans blue dye, and nanoparticle probes of different diameters in the living brain.

Walker-Samuel and co-workers [59] developed a protocol which combines appropriate mathematical modelling with in vivo imaging techniques to spatially map drug uptake on the tumour and monitor treatment response. The numerical modelling component accounts for the steady-state vascular and interstitial fluid transport and also the vascular and interstitial uptake of exogenously administered material. For the proof-of-concept, the uptake of a gadolinium-based MRI compound and of a vascular disrupting agent (VDA(OXi4503)) on tumour vasculature was determined.

A framework which produces realistic substrates for computational modelling of fluid dynamics in tumours microenvironment, allowing to perform computational experiments on tumours, considering their microstructure and its inherent heterogeneity and directly comparing the modelling solutions for tumour fluid dynamics and material delivery with experimental measurements performed on the same tumours, was recently proposed. It forms the 'realistic numerical image-based modelling of biological tissue substrates' (REANIMATE) protocol, for which an enlightening scheme is presented in Fig. 1 in Ref. [59].

In Ref. [14] the convention enhanced delivery (CED) of liposomes loaded with doxorubicin was studied through a multiphysics model applied to 3D brain tumour images obtained by magnetic resonance. The model examines the role of tumour and liposome properties (see Tables 1 and 2 in Ref. [14]) covering important steps such as the drug release from the liposomes, drug migration with interstitial fluid flow, diffusion in the interstitial space of tumour and the surrounding normal tissue, binding with proteins, drainage by blood and elimination due to metabolism and physical degradation. The numerical model divides the tumour and its surrounding normal tissue into three compartments: extracellular space, cell membrane and intracellular space. Among other assumptions, it considers that (i) brain tumour and surrounding normal tissue are porous media, (ii) drug delivery occurs under general conditions without the effect of the insertion of the catheter, which is (iii) considered to be located in the tumour centre without examining the impact of infusion location, and also (iv) the effect of cell density on convention enhanced delivery treatments can be disregarded. Simulation results showed that intracerebral infusion was effective in increasing the interstitial fluid velocity and inhibiting the fluid leakage from blood around the infusion site. The effect of each transport property on the delivery outcomes, allowing to establish and optimise the liposome properties and delivery regimen for enhancing treatment efficacy, was also illustrated.

In a completely different approach, Pellegrino and co-workers [60] used numerical simulations to complement their experimental work in which they studied the influence of the nanoparticles features such as surface charge, size, shape and composition in neuron activity and electrical responses. The numerical simulations were performed with the finite element method (Comsol Multiphysics) to estimate the effect of negative NPs on the membrane potential (see Fig. 5 in Ref. [60]). The model explained how a Coulombic potential on the neuron surface retains only negative NPs and simulations predicted membrane depolarisation in accordance with the experimental results. The NP surface charge is crucial for the modulation of neuronal electrical activity. Negatively charged NPs at low concentration (10 nM) interacted with the neuronal membrane, whereas positively and neutrally charged NPs never targeted on neurons, independently of the shape and material of the NPs.

Mathematical modelling and computer simulations have also been combined [61] to predict distribution patterns and efficacy of magnetic hyperthermia treatment in cancer tumour models. The 3D models of brain tumours were developed based on MRI and computed tomography scans. The effect of treatment duration and site of injection of the magnetic nanoparticles on the distribution patterns, temperature profile and the corresponding cell death rate were explored by simulations and validated experimentally on agarose gel tissue-mimicking phantom (AGTMP) models. The amount of cell death was calculated solving bioheat equations, correlating tissue temperature profile with the cell death rate.

It was found that the cell death rate was directly proportional to the amount of heat released from the nanoparticles. Figures 5 and 6 in Ref. [61] show the 3D temperature profiles and cell death profiles of four different distribution patterns in different injection scenarios, followed by mechanistic explanation.

There are also some studies in which numerical models are applied to alternative approaches to access the CNS. Tu and colleagues [62] used a computationally simulated fluid and particle dynamics approach to identify the suitable aerosol particle size and to establish the maximum inhaled dose, between two nasal drug delivery devices, a breath-powered bidirectional device and a standard open aerosol mask. Due to the complexity of the nasal structure the application of direct nose-to-brain drug delivery via the olfactory route is associated with an extremely low bioavailability. According to these predictions, the peak olfactory deposition efficiency (based on counted regional and total inhaled particle numbers) can be more than three times greater than reported dosage level when using conventional devices.

14.4 Optimising Drug Delivery to the Brain

In parallel with the development of a huge amount of mathematical models and simulations to describe, explain and compare tumour progression and treatment efficacy, there have been also a growing number of studies focused on the improvement of formulations and nanocarriers to more effectively cross the BBB and enhance anticancer activity of the formulations. Aspects such as nanoparticle formulation, shape, BBB transport, interaction between drugs and carriers [63, 64] and interaction between drugs and relevant biological receptors have been addressed by MD [65–67], in combination with docking or using ab initio calculations [68, 69]. Gao and co-workers [63] investigated the interaction between α-mangostin, a potential anticancer molecule and nanoparticles of methoxy polyethylene glycol (MPEG)-poly(lactide) (PLA) to be used against glioma cells. Through a joint approach combining experimental and computational characterisation, the results demonstrated the effective anticancer activity of α-mangostin and that the MPEG-PLA nanoparticles greatly improved the efficacy against malignant glioma.

In turn, Wei et al. [66] proposed a computational biology approach to investigate the interaction of different magnetic nanoparticles with α-synuclein. The aggregation of this protein has been related to several neurodegenerative disorders and can be inhibited by CeO_2 nanoparticles. The authors performed docking to inspect the best fitting in the active site of α-synuclein of CeO_2, Au, and Fe_2O_2 nanoparticles and L-DOPA drug molecules as standard control (see Figs. 2 and 3 in Ref. [66]) followed by MD to evaluate the stability of the complexes at two different temperatures, and predict the activity of the α-synuclein in the presence of selected nanoparticles (from docking) and compared to the drug control. The results showed the potential binding of L-DOPA and its interference with the function of with α-synuclein and also the substantial contacts and interaction of CeO_2 nanoparticles with α-synuclein at the active sites explaining its potential inhibitor effect of α-synuclein. Following a similar approach, Metwally et al. [67] used docking to inspect the potentiality of five curcumine analogues to treat Alzheimer's disease. Curcumin was proven to combat the Alzheimer's disease by binding to the amyloid beta plaques and blocking their self-assembly, besides exerting a potent anti-inflammatory effect through the inhibition of cyclooygenase enzyme (COX-2). In order to score the molecules, the authors considered as descriptors, the molecular weight, logP, total hydrophobic surface area, number of H-atoms donors and acceptors and the molecular flexibility. The best molecules possess high total hydrophobic surface area, high molecular flexibility and high log*P*. The construction of a poly(lactic-*co*-glycolic acid) (PLGA) carrier was done by MD.

Density functional theory (DFT) calculations were used [68] to investigate the potential of maghemite nanoparticle (γ-Fe_2O_3) as a delivery system for carmustine, an anticancer agent to brain tumours. Based on the DFT results and resorting to the analysis of electron densities, their Laplacian and natural bond analysis (NBO), the authors found that the interaction between the drug and the nanoparticle was weak, suggesting the adsorption of carmustine at the surface of the nanoparticle. It was found that hydrogen bonding between the drug and the nanoparticle stabilise the structure. The topological properties of the electron density reveal the presence of partial covalent interactions between the adsorbed molecule and the nanoparticle, while NBO analysis suggests a charge transfer from the drug to the nanoparticle. Contour maps and molecular graphs of the most stable structures were used for indicating critical points and bond paths.

Kopelman and co-workers [70] synthetised different nanoparticles with tuneable drug release. The polymer matrix density of amine or carboxyl functionalised hydrogel nanoparticles, loaded with cisplatin, was varied. It was shown that the NPs displaying the loose matrix, released more cisplatin, with a rate faster than 30 times. The relation between matrix density and drug release kinetics was detailed through Monte Carlo simulations. In short, the model consists of a 2D square lattice with $L \times L$ sites. Drug particles are randomly placed on the lattice sites and are allowed to diffuse with time, taking steps only to adjacent sites. When a drug molecule reaches the perimeter of the matrix, it is permanently removed from the system. Some sites were blocked with the aim of hindering particle motion. This means that if a drug particle diffuses towards a blocked site it must go back and find an open site to diffuse into. Particle diffusion was simulated by selecting particles at random and moving them randomly to one of the nearest-neighbour sites. A particle is removed from the system when it migrated through one of the perimeter sites. The number of particles released from the system was monitored as a function of time, approximated by Monte Carlo steps. Drug release was evaluated for different obstacle sites concentrations and different matrix densities. A good agreement between simulation and experiment was obtained (see Fig. 4 in Ref. [70]).

Wu et al. [71] used MD to evaluate the potential of propionylated amylose to encapsulate hydrophobic drugs and release them by the interaction with POPE at concentrations similar to those found in the BBB. The release was promoted by the unfold of the helical structure of the amylose–hydrophobic drug complexes (see Scheme 1 in Ref. [71]). As hydrophobic model drug for the CNS the authors used propofol. The results showed that the nanoclusters exhibited high BBB permeability and specificity, rapid onset, short maintenance, quick recovery and reduced dosage. MD was used to inspect (i) drug encapsulation, (ii) the effect of propionylation on the stability of amylose–drug complexes and (iii) the release of propofol triggered by POPE solution, POPE and POPC bilayers. Results indicated that when nanoclusters contact with the membrane mimicking the BBB the helix unfolds and release the loaded drug, which crosses the BBB.

14.5 Concluding Remarks

Advanced computational modelling has critically facilitated the understanding of the mechanisms involved in brain-related diseases and has accelerated the optimisation of improved nanotherapies. However, it is still crucial to develop accurate computational models complementary to in vitro/in vivo information, enabling the so-called translational research.

In silico studies of glioblastoma multiforme are very demanding, with methodological trends moving towards advanced machine learning approaches. With regard to simulations, coarse-grained models and force fields will be essential for providing an oversimplification of the systems under scrutiny. These should be accompanied by innovative resources and theoretical concepts, serving as the basis of successful computations for brain delivery processes and also for the design of functional and cost-effective nanotherapies.

Despite several efforts, the design of drugs and nanodelivery systems remains a challenge in the case of the BBB. Computational approaches can strongly contribute to a definite solution. However, 'there is a never ending challenge between interpretability and predictive ability of models.'

References

1. de Lange, E. C. M., et al. (2017). Novel CNS drug discovery and development approach: model-based integration to predict neuro-pharmacokinetics and pharmacodynamics. *Expert Opin. Drug Discov.*, **12**(12), 1207–1218.
2. Shityakov, S., Förster, C. Y. (2018). Computational simulation and modeling of the blood–brain barrier pathology. *Histochem. Cell Biol.*, **149**(5), 451–459.
3. Hassanzadeh, P., Atyabi, F., Dinarvand, R. (2017). Application of modelling and nanotechnology-based approaches: the emergence of breakthroughs in theranostics of central nervous system disorders. *Life Sci.*, **182**, 93–103.
4. Shityakov, S., et al. (2017). In silico models for nanotoxicity evaluation and prediction at the blood-brain barrier level: a mini-review. *Comput. Toxicol.*, **2**, 20–27.
5. Joanna, K., et al. (2018). Essentials and perspectives of computational modelling assistance for CNS-oriented nanoparticle-based drug delivery systems. *Curr. Med. Chem.*, **25**(42), 5894–5913.
6. Bramini, M., et al. (2018). Interfacing graphene-based materials with neural cells. *Front. Syst. Neurosci.*, **12**, 12.
7. Bourganis, V., et al. (2018). Recent advances in carrier mediated nose-to-brain delivery of pharmaceutics. *Eur. J. Pharm. Biopharm.*, **128**, 337–362.
8. Yan, X., et al. (2019). In silico profiling nanoparticles: predictive nanomodeling using universal nanodescriptors and various machine learning approaches. *Nanoscale*, **11**(17), 8352–8362.

9. Xiong, S., et al. (2019). Oral delivery of puerarin nanocrystals to improve brain accumulation and anti-Parkinsonian efficacy. *Mol. Pharmaceutics*, **16**(4), 1444–1455.
10. Teleanu, D. M., et al. (2019). Nanomaterials for drug delivery to the central nervous system. *Nanomaterials (Basel)*, **9**(3), 371.
11. Sakai, K., Yamada, K. (2019). Machine learning studies on major brain diseases: 5-year trends of 2014–2018. *Jpn. J. Radiol.*, **37**(1), 34–72.
12. Kopec, B. M., et al. (2019). Methods of delivering molecules through the blood-brain barrier for brain diagnostics and therapeutics, in *Blood-Brain Barrier*, Barichello, T., ed., Springer New York, New York, NY, pp. 9–43.
13. Chen, X. (2019). Application of nanoparticles for brain and lung cancer therapeutics. *J. Drug Deliv. Ther.*, **9**(1-s), 384–386.
14. Zhan, W., Wang, C.-H. (2018). Convection enhanced delivery of liposome encapsulated doxorubicin for brain tumour therapy. *J. Control. Release*, **285**, 212–229.
15. Mendes, M., et al. (2018). Modeling of ultra-small lipid nanoparticle surface charge for targeting glioblastoma. *Eur. J. Pharm. Sci.*, **117**, 255–269.
16. Kaushik, A. C., et al. (2018). Nano-particle mediated inhibition of Parkinson's disease using computational biology approach. *Sci. Rep.*, **8**(1), 9169.
17. Li, X., et al. (2017). Nano carriers for drug transport across the blood–brain barrier. *J. Drug Targeting*, **25**(1), 17–28.
18. Payne, C. K. (2019). A protein corona primer for physical chemists. *J. Chem. Phys.*, **151**(13), 130901.
19. Miranda, A., et al. (2017). Computational modeling in glioblastoma: from the prediction of blood–brain barrier permeability to the simulation of tumor behavior. *Future Med. Chem.*, **10**(1), 121–131.
20. Żołek, T., et al. (2019). Evaluation of blood-brain barrier penetration and examination of binding to human serum albumin of 7-O-arylpiperazinylcoumarins as potential antipsychotic agents. *Bioorg. Chem.*, **84**, 211–225.
21. McCarthy, D. J., et al. (2015). Nanoparticles and the blood-brain barrier: advancing from in-vitro models towards therapeutic significance. *Pharm. Res.*, **32**(4), 1161–1185.
22. Md, S., et al. (2018). Nano-carrier enabled drug delivery systems for nose to brain targeting for the treatment of neurodegenerative disorders. *J. Drug Deliv. Sci. Technol.*, **43**, 295–310.

23. Agarwal, S., et al. (2018). Vesicular systems employing natural substances as promising drug candidates for MMP inhibition in glioblastoma: a nanotechnological approach. *Int. J. Pharm.*, **551**(1), 339–361.

24. Lanevskij, K., Japertas, P., Didziapetris, R. (2013). Improving the prediction of drug disposition in the brain. *Expert Opin. Drug Metab. Toxicol.*, **9**(4), 473–486.

25. Langhoff, W., Riggs, A., Hinow, P. (2018). Scaling behavior of drug transport and absorption in in silico cerebral capillary networks. *PLoS One*, **13**(7), e0200266.

26. Zhang, Y.-Y., et al. (2016). Integrating in silico and in vitro approaches to predict drug accessibility to the central nervous system. *Mol. Pharmaceutics*, **13**(5), 1540–1550.

27. Oller-Salvia, B., et al. (2016). Blood–brain barrier shuttle peptides: an emerging paradigm for brain delivery. *Chem. Soc. Rev.*, **45**(17), 4690–4707.

28. Li, Y., Zhang, X., Cao, D. (2015). Nanoparticle hardness controls the internalization pathway for drug delivery. *Nanoscale*, **7**(6), 2758–2769.

29. Ding, H.-m., Ma, Y.-q. (2015). Theoretical and computational investigations of nanoparticle–biomembrane interactions in cellular delivery. *Small*, **11**(9–10), 1055–1071.

30. Cova, T. F. G. G., et al. (2018). Drastic stabilization of junction nodes in supramolecular structures based on host–guest complexes. *Macromolecules*, **51**(7), 2732–2741.

31. Alagia, A., et al. (2018). Exploring PAZ/3′-overhang interaction to improve siRNA specificity. A combined experimental and modeling study. *Chem. Sci.*, **9**(8), 2074–2086.

32. Cova, T. F., Milne, B. F., Pais, A. A. C. C. (2019). Host flexibility and space filling in supramolecular complexation of cyclodextrins: a free-energy-oriented approach. *Carbohydr. Polym.*, **205**, 42–54.

33. Becton, M., Averett, R., Wang, X. (2017). Effects of nanobubble collapse on cell membrane integrity. *J. Micromech. Mol. Phys.*, **2**(2), 1750008.

34. Goliaei, A., Adhikari, U., Berkowitz, M. L. (2015). Opening of the blood-brain barrier tight junction due to shock wave induced bubble collapse: a molecular dynamics simulation study. *ACS Chem. Neurosci.*, **6**(8), 1296–1301.

35. Theodorakis, P. E., et al. (2017). Physical insights into the blood–brain barrier translocation mechanisms. *Phys. Biol.*, **14**(4), 041001.

36. Shamloo, A., et al. (2016). Computing the blood brain barrier (BBB) diffusion coefficient: a molecular dynamics approach. *J. Magn. Magn. Mater.*, **410**, 187–197.

37. Pedram, Z. M., et al. (2016). Optimal magnetic field for crossing super-para-magnetic nanoparticles through the brain blood barrier: a computational approach. *Biosensors*, **6**(2), 25.

38. Mehdipour, A. R., Hamidi, M. (2009). Brain drug targeting: a computational approach for overcoming blood–brain barrier. *Drug Discov. Today*, **14**(21), 1030–1036.

39. Miao, R., et al. (2019). Improved classification of blood-brain-barrier drugs using deep learning. *Sci. Rep.*, **9**(1), 8802.

40. Jiang, L., et al. (2015). A method to predict different mechanisms for blood–brain barrier permeability of CNS activity compounds in Chinese herbs using support vector machine. *J. Bioinf. Comput. Biol.*, **14**(01), 1650005.

41. Andres, C., Hutter, M. C. (2006). CNS permeability of drugs predicted by a decision tree. *QSAR Comb. Sci.*, **25**(4), 305–309.

42. Zhang, L., et al. (2008). QSAr modeling of the blood–brain barrier permeability for diverse organic compounds. *Pharm. Res.*, **25**(8), 1902.

43. Winkler, D. A., Winkler, D. A., Burden, F. R. (2004). Modelling blood-brain barrier partitioning using Bayesian neural nets. *J. Mol. Graphics Modell.*, **22**(6), 499–505.

44. Hemmateenejad, B., et al. (2006). Accurate prediction of the blood–brain partitioning of a large set of solutes using ab initio calculations and genetic neural network modeling. *J. Comput. Chem.*, **27**(11), 1125–1135.

45. Shamsipur, M., Hemmateenejad, B., Akhond, M. (2002). Multicomponent acid–base titration by principal component-artificial neural network calibration. *Anal. Chim. Acta*, **461**(1), 147–153.

46. Gao, Z., et al. (2016). Predict drug permeability to blood–brain-barrier from clinical phenotypes: drug side effects and drug indications. *Bioinformatics*, **33**(6), 901–908.

47. Venkatasubramanian, V. (2019). The promise of artificial intelligence in chemical engineering: is it here, finally? *AIChE J.*, **65**(2), 466–478.

48. LeCun, Y., Bengio, Y., Hinton, G. (2015). Deep learning. *Nature*, **521**, 436.

49. Mater, A. C., Coote, M. L. (2019). Deep learning in chemistry. *J. Chem. Inf. Model.*, **59**(6), 2545–2559.

50. Goh, G. B., Hodas, N. O., Vishnu, A. (2017). Deep learning for computational chemistry. *J. Comput. Chem.*, **38**(16), 1291–1307.

51. Gawehn, E., Hiss, J. A., Schneider, G. (2016). Deep learning in drug discovery. *Mol. Inf.*, **35**(1), 3–14.

52. Zhang, L., et al. (2017). From machine learning to deep learning: progress in machine intelligence for rational drug discovery. *Drug Discov. Today*, **22**(11), 1680–1685.

53. Wang, Z., et al. (2018). In silico prediction of blood–brain barrier permeability of compounds by machine learning and resampling methods. *ChemMedChem*, **13**(20), 2189–2201.

54. Ozdemir-Kaynak, E., Qutub, A. A., Yesil-Celiktas, O. (2018). Advances in glioblastoma multiforme treatment: new models for nanoparticle therapy. *Front. Physiol.*, **9**, 170.

55. Wijeratne, P. A., Vavourakis, V. (2019). A quantitative in silico platform for simulating cytotoxic and nanoparticle drug delivery to solid tumours. *Interface Focus*, **9**(3), 20180063.

56. Khan, A. I., et al. (2018). Quantification of kinetic rate constants for transcytosis of polymeric nanoparticle through blood-brain barrier. *Biochim. Biophys. Acta Gen. Subj.*, **1862**(12), 2779–2787.

57. Arvanitis, C. D., et al. (2018). Mechanisms of enhanced drug delivery in brain metastases with focused ultrasound-induced blood–tumor barrier disruption. *Proc. Natl. Acad. Sci.*, **115**(37), E8717.

58. Hersh, D. S., et al. (2018). MR-guided transcranial focused ultrasound safely enhances interstitial dispersion of large polymeric nanoparticles in the living brain. *PLoS One*, **13**(2), e0192240–e0192240.

59. d'Esposito, A., et al. (2018). Computational fluid dynamics with imaging of cleared tissue and of in vivo perfusion predicts drug uptake and treatment responses in tumours. *Nat. Biomed. Eng.*, **2**(10), 773–787.

60. Dante, S., et al. (2017). Selective targeting of neurons with inorganic nanoparticles: revealing the crucial role of nanoparticle surface charge. *ACS Nano*, **11**(7), 6630–6640.

61. Saeedi, M., et al. (2017). A new prospect in magnetic nanoparticle-based cancer therapy: taking credit from mathematical tissue-mimicking phantom brain models. *Nanomed. Nanotechnol. Biol. Med.*, **13**(8), 2405–2414.

62. Dong, J., et al. (2017). Numerical comparison of nasal aerosol administration systems for efficient nose-to-brain drug delivery. *Pharm. Res.*, **35**(1), 5.

63. Zheng, S., et al. (2018). Novel chemically synthesized, alpha-mangostin-loaded nano-particles, enhanced cell death through multiple pathways against malignant glioma. *J. Biomed. Nanotechnol.*, **14**(11), 1866–1882.

64. Mousavi, S. V., Hashemianzadeh, S. M. (2018). Poly (n-butyl cyanoacrylate) as a nanocarrier for rivastigmine transport across the blood–brain barrier in Alzheimer's disease treatment: a perspective from molecular dynamics simulations. *J. Mol. Model.*, **24**(9), 252.

65. Lawal, M., Olotu, F. A., Soliman, M. E. S. (2018). Across the blood-brain barrier: neurotherapeutic screening and characterization of naringenin as a novel CRMP-2 inhibitor in the treatment of Alzheimer's disease using bioinformatics and computational tools. *Comput. Biol. Med.*, **98**, 168–177.

66. Kaushik, A. C., et al. (2018). Nano-particle mediated inhibition of Parkinson's disease using computational biology approach. *Sci. Rep.*, **8**(1), 9169–9169.

67. Hathout, R. M., El-Ahmady, S. H., Metwally, A. A. (2018). Curcumin or bisdemethoxycurcumin for nose-to-brain treatment of Alzheimer disease? A bio/chemo-informatics case study. *Nat. Prod. Res.*, **32**(24), 2873–2881.

68. Khorram, R., et al. (2019). The computational study of the γ-Fe2O3 nanoparticle as Carmustine drug delivery system: DFT approach. *J. Biomol. Struct. Dyn.*, **37**(2), 454–464.

69. Hajareh Haghighi, F., et al. (2018). Stabilization of DOPA zwitterions on laser-generated gold nanoparticles: ONIOM computational study of the charge-dependent structural and electronic changes of DOPA adsorbed on the gold nanosurface. *J. Phys. Chem. C*, **122**(15), 8680–8692.

70. Shirakura, T., et al. (2017). Matrix density engineering of hydrogel nanoparticles with simulation-guided synthesis for tuning drug release and cellular uptake. *ACS Omega*, **2**(7), 3380–3389.

71. Gao, W., et al. (2017). Rapid and efficient crossing blood-brain barrier: hydrophobic drug delivery system based on propionylated amylose helix nanoclusters. *Biomaterials*, **113**, 133–144.

Chapter 15

Translational Challenges

Bárbara Rocha,[a] Nelson Pacheco Rocha[b] and Bruno Gago[c]
[a]*Faculty of Pharmacy and Center for Neuroscience and Cell Biology, University of Coimbra, Health Sciences Campus, Azinhaga de Santa Comba, 3000-548 Coimbra, Portugal*
[b]*Institute of Electronics and Informatics Engineering of Aveiro, Medical Sciences Department, University of Aveiro, Campus Universitário de Santiago, Agra do Crasto – Edifício 30, 3810-193 Aveiro, Portugal*
[c]*Institute for Biomedicine – iBiMED, Medical Sciences Department, University of Aveiro, Campus Universitário de Santiago, Agra do Crasto – Edifício 30, 3810-193 Aveiro, Portugal*
bmgago@ua.pt

Translational medicine is currently recognised as a multidisciplinary branch of biomedical research which aims to transfer basic research knowledge to clinical practice. This concept gained consistency, in the past decades, as a consequence of the urgency to transform laboratory findings in useful and effective clinical tools. In the field of nanoparticles, the feasibility of clinical translation is particularly important due to the enormous variety of materials which are emerging, with the promise of becoming novel therapeutic tools.

This chapter aims to present an overview of the translational challenges related to the clinical application of nanoparticles. The

Nanoparticles for Brain Drug Delivery
Edited by Carla Vitorino, Andreia Jorge and Alberto Pais

ISBN 978-981-4877-31-2 (Hardcover), 978-1-003-11932-6 (eBook)
www.jennystanford.com

discussion is focused on the role of nanoparticles as carriers of drugs, the importance of nanotechnology for the diagnosis and treatment of neurological disorders and for the management of brain tumours and also on the challenges of the regulatory pathway.

In terms of clinical applications, nanoparticles are being presented for chemotherapeutic drug delivery for the treatment of aggressive brain tumours and their advantages on the management of diseases with poor prognosis, such as central nervous system (CNS) tumours, are consensual. With this, researchers are now facing challenges regarding the safety and toxicity of the novel systems.

All these demands can only be attended if all the stakeholders – manufacturers, academia, researchers, governments and regulatory entities – actuate under the same base of principles and according to the same rules. Thus, new regulations must be created to increase transparency, traceability and safety, while demanding more clinical evidence and the involvement of experts in the approval process.

15.1 Introduction

Basic research is crucial to understand the principles and mechanisms of biological processes and to characterise the impact of novel therapeutic strategies on the human body. However, frequently, the findings of basic research do not lead to real outcomes in clinical practice. This can be a consequence of multiple challenges, such as (i) current basic research setup and research metrics used by academia; (ii) lack of appropriate planning of research and funding; (iii) communication/collaboration between academia, research and industry; (iv) spin-off policies in academia; (v) uneven profit distribution (with prejudice for universities in benefit of industry); (vi) adequate clinical trial's design; (vii) dissemination of new clinical knowledge into clinical practice; and (viii) modification of populations' behaviours (through information and education) to change paradigms of disease prevention. Ultimately, this state of affairs leads to enormous loss of potential from scientific, economic, and societal points of view.

The concept of translational medicine was first mentioned in the 1990's – but only gained consistency in the early 2000's – as a consequence of the urgency to optimise drug development processes and transform laboratory findings in useful clinical tools.

Translational medicine is generally recognised as a multidisciplinary branch of biomedical research which aims to transfer basic research knowledge to clinical practice – from bench-to-bedside – to improve diagnosis, treatment, and prevention of human disease [1]. In the process, findings from molecular biology are applied in the discovery of novel treatment strategies and integrated within clinical trials, leading to the introduction of therapeutic innovation in a continuous bidirectional flow of information.

The issue of translation has gained importance in the field of nanomedicines due to the exponential growth in discovery, in the last decade, – with uncountable types and combinations of materials – and to the urgency of transforming academic knowledge on valid therapeutic options. Several questions emerge while considering the real-life utilisation of nanoparticles for drug delivery but safety and toxicity are the major aspects to evaluate.

This chapter aims to present an overview of the translational challenges related to the clinical applications of nanoparticles. The following sections will cover: the concept of translational medicine, the role of nanoparticles as carriers of drugs and the importance of nanotechnology for the diagnosis and treatment of neurological disorders and for the management of brain tumours. Finally, the challenges of clinical applications of nanoparticles will be discussed, including the regulatory pathway challenges.

15.2 Translational Medicine

Translational medicine can be divided into four stages: T1, translation to humans; T2, translation to patients; T3, translation to practice; and T4, translation to population (Fig. 15.1). All these address the major hurdles commonly found in the making sure that relevant findings from basic research actually reach the potential beneficiaries [2].

According to the principles of translational medicine, basic research must be carefully planned and conducted in a manner which supports future development needs. At this stage, scientists must be aware of the demands and challenges – related to either technical support, costs, good practices or logistics – inherent to the translation of their results to humans, specifically to clinical trials of medicines and medical devices. Several aspects must be considered and debated at an early stage and with adequate planning: animal models, stability, mechanism of action, target population and administration route, among others. This will determine whether a promising treatment or device will be able to cross 'the valley of death' with sufficient and adequate conditions to be integrated in a clinical trial [2, 3].

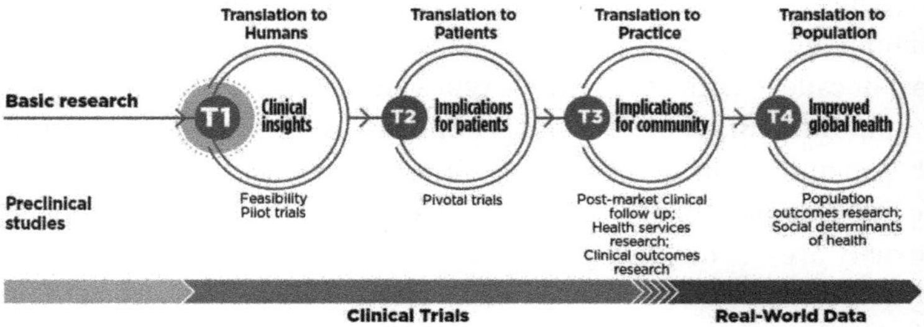

Figure 15.1 Stages of translational medicine (T1 to T4). Reprinted by permission from Springer Nature: Springer, Ambient Assisted Living as Medical Devices: A European Perspective by Bruno Gago, Copyright (2018).

The translation process itself begins with the early transfer of basic research to humans with the primary objective of assessing clinical effect and viability – T1, translation to humans. This is a critical step in which the first clinical insights of the drug/device candidate are collected in phase I/IIa clinical trials, usually conducted in healthy volunteers (although not always).

The evidence of clinical effect in humans must then be confirmed in patients, treated in controlled environments during phase IIb/III clinical trials – T2, translation to patients. At the end of this stage researchers will have insights about the clinical application, efficacy and safety. Marketing authorisation can be obtained at this stage.

Next, research will be focused on the best strategies to apply clinical research outcomes, including patient-reported outcomes, to define recommendations for routine clinical practice – T3, translation to practice. At this point, research is no longer conducted in controlled environments but is rather implemented in 'real-world' conditions, amongst a variety of uncontrollable and unpredictable factors. The main implications of the drug/device candidate for the community will arise at this stage as a result of phase IV trials and health services research.

But, considering the ultimate goals of translational medicine, the process cannot be closed with the translation of results to patients: a global approach regarding whole populations is mandatory [1]. Outcomes must be integrated in the search for the factors and interventions which affect the daily life and health of a population - T4, translation to population. This can be achieved through cost–benefit evaluations, surveillance studies and policy analysis. The major objective of this stage, and of the whole translation process, is to improve global health through the integration of the research outcomes collected during basic research and stages T1, T2 and T3. Improvements can arise both from the generated clinical outcomes but also from policy development in the sequence of the translation process.

The success of the translation of knowledge from laboratories to clinical practice, with the aim of improving the health of populations, depends on solid and continuous communication between academia and industry. Their philosophies and expectations are distinct, but cooperation is the only channel which guarantees the bidirectional flow of data which is essential for a successful process in which a drug/device candidate is transformed into a valuable therapeutic tool.

15.3 Nanoparticles as Carriers of Drugs

The limitations associated with the current treatment options for many progressive and fatal disorders, such as malignant neoplasms, stroke and neurodegenerative diseases, lead to an urgent need to develop new drugs and technological tools which can truly provide adequate support to these patients [4–6]. In this context, nanoparticles emerge as a powerful and promising strategy for disease prevention and management by delivering drugs in the optimal dose range, at the desired organ site and without major adverse effects [7, 8].

However, and regardless of their chemical and physical properties, most nanoparticles face common challenges: first, these particles must have a satisfactory blood residence time and biodistribution profile. In fact, one important drawback of these delivery devices is their rapid clearance upon systemic administration, particularly when the surface is functionalised with other biomolecules [9]. For instance, proteins adsorbed at the surface are recognised by endogenous opsonins, inducing particle aggregation and removal from the bloodstream by phagocytes in the liver and spleen [10–12]. Second, the specific interaction with target cells at the desired tissue is crucial for the overall success of nanotherapies and thus it is mandatory to reduce nonspecific distribution and cell interactions. Once again, surface functionalisation can be performed to enhance specific cell binding, being even possible to target a cell surface antigen with a specific ligand, thereby significantly improving the specificity of these nanosystems [13, 14]. Third, an efficient drug delivery system must be able to navigate the bloodstream and deliver therapeutics in a controlled and programmable fashion. To accomplish this objective, the nanoparticle must be stable enough to resist biological attacks from the immune system and physical obstacles such as turbulent blood flow and cell membranes. This requires not only the development of stable drugs but also the design of the most suitable architecture to allow optimal navigation and anchoring [15, 16]. Finally, one cannot ignore the discrepancy between the basic and preclinical research published regarding the synthesis, development and biomedical applications of nanoparticles and the few drugs or devices which actually reach the patient bedside [17–19].

15.4 Nanotechnology: From the Diagnosis to the Treatment of Neurological Disorders

The potential biological applications of nanoparticles go far beyond drug delivery. The ability to manipulate materials at the nanoscale level (1–100 nm), roughly the size of a virus, and to encapsulate drugs within these structures, creates new and exciting therapeutic opportunities (e.g. to promote accurate laser photothermal therapy in cancer which may also exhibit antimicrobial properties) [20–22]. Indeed, in addition to targeted drug delivery, nanoparticles may also be used in bioimaging and biosensing as well as gene delivery, artificial implants and bacterial eradication [23–26].

The biomedical applications of nanoparticles appear to be so wide that the use of nanosystems in the diagnosis, treatment and disease monitoring launched the foundations for a new medical field, coined 'nanomedicine' [27].

The clinical applications of nanoparticles are very significant for early diagnosis and therapy monitoring of disorders such as cancer and neurodegenerative diseases, being an indispensable asset both for the clinician, by aiding in patient management, and for patients, by increasing the odds of survival and quality of life [27]. In fact, nanoparticles are already being used in several bioimaging techniques such as positron emission tomography (PET), magnetic resonance imaging (MRI) and ultrasound (US) [28–30]. In this context, nanoparticles can be used as contrast agents allowing, for instance, the characterisation of early atherosclerotic lesions in the arterial intima of an animal model of the disease [31]. Also, different types of nanoparticles (core–shell structures, matrix-dispersed, self-assembled and micelle-/liposome-like nanoparticles) may be used to detect tumour hypoxia through optical hypoxia imaging [32]. The decrease of pO_2 is a common feature of solid tumours and increases with tumour progression. Hence, the possibility to detect hypoxic regions, combining optic hypoxic imaging with more sensitive techniques such as MRI appears to be a powerful tool to detect early-stage cancer [33].

Another example of the translational opportunities for nanoparticles is the early diagnosis and treatment of Alzheimer's disease [6]. By using sensors based on nanotubes, cantilevers or nanowires, with increased magnetic and optic properties, it is possible to detect Aß-plaques at early stages of the disease, even before the decline in memory and cognition [6, 27]. Furthermore, these nanoparticles may be used to encapsulate rivastigmine (a gold standard treatment for alleviating dementia symptoms), promoting the passage through the blood–brain barrier (BBB) and the targeted and controlled release of the drug in the central nervous system (CNS). In fact, polymeric nanoparticles delivering rivastigmine have been shown to accelerate memory recovery in Alzheimer's disease patients and improved delivery into the brain of a murine model of the disease [6, 34].

The most appealing application of nanoparticles and nanoystems in the medical field is the targeted delivery of chemotherapeutic agents due to the precise drug release at the tumour mass, while preserving the surrounding tissue and avoiding the toxicity and adverse symptoms of classic chemotherapeutic drugs. However, the applications of nanoparticles in cancer go far behind targeted drug delivery. One very interesting example is the ability to design nanoparticles which allow the surgeon to visually identify the tumour during excision, thereby aiding in precise tumour resection [27]. Chitosan particles encapsulating quantum dots, with the ability to immobilise at the surface both the tumour-targeting ligand and chemokines, allow the visualisation of the mass under an optical microscope because of the interaction between tumour and immune cells. In fact, by glowing when exposed to UV light, quantum dots allow the surgeon to actually see the tumour during the procedure [35].

15.5 Clinical Applications of Nanoparticles in the Management of Brain Tumours

Gliomas, malignant tumours of the glia cells, are the most common primary tumours of the CNS. More than 50% of gliomas are glioblastoma multiforme (GBM), a grade IV astrocytoma, with quite poor prognosis (average survival of 15 months after the diagnosis) [36]. The current standard of care includes careful surgical resection followed by the oral administration of temozolomide with simultaneous radiotherapy but without significant improvement of disease progression [37]. As one of the most common and fatal primary tumours of the CNS in adults, the need for novel therapeutic strategies is imperious. In recent years, polymeric nanoparticles carrying paclitaxel, a chemotherapeutic agent, have been used by taking advantage of one of the few known biological features of this type of tumours. GBM is a highly angiogenic mass but the tumoural blood vessels exhibit dysfunctional junctions between the endothelial cells. In fact, both within the tumoural mass and at the BBB there is a downregulation of claudin-1, a key tight junction protein which holds endothelial cells together [38]. The disruption of tight junction architecture increases vessel permeability and promotes the passage of systemic compounds into the cerebral parenchyma. Circulating nanoparticles containing paclitaxel can therefore cross the BBB and accumulate in the tumour [5]. In this particular case, the BBB, which in theory could be an obstacle for drug delivery, even facilitates the access to the CNS. Also, the infiltrative nature of GBM, disrupts the lymphatic drainage, which further promotes drug accumulation at the tumour site [39]. To promote even further the delivery and retention of paclitaxel-containing nanoparticles within the tumour and inhibit the capture by the reticuloendothelial system, CED, a method to maintain a pressure gradient during infusions, may be applied. Although showing promising results, with prolonged survival time, these, and similar devices, have only been tested in animals [40, 41].

Similar approaches, encapsulating paclitaxel with carbon nanoparticles, have been shown to improve the outcome of head and neck tumours, but again, no data on human volunteers has been demonstrated [42]. Other studies exploit the advantages of using targeted chemotherapeutical drugs incorporated in 'minicells' but most of them are still at the preclinical level [43, 44]. One rewarding example comes from a multicentric study in Australia where 28 patients with advanced cancer were treated with 'minicells' containing paclitaxel and coated with epidermal growth factor receptor (EGFR), which is usually expressed by the tumour cells [45]. Ten of these patients had stable disease at 6 weeks, and importantly, these biodevices have been shown to be safe, with only minor symptoms (fever) at the day of administration and without significant toxicity [45]. Human clinical trials are now on course using a doxorubicin delivery system to target EGFR in patients with glioblastoma [46]. In this context, the 'minicells' have been shown to be well tolerated, inducing mild symptoms such as fever, nausea and chills. Regarding the efficacy on tumour progression, a recommended phase two dose was suggested by the authors [46].

15.6 Challenges of Clinical Applications of Nanoparticles

Despite the use of nanoparticles in the diagnosis of neurological diseases through bioimaging techniques, where nanoparticles are used as contrast agents, and in chemotherapeutic drug delivery for the treatment of aggressive brain tumours, such as gliomas, as well as the unanimous consensus on the advantage of nanoparticles to manage diseases with poor prognosis, such as CNS tumours, Alzheimer's or Parkinson's disease, one cannot point but a few examples of the clinical applications of nanoparticles [5, 45–49].

The scarce examples of nanoparticles application at the patient bedside should not harm the expectations of researchers, clinicians and patients. In fact, the basic, methodological research on nanomaterials and devices is fine tuning the biological properties of nanoparticles to allow their use in the clinical practice. Our expectations must be high for the next few years, when the time has come to test new materials, new nanoarchitectures and, hopefully, new drugs, at the preclinical and clinical levels. It is quite clear that nanotechnology will be a future cornerstone in the diagnosis, treatment and follow-up of neurological disorders with still poor prognosis.

Several reasons may justify the difficulties in translating the preclinical knowledge of nanoparticles into clinical practice, but safety, toxicity (both general and organ-specific) and administration, distribution, metabolism and excretory pathways are major issues which halt the application of most nanoparticles in humans (for a critical review see Ref. [50]). Of note, the clinical applications of nanotechnologies are highly dependent on the chemical and biophysical characteristics of the particles, such as the nanomaterials composing the core and corona (nanocrystals, polymeric or nonpolymeric nanostructures), as well as the size, shape, charge and optical properties of the whole particle [7–9].

One cannot escape from pointing the finger to the technical and biological problems regarding the design of nanoparticles, but it is important to highlight the additional challenges which these particles face to reach the CNS. In fact, the delivery of drugs into the CNS is not a straightforward task. First, nanoparticles have to cross the BBB, the semipermeable border, comprising endothelial cells, astrocytes end-feet and perycites, which separates the systemic bloodstream from the brain. Then, these nanosystems must retain the most suitable chemical and biophysical characteristics to concentrate in the affected region, whether it may be a tumoural mass, an ischaemic lesion or defected neuronal area.

The BBB is a dynamic structure comprising different cells and membranes which selects the molecules, exogenous or endogenous, which reach the cerebrospinal fluid and nervous tissue. This holds true for our own benefit, preventing the passage of toxins or pathogens, but at the same time inhibits the passage of drugs with therapeutic value. The BBB may be an obstacle for nanoparticles but these nanosystems may also be envisioned as means to overcome this biological fence. Nanocarriers, while being small enough, may also be engineered at their surface, to facilitate the selective passage through the BBB and deliver onsite and in a programmed fashion, the active drugs. In fact, they may be used to allow the passage of hydrophilic or charged drugs which, as free molecules, could not reach the brain. Several mechanisms, including endocytosis and transcytosis have been suggested to mediate the selective passage of nanocarriers (for a recent review see Ref. [7]). Furthermore, these nanosystems may also be shielded against enzymatic cleavage, increasing the bioavailability of the drugs in the CNS (reviewed in Ref. [6]). This is precisely the main advantage in encapsulating rivastigmine within polymeric nanoparticles in an attempt to improve Alzheimer's disease outcomes. But is not only Alzheimer's disease which may benefit from the use of nanoparticles. Brain tumours, human immunodeficiency virus (HIV) encephalopathy and acute ischaemic events may also be managed by using specific drug delivery shielded by nanostructures [7].

The gap between the galloping rhythm of basic research on the biomedical applications of nanoparticles and its objective use in clinical practice is undeniable. However, it should be noted that the technological advancements regarding nanodevices and nanoparticles which overcome most of the recognised physiological barriers (such as the BBB) are being reported quite recently at impressive high rate and therefore one needs to be patient before making any comments on their translational potential.

15.7 The Importance of the Regulatory Pathway

In a context of continuous growth and constant innovation, the pharmaceutical technology sector faces big challenges, especially in what concerns to the safety of products. Scientists and manufacturers have the responsibility of creating quality products, according to the market needs, while guaranteeing safety for users. Nanoparticles as carriers of drugs add strains to this context, as qualification and research demands might be unclear or misinterpreted.

In the scope of new drug delivery technologies, this becomes even more significant as products shall not only fulfil the needs of the drug they carry, but also be designed and manufactured in a way which reduces potential risks, while always guaranteeing the expected benefit–risk balance to the patient.

These demands can only be attended if all the stakeholders – manufacturers, academia, researchers, governments and regulatory entities – actuate under the same base of principles and according to the same rules.

The medical application of nanomaterials contributes to the development of drug delivery systems both on the pharmaceutical and medical technology level. While out of the scope of the book, the field of nanomaterial in the medical device sector evidences how compliance with the regulatory obligations is fundamental to cross the valley of death when bringing new technologies to the patient bedside.

Existing regulations, provided by regulatory agencies of each country, are no longer adequate to guarantee the quality, safety, efficacy and environmental safety of nanoparticles in medicine technologies. In medicines, this is mainly related to the chemical variability and structural complexity of these systems which determine their pharmacodynamics, pharmacokinetics and preferential administration route, while hindering an approximate prediction of cell interaction and safety profiles, posing unknown risks for patients and manufactures.

For medical devices, in Europe, the old regulatory environment, Council Directives 90/385/EEC (active implantable medical devices) [51] and 93/42/EEC (medical devices) [52], as well as Directive 98/79/EC of the European Parliament and of the Council (on in vitro diagnostic medical devices) [53] do not contain explicit requirements regarding nanomaterials.

In this context, in 2007, the Working Group on New and Emerging Technologies in Medical Devices (N&ET Working Group) presented a report with findings and recommendations on medical devices manufactured resorting to nanotechnology. The group considered that, even though the medical devices legislation is suitable for the particularities of nanomaterial-based medical devices, it would be appropriate to develop regulatory guidance for risk evaluation of products covered by the abovementioned directives. It was also considered that particular attention must be devoted to the postmarketing period with effective surveillance systems. [54]

As a consequence, on January 2015, the EU Scientific Committee on Emerging and Newly Identified Health Risks (SCENIHR) emitted an Opinion on the 'Guidance on the determination of potential health effects of nanomaterials used in medical devices', which 'addresses the use of nanomaterials in medical devices and provides information for risk assessors regarding specific aspects which need to be considered in the safety evaluation of nanomaterials' considering the various possible formats and combinations. The document recommends a phased risk evaluation approach – considering cover particle release (phase 1), particle distribution and persistence (phase 2), hazard assessment (toxicological evaluations) (phase 3), risk characterisation/risk assessment (phase 4) – to avoid unnecessary testing [55].

Regarding procedures standardisation, this area is supported by ISO/TR 10993, specifically by Chapter 22 of 2017 – Guidance on nanomaterials – which includes extensive considerations for the biological evaluation of medical devices based on nanomaterials, including aspects like characterisation, samples preparation, release profile, toxicokinetics and risk assessment. This document is considered a good basis for the development of protocols for nanomaterials evaluation [56].

The availability of standards for the development of nanomedicine technology is crucial for the development of safety and effective products with high quality standards allowing the mutual acceptance of data on various markets and sectors.

The emerging nanotechnologies in the field of drug delivery will benefit from a close collaboration with other health sectors in which regulatory science is already producing standardisation guidelines to help scientists in the planning of their regulatory roadmap to quick and efficiently get into the market.

The analysis of the global framework of standards for nanotechnologies evidences which medical devices area is in the lead of regulatory science, with very specific legal obligations under the new regulations and legislation (mainly in Europe), and with specific ISO standards for the biological evaluation of medical devices incorporating nanomaterials.

However, and unfortunately, major gaps exist at the nanomedicines level, namely in the areas of drug loading, drug release and detection of nanomaterial in biological tissues. This is well evidence in a recent research which compiled the existing documentation and requirements regarding standardisation of nanomaterials for nanomedicines including: methods for physicochemical characterisation, methods for safety evaluation, nanoscale reference materials, and drug loading and drug release evaluation [57]. In most cases, the methods address a specific type of nanomaterial being of very limited application, considering the chemical variability of these materials. It was also evidenced that standardisation is not totally focused on the biological activity of the nanomaterials so that in many cases guidance on the evaluation of their suitability for nanomedicine is still lacking [57].

In this context, it is necessary to look for all existing scientific evidence and also to the one which will be generated in the future, for nanomedicines, in order to help regulatory scientist to develop sets of guidelines which will reduce the uncertainty of product development, allowing novel ideas to cross the valley of death, with success [57].

Still, as already mentioned, several other questions need to be addressed and so a solid, comprehensive regulatory basis embracing aspects like manufacturing, quality control (including adequate/novel standardised analytical tools), safety (human and environmental), clinical evaluation and patent protection must be available and its application shall be guaranteed and inspected. During this process, competent authorities are obliged to closely monitor the evolution of research and of the market, supporting/inspecting manufacturers during the development and commercialisation processes.

New regulations should adopt strict measures to increase transparency, traceability and safety, while demanding more clinical evidence and the involvement of experts in the approval process.

References

1. Mirvis, D. M. (2009). From research to public policy: an essential extension of the translation research agenda. *Clin. Transl. Sci.*, **2**, 379–381.
2. (a) Waldman, S. A., Terzic, A. (2010). Clinical and translational science: from bench-bedside to global village. *Clin. Transl. Sci.*, **3**, 254–257. (b) Gago, B. (2018). Ambient Assisted Living as Medical Devices: A European Perspective, Springer.
3. Hudson, J., Khazragui, H. F. (2013). Into the valley of death: research to innovation. *Drug Discov. Today*, **18**, 610–613.
4. Wong, H. L., Wu, X. Y., Bendayan, R. (2012). Nanotechnological advances for the delivery of CNS therapeutics. *Adv. Drug Deliv. Rev.*, **64**, 686–700.
5. Michael, J. S., Lee, B.-S., Zhang, M., Yu, J. S. (2018). Nanotechnology for treatment of glioblastoma multiforme. *J. Transl. Intern. Med.*, **6**, 128–133.
6. Leszek, J., et al. (2017). Nanotechnology for Alzheimer disease. *Curr. Alzheimer Res.*, **14**(11), 1182–1189.
7. Nikalje, A. P. (2015). Nanotechnology and its applications in medicine. *Med. Chem.*, **5**, 2.
8. Petros, R. A., Desimone, J. M. (2010). Strategies in the design of nanoparticles for therapeutic applications. *Nat. Rev. Drug Discov.*, **9**, 615–627.
9. Alexis, F., Pridgen, E., Molnar, L. K., Farokhzad, O. C. (2008). Factors affecting the clearance and biodistribution of polymeric nanoparticles. *Mol. Pharm.*, **5**, 505–515.
10. Romberg, B., Hennink, W. E., Storm, G. (2008). Sheddable coatings for long-circulating nanoparticles. *Pharm. Res.*, **25**, 55–71.
11. Owens, D. E., Peppas, N. A. (2006). Opsonization, biodistribution, and pharmacokinetics of polymeric nanoparticles. *Int. J. Pharm.*, **307**, 93–102.
12. Moghimi, S. M., Hunter, A. C., Murray, J. C. (2001). Long-circulating and target-specific nanoparticles: theory to practice. *Pharmacol. Rev.*, **53**, 283–318.
13. Avgoustakis, K. (2004). Pegylated poly(lactide) and poly(lactide-co-glycolide) nanoparticles: preparation, properties and possible applications in drug delivery. *Curr. Drug Deliv.*, **1**, 321–333.

14. Otsuka, H., Nagasaki, Y., Kataoka, K. (2003). PEGylated nanoparticles for biological and pharmaceutical applications. *Adv. Drug Deliv. Rev.*, **55**, 403–419.

15. Poon, Z., Lee, J. B., Morton, S. W., Hammond, P. T. (2011). Controlling in vivo stability and biodistribution in electrostatically assembled nanoparticles for systemic delivery. *Nano Lett.*, **11**, 2096–2103.

16. Ferrara, K. W., Seo, J. W., Zhang, H. (2009). Imaging nanoparticle stability and activation in vivo. *Conf. Proc. IEEE Eng. Med. Biol. Soc.*, **2009**, 4580–4581.

17. Li, C. (2014). A targeted approach to cancer imaging and therapy. *Nat. Mater.*, **13**, 110–115.

18. Duncan, R., Gaspar, R. (2011). Nanomedicine(s) under the microscope. *Mol. Pharm.*, **8**, 2101–2141.

19. Skotland, T., Iversen, T.-G., Sandvig, K. (2010). New metal-based nanoparticles for intravenous use: requirements for clinical success with focus on medical imaging. *Nanomedicine*, **6**, 730–737.

20. Calvo, P., Remuñan-López, C., Vila-Jato, J. L., Alonso, M. J. (1997). Chitosan and chitosan/ethylene oxide-propylene oxide block copolymer nanoparticles as novel carriers for proteins and vaccines. *Pharm. Res.*, **14**, 1431–1436.

21. Abadeer, N. S., Murphy, C. J. (2016). Recent progress in cancer thermal therapy using gold nanoparticles. *J. Phys. Chem. C*, **120**, 4691–4716.

22. Wang, L., Hu, C., Shao, L. (2017). The antimicrobial activity of nanoparticles: present situation and prospects for the future. *Int. J. Nanomed.*, **12**, 1227–1249.

23. Farokhzad, O. C., et al. (2006). Targeted nanoparticle-aptamer bioconjugates for cancer chemotherapy in vivo. *Proc. Natl. Acad. Sci.*, **103**, 6315–6320.

24. Langer, R. (2001). Drug delivery: drugs on target. *Science*, **293**, 58–59.

25. Stoimenov, P. K., Klinger, R. L., Marchin, G. L., Klabunde, K. J. (2002). Metal oxide nanoparticles as bactericidal agents. *Langmuir*, **18**, 6679–6686.

26. Vaseashta, A., Dimova-Malinovska, D. (2005). Nanostructured and nanoscale devices, sensors and detectors. *Sci. Technol. Adv. Mater.*, **6**, 312–318.

27. Nasimi, P., Haidari, M. (2014). Medical use of nanoparticles. *Int. J. Green Nanotechnol.*, **1**, 194308921350697.

28. Margolis, D. J. A., et al. (2007). Molecular imaging techniques in body imaging. *Radiology*, **245**, 333–356.
29. Kircher, M. F., Mahmood, U., King, R. S., Weissleder, R., Josephson, L. (2003). A multimodal nanoparticle for preoperative magnetic resonance imaging and intraoperative optical brain tumor delineation. *Cancer Res.*, **63**, 8122–8125.
30. Weissleder, R. (2002). Scaling down imaging: molecular mapping of cancer in mice. *Nat. Rev. Cancer*, **2**, 11–18.
31. Ruehm, S. G., Corot, C., Vogt, P., Kolb, S., Debatin, J. F. (2001). Magnetic resonance imaging of atherosclerotic plaque with ultrasmall superparamagnetic particles of iron oxide in hyperlipidemic rabbits. *Circulation*, **103**, 415–422.
32. Liu, J., Liu, Z., Wu, D. (2019). Multifunctional hypoxia imaging nanoparticles: multifunctional tumor imaging and related guided tumor therapy. *Int. J. Nanomed.*, **14**, 707–719.
33. Lee, D.-E., et al. (2012). Multifunctional nanoparticles for multimodal imaging and theragnosis. *Chem. Soc. Rev.*, **41**, 2656–2672.
34. Joshi, S. A., Chavhan, S. S., Sawant, K. K. (2010). Rivastigmine-loaded PLGA and PBCA nanoparticles: preparation, optimization, characterization, in vitro and pharmacodynamic studies. *Eur. J. Pharm. Biopharm.*, **76**, 189–199.
35. Chatterjee, D. K., Zhang, Y. (2007). Multi-functional nanoparticles for cancer therapy. *Sci. Technol. Adv. Mater.*, **8**, 131–133.
36. Ostrom, Q. T., et al. (2013). CBTRUS statistical report: primary brain and central nervous system tumors diagnosed in the United States in 2006–2010. *Neuro. Oncol.*, **15**, ii1–ii56.
37. Stupp, R., et al. (2005). Radiotherapy plus concomitant and adjuvant temozolomide for glioblastoma. *N. Engl. J. Med.*, **352**, 987–996.
38. Liebner, S., et al. (2000). Claudin-1 and claudin-5 expression and tight junction morphology are altered in blood vessels of human glioblastoma multiforme. *Acta Neuropathol.*, **100**, 323–331.
39. Maeda, H. (2001). The enhanced permeability and retention (EPR) effect in tumor vasculature: the key role of tumor-selective macromolecular drug targeting. *Adv. Enzyme Regul.*, **41**, 189–207.
40. Zhou, J., et al. (2013). Highly penetrative, drug-loaded nanocarriers improve treatment of glioblastoma. *Proc. Natl. Acad. Sci.*, **110**, 11751–11756.
41. Inoue, T., et al. (2009). Therapeutic efficacy of a polymeric micellar doxorubicin infused by convection-enhanced delivery against intracranial 9L brain tumor models. *Neuro. Oncol.*, **11**, 151–157.

42. Sano, D., et al. (2012). Noncovalent assembly of targeted carbon nanovectors enables synergistic drug and radiation cancer therapy in vivo. *ACS Nano*, **6**, 2497–2505.

43. Elvidge, S. (2012). Bacterial 'minicells' deliver cancer drugs straight to the target. *Fierce Drug Deliv.*

44. Haque, F., et al. (2012). Ultrastable synergistic tetravalent RNA nanoparticles for targeting to cancers. *Nano Today*, **7**, 245–257.

45. Solomon, B. J., et al. (2015). A first-time-in-human phase i clinical trial of bispecific antibody-targeted, paclitaxel-packaged bacterial minicells. *PLoS One*, **10**, e0144559.

46. Whittle, J. R., et al. (2015). First in human nanotechnology doxorubicin delivery system to target epidermal growth factor receptors in recurrent glioblastoma. *J. Clin. Neurosci.*, **22**, 1889–1894.

47. Nichols, J. W., Bae, Y. H. (2012). Odyssey of a cancer nanoparticle: from injection site to site of action. *Nano Today*, **7**, 606–618.

48. Gozzard, D. (2011). When is high-dose intravenous iron repletion needed? Assessing new treatment options. *Drug Des. Devel. Ther.*, **5**, 51–60.

49. Parveen, S., Misra, R., Sahoo, S. K. (2012). Nanoparticles: a boon to drug delivery, therapeutics, diagnostics and imaging. *Nanomedicine*, **8**, 147–166.

50. Skotland, T., Iversen, T.-G., Sandvig, K. (2014). Development of nanoparticles for clinical use. *Nanomedicine*, **9**, 1295–1299.

51. European Council (1990). Council Directive 90/385/EEC of 20 June 1990 on the approximation of the laws of the Member States relating to active implantable medical devices. *OJEU.*

52. European Council (1993). Council Directive 93/42/EEC of 14 June 1993 on concerning medical devices. *OJEU.*

53. European Parliament & European Council (1998). Directive 98/79/EC of the European Parliament and of the Council of 27 October 1998 on in vitro diagnostic medical devices. *OJEU.*

54. Working Group On New and Emerging Technologies in Medical Devices (2007). Report on Nanotechnology to the Medical Devices Expert Group - Findings and Recommendations.

55. SCENIHR (Scientific Committee on Emerging and Newly-Identified Health Risks). The appropriateness of the risk assessment methodology in accordance with the Technical Guidance Documents for new and existing substances for assessing the risks of nanomaterials.

56. International Organization for Standardization (2017). ISO/TR 10993–22:2017 - Biological evaluation of medical devices - Part 22: Guidance on nanomaterials.

57. Halamoda-Kenzaoui, B., Holzwarth, U., Roebben, G., Bogni, A., Bremer-Hoffmann, S. (2019). Mapping of the available standards against the regulatory needs for nanomedicines. *Wiley Interdiscip. Rev. Nanomed. Nanobiotechnol.*, **11**, 1–17.

Index

For Product Safety Concerns and Information please contact our EU
representative GPSR@taylorandfrancis.com
Taylor & Francis Verlag GmbH, Kaufingerstraße 24, 80331 München, Germany

www.ingramcontent.com/pod-product-compliance
Ingram Content Group UK Ltd.
Pitfield, Milton Keynes, MK11 3LW, UK
UKHW021502240926
475702UK00035B/123
* 9 7 8 9 8 1 4 8 7 7 3 1 2 *